fesh oil

Aging Without Growing Old

BY

Judy Lindberg McFarland

with Laura Gladys McFarland

AGING WITHOUT GROWING OLD by Judy Lindberg McFarland
Published by Siloam Press
A part of Strang Communications Company
600 Rinehart Road
Lake Mary, Florida 32746
www.charismahouse.com

Unless otherwise noted, all Scripture quotations are from the King James Version of the Bible.

This book is not intended to provide medical advice or to take the place of medical advice and treatment from your personal physician. Readers are advised to consult their own doctors or other qualified health professionals regarding the treatment of their medical problems. Neither the publisher nor the author takes any responsibility for any possible consequences from any treatment, action or application of medicine, supplement, herb or preparation to any person reading or following the information in this book. If readers are taking prescription medications, they should consult with their physicians and not take themselves off of medicines to start supplementation without the proper supervision of a physician.

Portions of this book were previously published as *Aging Without Growing Old,* ISBN 1-888848-08-1, by Western Front, Ltd., copyright © 2000.

Library of Congress Catalogue Card Number: 2002092656
International Standard Book Number: 0-88419-969-X

03 04 05 06 — 8 7 6 5 4 3 2
Printed in the United States of America

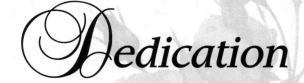

Dedication

I dedicate this work to the memory of my Mother,
Gladys Melcher Lindberg, a pioneer in the field
of nutrition whose incredible insights and loving counsel
put thousands on the path to robust health.

And to the memory of my father,
Walter Harold Lindberg, whose vision,
brilliance and hard work gave Mother
a platform from which to teach.

Acknowledgments

My precious family has been supportive throughout the writing of this book, reading and re-reading chapters, proofing drafts and making suggestions. I first want to thank my husband, Don, for his unconditional love, encouragement and support for this project.

I also thank my son Douglas, who has given me critical medical advice on several chapters. He was raised in a family believing in and using nutritional supplements, even though he was not taught this type of preventive or nutritional medicine at the university or medical school.

My daughter Laura will always have a special place in my heart for sticking with me to the final word of the final chapter. She really knows how to get a job done. Not only has she been by my side as we attended many educational seminars and conferences, she has worked in our business and stayed abreast of the most recent nutritional information. I am forever indebted to you, Laura.

Several others have helped me in writing this book. I want to thank Helen Hosier and Norm Rohrer for getting me started in the very early stages, and Frank Murray for his contribution toward the first manuscript. Thank you, Dr. Jan Dargatz, a very professional and patient editor who put up with so many changes. I also want to acknowledge and thank Marcia Zimmerman, C.N., Richard Passwater, Ph.D., Dan McFarland, B.A., and Carol McFarland, B.A., M.Ed., for taking time out of their busy schedules to read the initial manuscript and offer their suggestions.

There is a very special group of my dear friends that have been praying for the message in this book and for me, as I completed this project. May God bless all of you.

There are many to whom I have looked for authority that I have had the honor of knowing. These experts, from Mother's generation, are gone now, but I want to acknowledge them: Adelle Davis (author); Carlton Fredericks, Ph.D. (author); Gaylord Hauser (pioneering nutritionist); Lester Morrison, M.D., D.Cs., F.A.C.P. (arteriosclerosis research);

Linus Pauling, Ph.D. (vitamin C); Evan Shute, M.D. (vitamin E); Broda Barnes, M.D., Ph.D. (thyroid); Robert Bingham, M.D. (arthritis); and Robert Mendelsohn, M.D. (author). We all have benefited from their numerous accomplishments and their pioneering spirit.

Now there are new "stars" from my generation, experts in the field of health, who have become family friends or friends I have made from our industry. They include: Jeffrey Bland, Ph.D.; Eric Braverman, M.D.; Richard Casdorph, M.D.; Michael Corrigan; Dr. William Crook; Udo Erasmus; Ann Louise Gittleman; Abram Hoffer, M.D., Ph.D.; Betty Kamen; Hans Kugler, Ph.D.; William Lane, Ph.D.; Stephen Langer, M.D.; Earl Mindell, R.Ph., Ph.D.; Michael Murray, N.D.; Richard Passwater, Ph.D.; Walter Pierpaoli, M.D., Ph.D., Joseph Pizzorno, N.D.; Dr. Patrick Quillin; William Regelson, M.D.; Maureen Salaman; Steven Schechter, N.D.; James F. Scheer; Lendon Smith, M.D.; Dana Ullman; Frank Varese, M.D.; Julian Whitaker, M.D.; Janet Zand, L.Ac, O.M.D.; Marcia Zimmerman; and many, many others.

These are the new stars, the ones from whom I still have the opportunity to learn. You will find many of them referenced in this book.

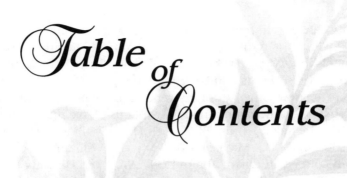

Table of Contents

Foreword

Douglas Walter McFarland, M.D.

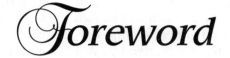

Growing up in the McFarland household was not your average experience. Nowhere in the cupboard would you find cookies, candy, white bread or processed foods. The refrigerator had no bologna, American cheese, soft drinks, margarine or ice cream. My friends would say that there was nothing to snack on at my house! Instead, I snacked on fruits, nuts, trail mix and an occasional treat such as homemade peanut butter candy or powdered milk candy.

The importance of health and of eating right was impressed upon me by my family at an early age, but most other people I encountered never appeared concerned about nutrition. It seemed that people were only interested in their health when they became ill. If one tried to eat good foods or take vitamins, he or she was considered a "health nut."

Our summer vacations were also different. As part of our vacations, we often went to various cities to attend nutrition conventions. During each convention, so many people would want to talk to my grandmother, Gladys Lindberg, that they often stood in line! I concluded that she must be famous, and I was right—my grandmother was famous in nutrition circles. I came to realize that being a McFarland was unique, from the food we ate to the fact that my grandmother always wore pink.

I learned at a young age about taking vitamins and drinking protein shakes, but it was while I was a teenager that I began to recognize the depth of my grandmother's convictions about healthy eating. As I drove her home from work every Saturday, she told me about the people she had counseled that day and about their terrible physical problems for which physicians had no cure. The hours she spent speaking with people at the nutrition store were more than mere business hours to her—she was deeply concerned about the good health of her clients.

Mother and grandmother worked closely together in their crusade for good health. On many occasions, Mother would read to me the thank you letters that she and my grandmother had received from people whose lives and health had been turned around as the result of following the program my grandmother and Mother had developed. The secret of the program created by my grandmother and Mother was simple, and it is something I experienced firsthand in my childhood and teen years: a variety of good natural foods, vitamins and mineral supplementation, and no junk foods.

In college I began to realize why people such as Mother and grandmother had a difficult time reaching and convincing a wide audience about the benefits of nutrition and supplements. Physicians, scientists, professors, and educators would not accept evidence and arguments that foods and vitamins could improve one's health, and this is an attitude that has been perpetuated by the popular press as well. I was often surprised at how my professors would deride brilliant scientists, such as Linus Pauling, for their "unconventional" views on vitamins.

In medical school, I again was surprised at how little time was spent on nutrition and preventive medicine. Although my medical interests led me to the field of Emergency Medicine, I readily understand how people can be frustrated with modern medicine. After years of living unhealthy lives, so many people are terrified to see their health fall apart in the "golden years"—and this is compounded when they see no effective treatments or cures offered by their doctors. As a physician, I realize that modern medicine has provided me with an education in diseases and how to treat them, but far less information on how to prevent them. In my work within the Emergency Department, I see patients with strokes, heart attacks, emphysema, cirrhosis of the liver, diverticulitis, and many other problems that are testament to poor prevention.

Modern medicine in the U.S. has focused on the treatment of disease with surgery or medications but has left the "achievement of optimal health" largely unresearched. The average American's high fat diet, inadequate exercise, and abuse of alcohol and tobacco have prevented millions from achieving their full health potential. As a nation, we are now beginning to recognize the importance of weight loss, exercise, a healthy diet, and the value of vitamins, minerals, and herbal supplements. We are also realizing the limitations of current medical treatments to cure disease and help us reach optimal health. I believe real breakthroughs in medicine will come in the field of prevention and how to obtain optimal health, not from new surgical or drug treatments after a disease is diagnosed. I also believe that people like my grandmother, who began her pioneering work in nutrition more than 50 years ago, are to be thanked for enlightening and empowering us to live healthier lives.

This book is easy to read and it should be easily understood by people of all backgrounds. Thousands of people have benefited tremendously from the Lindberg Nutrition Program with results that confirm the nutritional basis for many of their ailments.

The Lindberg Nutrition Program is not a new fad that will be gone tomorrow, but is based on classic and current medical and nutritional studies. Skeptics will say that a few anecdotal reports of success on this program prove nothing, and they are correct. But the hundreds of "anecdotes" over the years who have had seemingly miraculous improvements in their health are compelling and cannot be ignored. I believe you will be surprised at the amount of current scientific findings on vitamins and supplements that has never reached the popular media—findings that support the program recommended in this book.

For anyone seeking to take charge of their health—and to optimize their health—this book is an excellent resource for years to come.

—DOUGLAS WALTER MCFARLAND, M.D.

Preface

"I believe the most important investment you can make is the investment in your health." I appeared on a financial network television program here in southern California, with the stock quotes racing across the screen below me, and that's how I started the program. I also said, "We often do not appreciate our health until we lose it. Then not all the money in the world may enable us to regain it."

Aging Without Growing Old is meant to provide practical, easy-to-follow suggestions for maintaining good health and the sense of well-being, both physical and mental; I believe it's our birthright! I want to help you prevent all the degenerative diseases and illnesses that accompany aging, and the heartaches resulting from the loss of one's health. I hope to teach you how to prevent some of the suffering that characterizes so many lives. Since my Mother Gladys Lindberg's time, there has been a tremendous amount of new, scientifically substantiated nutrition information, much of which is included in this book. However, my basic understanding of good nutrition still emanates from my precious Mother.

Many times my thoughts flashed back to her life, with her amazing wisdom and scientific mind placing her over 50 years ahead of her time in the field of applied nutrition. I can still visualize her beauty, grace, and charm, always elegantly dressed in her favorite color, pink, surrounded by familiar groups of clients. As always, she patiently listened to each health complaint and then stated to everyone: "I am not a doctor and cannot treat disease, but healthy people don't have that, so let's make you healthy."

Mother once had a desire deep in her heart to be a physician and have the ability like her grandson, Douglas, to go to medical school and be able to treat disease, but that was not her lot in life. Instead, she raised three sickly children through the 1930s Depression and World War II. Her experiences not only compelled her to want to see people well, but also made her a more understanding and compassionate person.

What happened next was to change drastically the course of all our lives. My sister Janice had one of her frequent bouts with a high fever. She had them frequently, and Mother couldn't seem to resolve what was causing these fevers. One evening, Mother knelt beside her bed and prayed for knowledge and wisdom on how to keep her feverish child well. She fell asleep beside her, and in the morning, Janice's body was cool. Mother knew her prayers had been answered and realized almost instantly that nearly all the food we ate had been highly processed, preserved or devitalized in some way. As she would say, "Everything we were eating came from a tin can or paper bag." She had been raised in the little town of Peck, Idaho, and everything her family ate was natural and they raised it themselves. Thus, with an insatiable drive, she began the quest of her life—to make and keep her family healthy. During World War II she started with an organic "victory" garden in our backyard, as her parents had.

Mother was an avid reader of scientific journals. She attended scientific lectures and conventions on all aspects of nutrition, and luckily for me she did not drive. I was able to attend many of them as her chauffeur! She loved reading about the tremendous scientific work of unsung medical heroes and their results with nutritional substances. She always shared the great stories of these wonderful pioneering doctors with me. In surveying the past, Mother set about to glean the best nutritional practices of the past and to apply them to the present and future of her family. She had no desire to go back to her "hard life," nor to revert to a primitive lifestyle, but she did desire to bring the best nutritional qualities of the past into modern-day living.

As she read, she classified and compiled information to use in developing a successful nutritional program for her own family. When neighbors saw the remarkable change in our lives, word began to spread quickly. Soon, Mother had relatives, neighbors, and friends coming to our home regularly for advice on what to do to help their children and themselves become healthier.

Word of her program spread across the Los Angeles area. She was asked so often about the vitamins and minerals she was giving us that she began to buy them in quantities of a thousand at a time. There were very few nutrition stores in that era. Then, when friends stopped in for advice, she would hold classes around the dining room table. They all wanted to try what Mother was discussing, so they would count out their own vitamins, put them into white envelopes, and pay Mother exactly what the vitamins had cost her. Mother had great satisfaction in seeing people's health improve from month to month, as her "clients" came back for more.

The Beginning of the Vitamin and Mineral Packs

One of Mother's clients was a blind woman who couldn't distinguish between the envelopes of the various vitamin and mineral tablets. So Mother spread out a hundred small squares of wax paper on the dining room table and placed a daily supply of about six vitamins and minerals on each square. Then she twisted the squares into packets so the woman could take just one packet a day. The woman loved the idea, and so did her friends.

It became a popular way of packaging the vitamins and minerals. We had tried many ways of producing these vitamin and mineral packets by hand, for over 15 years. My brother Bob, who was a brilliant engineer, finally designed a machine that allowed the tablets and capsules to drop into little cellophane packets, which were then sealed. This was the beginning of our very popular *Lindberg Vitamin and Mineral Packs*. Today this kind of packaging is everywhere, but now you know where this concept all started—around our dining room table in the mid-1940s!

Why multiple tablets in a packet? Mother always believed no single vitamin or mineral could contain a high enough potency for her formulas without becoming too large to swallow. She never agreed with the one-tablet-a-day or two or three-a-day concept.

Our First Store Opened in 1949 by Walter Harold Lindberg

Finally the day came when, after observing for a long time what was happening in our home, my father said, half jokingly, "Gladys, this has become a business. You must get this out of the house." And get it out of the house he did, in 1949. My father, Walter Harold Lindberg, had a unique business ability, coupled with perseverance and hard work. He took the initiative and found the location for our first store. It was his idea to call it the Lindberg Nutrition Service. He said, "Our service will be Gladys giving her time to help people become nutrition-wise, and it will be free advice." Our motto was "Keep in the Pink"—referring to the natural color of good health and, of course, Mother's favorite color. Our stores and labels were all pink in color. Mother wore only pink clothes and was driven in a pink car. In later years when her grandsons were her designated drivers, they weren't too happy about driving her in "that pink Cadillac."

We were the first tenants in a new building in southwest Los Angeles, unaware that this modest beginning was the forerunner of a chain of the new concept of nutrition supermarkets in southern California. At that time nutrition stores were small "holes in the wall," and ours was a completely different concept. The business grew so quickly that my father left his management position with Earl M. Jorgensen steel company.

In 1955 we opened our second store, with more than 10,000 square feet in the new Baldwin Hills shopping center in Los Angeles. This store and the store next to it eventually became our headquarters. In the mid-'60s, we opened a beautiful store on Wilshire Boulevard in West Los Angeles, next to Beverly Hills. I loved going to this store because of all the activity and the movie stars and celebrities I would meet.

Our Store on Wilshire Boulevard— Where the Stars Met

One day, as I walked into our Wilshire store, Mother was having a consultation with the talented *Doris Day* and her husband, *Marty Melcher.*

Another day I recognized *Robert Stack* of the *Untouchables* fame. His wife at that time, Rosemarie, often visited with Mother. They were on Mother's program for many years.

The actress *Jennifer Jones,* of *Song of Bernadette* and *Duel in the Sun* fame, had Mother come to her home in Beverly Hills to help her with her then ill husband, *David O. Selznick,* director of *Gone with the Wind.*

The classic, old-time actress, *Marjorie Main* of *Ma and Pa Kettle* movie fame, would come to the store and consult with Mother. She bought all her nutritional groceries and fresh organic produce each time. It was fun to help her out to her car with all of her packages.

The great beauty, *Arlene Dahl,* was another film star who benefited from Mother's program.

One day while at the Wilshire store, actress *Gloria Swanson* came in to shop. She was a strict vegetarian and would eat only organically grown vegetables. She found something in our produce area that wasn't marked "organic" and created a real scene. My darling father happened to be there and had a great time settling her down and charming her with his Swedish, very blue eyes. She became a very good customer.

Our sales gals at the vitamin department loved it when *Rock Hudson* would come and shop in our store. He was always so charming to everyone, they almost fought over who was going to wait on him. Sometimes I even volunteered.

Merle Oberon of *Wuthering Heights* fame had Mother up to her gorgeous home to help her with her nutrition. She was a strikingly beautiful woman and knew the importance of taking care of herself. When we would go to see *Katherine Kuhlman,* the well-known Christian evangelist, at the Shrine Auditorium in Los Angeles, we would see Merle Oberon backstage.

Mother was fascinated, witnessing these great healings at the Shrine, and she was invited backstage to have a private audience with Miss Kuhlman. Among other things, they discussed Miss Kuhlman's health, and she promised Mother she would start taking our vitamin packs. We sent her the vitamin packs for years and always received a personal thank you note from her.

Art and Lois Linkletter used our supplements and were customers at our Wilshire store for years. I saw Art Linkletter on Dr. Robert Schuller's television program. He was so mentally sharp and looked great, and said he was over 86. He had been doing something right.

Mahalia Jackson, considered one of the greatest gospel singers of all time, would come after hours to our Crenshaw store in her chauffeur-driven limousine. Mother would stay for hours to counsel with her. My husband, Don, would wait to lock up the store when the consultation was finished.

Opera star *Mary Costa* had been on Mother's program for years, often having products sent to her in New York and Florida.

In the World of Sports, *Gladys Lindberg* was also recognized as an authority. She worked with the Occidental College Track Team in Los Angeles in the early 50s. Coached by *Chuck Coker,* they had stunning results.

Many track athletes would reach their peak performance mid-season and start to decline thereafter. Under the Lindberg program, these track athletes continued to better their record through the year! Since track is an individual achievement sport, measured by time and distance, their improvement was easy to record and study. As word of their success spread, it began the era of athletes training and using vitamin and mineral supplements to improve their performance.

Bill Toomey came to see Mother, and she placed him on a nutrition program that included the Varsity Pack 2, our vitamin-mineral packet. He was training for the 1968 Olympic Games in Mexico City and went on to win the Gold Medal in the grueling decathlon championship event. How proud we were of his accomplishment!

My husband, *Don McFarland,* played football at U.S.C. from 1953 to 1955 and had the thrill of playing in the Rose Bowl in 1955, the year we were married. A few years later, U.S.C.'s head football coach, *Don Clark,* along with his then assistant coach, *Al Davis*, had a nutritional meeting with Mother at our Crenshaw store. They applied her nutrition program to their training table. We provided the football team with the Varsity Pack 2 packets of vitamins and minerals for the season. Coach Clark often reported how his team statistically had one of the lowest injury rates, with less bruising, muscle pulls, sprains, breaks, etc., of any of his other teams. They ended the season in better health than when they started. He felt that the Lindberg Nutrition Program contributed greatly to it, and was so impressed that he and his wife, Dorothy, became faithful customers, providing the vitamin packs for each of their eight children!

Al Davis went on to become head coach of the professional football team, *Oakland Raiders,* and became owner shortly thereafter. While located in both Oakland and Los Angeles, *George Anderson,* head trainer, used the same vitamin-mineral products with the Raiders that *Don Clark* used at U.S.C. The Raiders at that time claimed the best win-loss record of any modern-day professional team. They ordered the Varsity Pack 2 for their team for over 20 years.

Best-selling author heeded the Lindberg advice

As a young reporter, *Helen Gurley Brown,* editor of *Cosmopolitan* magazine for many years, had an encounter with Mother that changed her life. She reported the story in *Sex and the Single Girl*, a worldwide best-seller, and in *Sex in the Office,* both somewhat risqué books published in the late '50s and early '60s.

In writing about Mother she said, "I didn't start thinking nutrition even a little until one summer day 12 years ago when, at age 36, I'd been working at the Miss Universe pageant in Long Beach for two weeks and was feeling like the invisible woman from being around all that teenage pulchritude, totally ignored by anybody male over the age of seven. I passed Gladys Lindberg's nutrition store. It's hard to miss Gladys' if you're anywhere in the neighborhood. Wired with neon, it would look right at home on the Las Vegas Strip. Gladys doesn't think health foods have anything to hide their heads about.

"Friends had suggested I see her years before when I complained of feeling lower than an earthworm. I did telephone one day to see if she'd send over some vitamins, but she wanted to know what I'd had for breakfast. I didn't think it was any of her business and the conversation ended. This morning her store looked like Mecca," Helen said. "I parked and went in."

"Since Gladys holds court sort of like Gandhi—too many people to see and too few hours to see them in—I explained to a cast of about 30 that I was suffering from an acute case of jealousy as well as symptoms of disappearance. Gladys had me stick out my tongue, which she said was purplish, heavily coated, and had a deep groove down the center. Since these were the first words of a personal nature anybody had spoken to me in 14 days, I started to cry all over her blood sugar manuals. She said what I was really suffering from was acute fatigue and probably a vitamin deficiency brought on by years of lousy eating habits.

"I went home with the makings of Serenity Cocktail, several whole-wheat grains to cook with, the Varsity Pack (a technicolored collection of vitamins and minerals Gladys feeds athletes), and pounds and pounds of soy pancake mix. Health nuts always placate you with something that *sounds* like what you used to eat that actually bears no resemblance to it. *Delicious*, though!

"I won't bore you with my deficiencies and how they didn't grow after that. Just suffice to say I used to spend half my life in doctors' offices, which is very expensive on a secretary's salary, and I don't anymore."

Helen Gurley Brown wrote as she said of her "life changing encounter" in her later book, *The Late Show*, for women over 50. This version is just a little different, but really dear. Let me quote a part for you: "Gladys also began the more arduous task of separating me from a lifelong sugar addiction, a chore roughly as challenging as separating a tree from its bark with your fingernails (I'm not separated yet!). Dear

Gladys. I'm almost glad she isn't still here to see what's happened to her beloved protein. Gladys said a girl who didn't have at least 54 grams a day would probably die. Current guidelines suggest 44 and the figure is still dropping." Helen Gurley Brown is obviously a very clever writer.

Knowing the Pioneers in the Field of Nutrition

Being raised around the great pioneers in the nutrition field was an exciting part of my growing-up years. It certainly contributed to helping me form many of my own nutritional beliefs.

Adelle Davis—author, fellow pioneer, and Mother's friend

Perhaps one of the most significant events in Mother's early years of searching occurred when she heard Adelle Davis lecture at a department store in downtown Los Angeles. Adelle was giving a series of lectures while promoting her book, *Vitality Through Planned Nutrition.*

After the lecture, Mother introduced herself and enthusiastically shared with Adelle her own experiences, subsequent findings, and the results of her children's lives. She concluded, "I've been doing with my family all the things you talked about."

Thus began a lifelong friendship with Adelle. Mother and Adelle got together frequently for discussions on what was new in the field of health. Both were pioneers in applied nutrition and learned much from each other. Both had a commitment to raising people's consciousness about nutrition. Good health was the passion of their lives.

I often went to Adelle's home on Sundays with Mother and Dad while Adelle was writing her best-selling book, *Let's Eat Right to Keep Fit.* Mother happily contributed many examples for Adelle. In fact, when I read Adelle's book, it sounds like Mother talking. Adelle wanted to dedicate the book to Mother, but my father wouldn't allow it, desiring to protect Mother from some of the very negative press Adelle was receiving. Adelle was highly controversial in those days with her revolutionary ideas. She was promoting the use of vitamins, little-known and little-discussed at that time.

I feel more people around the world in those early years were turned on to nutrition by reading Adelle Davis' books than by any other author. Mutual affection and admiration always characterized our family's relationship with Adelle.

Gayelord Hauser—Author of *Look Younger, Live Longer.*

He was a tall, handsome German who came to Hollywood and gave what was then considered to be unorthodox diet advice to many of the stars in the late '30s and early '40s.

Hauser coined the words "wonder foods" to describe yogurt, dried skim milk, brewer's yeast, blackstrap molasses and wheat germ. During this time Mother added these foods to our diet. He emphasized the need to supplement one's diet with vitamins and minerals, and was especially fond of fresh fruit and vegetable juices. He was far ahead of his time. In the '50s, Gayelord Hauser's book, *Look Younger, Live Longer,* came out. It went on to become a very popular, international bestseller.

In the '60s, *Mirror, Mirror on the Wall* was published, which was a great book with beauty secrets for the stars. This book also discussed how the American diet is too high in fat and that we eat too little of the good, life-giving, beauty-giving foods. "We have refined the vitamins and minerals out of our clean, sanitary, packaged foods. And we have put in other additives that may keep our food from spoiling—for that is the purpose of them—but do us harm that we hardly know."

As you see, these pioneers were ahead of their time. We were able to spend time with Gayelord Hauser, and he graciously described us as *the first family of nutrition.*

The Swedish-born star, Greta Garbo

One of Gayelord Hauser's famous clients was the glamorous, Swedish-born movie star Greta Garbo, from the old classic movies and the famous saying "I want to be alone." We were invited to several parties in his palatial, beautifully decorated Beverly Hills home. Years later, when Hauser died at the age of 89 of complications from pneumonia, we attended his funeral and were invited to his home, where we met Greta Garbo. I was shocked at how unkindly she had aged. With her deeply wrinkled face, my heart ached for her. Mother's complexion looked like a rosebud compared to Garbo's, and Mother at that time was even older. Looking at the two women, I knew nutrition worked. Upon questioning, I was told Garbo was a heavy smoker. Certainly there is a tremendous lesson here for smokers.

Carlton Fredericks, Ph.D., author of many excellent books

He was a great nutritional author; in addition, a radio broadcaster. Dr. Fredericks was also a special friend with whom we shared many enlightening times, both when dining out and at conventions. He was always on the cutting edge with the latest nutritional information, and I learned so much from him. At one time, we sponsored a radio program for him on KABC in southern California. He was an outspoken advocate of nutrition rights and fought the powers-to-be. You will see him quoted several times in this book.

Jack La Lanne, one of Hollywood's original "fitness experts"

His top-rated Los Angeles TV program, *The Jack La Lanne Show,* was a new kind of program. It was all about exercise, and Jack made it fun. My children were small in the '60s, crawling around the room as I tried to exercise with him. I would do jumping-jacks and then run and change a diaper! Mother was on his television program several times, discussing the value of nutrition, especially hypoglycemia, one of her favorite topics. Jack and Elaine La Lanne became special friends of our family.

Jack La Lanne has stayed with his body building and nutritional supplements all these years. The fitness clubs that bore his name eventually numbered well over a hundred. On his 88th birthday, my daughter Laura and I attended his birthday celebration, which included Jack receiving his star on the Hollywood Walk of Fame. He still looks incredible! Congratulations Jack!

He made body building acceptable, and even today I enjoy seeing young men in our store, inquiring about how to take care of their health. They have been motivated to work out and maintain good health. One mother called me to ask what I thought about the body building products her teenage son wanted, and "was it just a waste of money?" I told her she should be thrilled he wanted to take care of himself instead of being in the streets taking drugs. She said, "Oh! Thank you, I hadn't thought of that."

Television Greats Believe in Treating the Body Right

When our first book, *Take Charge of Your Health,* was published by Harper & Row in 1981, both Mother and I were invited to be on many television programs.

Dr. Pat Robertson, host of the TV program, *The 700 Club*

He did a feature story on Mother and Lindberg Nutrition Service. He showed our retail stores and the 100,000-square-foot warehouse of Nature's Best, our distribution company. The warehouse was fully computer-automated and very impressive. (Nature's Best is now owned by my brother's family.) I was on the program with her, and the first question Pat Robertson asked Mother was, "How did a little lady like you start such a fantastic business?" Pat Robertson is very interested in keeping the body, "God's temple," in good health and often brings nutritional information to his television audience.

I had the pleasure of a return visit to Virginia Beach in 1998 to appear again on the same television program with Pat Robertson. He is still a strong believer in the importance of keeping ourselves healthy. We discussed the first edition of *Aging Without Growing Old*. I enjoyed talking with him after the television program, hearing about all the nutritional supplements he takes. He does a wonderful job informing the public about many aspects of life, including proper nutrition.

I returned to *The 700 Club* in October 1999 and taped eight additional programs with Pat Robertson. There is always so much to say and so little time to say it, but we covered many areas of nutrition. I provided eight nutritional pamphlets on each subject we discussed, so his audience could have this free information. I always consider it an honor to appear on this tremendous television program and to have an opportunity to share my nutritional beliefs with the audience.

One morning as I was watching *The 700 Club*, Pat Robertson was making his *Age Defying Protein Shake*. As he was adding protein powders, then soy lecithin granules, he states, "My friend Judy Lindberg McFarland taught me about lecithin." Then after adding MSM, he made the same statement that I taught him about MSM. Of course, I was amazed and thrilled! When he finished making this incredibly healthy drink he said to his co-hostess, Terry Meeuwsen, "You can get these products wholesale by calling Judy Lindberg McFarland's company, *Nutrition Express* at 1-800-338-7979." With that statement I almost fell off the bed (it was early in the morning). My husband called the warehouse to tell them what had happened and all of the phone lines were already jammed. We had to switch to our off-hours answering service. Within a relatively short period of time we received over 10,000 calls for his *Age-Defying Protein Shake* recipe. I understand *The 700 Club* had more responses to this segment than any other. If I hadn't seen this program we would have had no idea what was happening. Pat Robertson has been a blessing to me and of course to his huge audience. He wants them to be healthy! His *Age-Defying Protein Shake* recipe is very similar to my recipe listed in the *Let's Put it All Together* chapter.

Dr. Robertson also presented an article for his viewing audience called, "Age-Defying Antioxidant Program." Much to my surprise, he quoted me several times from this book, in his article. Our Lindberg Varsity Pack 2 was also recommended as having adequate levels of all the important antioxidants in high enough potencies, "to do you some good." He also suggested taking coenzyme Q10 and alpha-lipoic acid, two excellent products you will be reading about in several places in this book. After you learn about them, I am sure you will consider adding them to your nutritional program. Five hundred thousand requests for this article have been made.

The *Live With Regis* Show

In the early '80s Mother and I appeared on television with the dynamic Regis Philbin when our first book, *Take Charge of Your Health,* was released. We prepared a Serenity Cocktail drink with brewer's yeast, protein, whey, lecithin and a banana, all mixed together in certified raw milk. Regis was so dear, he drank it and even said it tasted good!

Regis was the popular co-host on *Live with Regis and Kathie Lee,* now (*Regis and Kelly*) and was the host of *Who Wants to Be a Millionaire?* He has always been an advocate of good nutrition, especially vitamin and mineral supplements, and takes our Lindberg Varsity Pack 2 vitamin and mineral packets along with his wife, Joy, who takes the Pink Pack for Women.

I was in New York in September 1999 with my daughter-in-law, Gabrielle, and visited Regis and Kathie Lee's "live" show. Regis really looks great and has not aged in all of these years; he's doing something right! He was so kind to introduce me on camera and tell the audience how he has been taking our Lindberg Varsity Pack vitamins every day, for almost 20 years. Kathie Lee Gifford asked me, "If you could only take one vitamin what would it be?" I said, "Probably vitamin E that is not only an antioxidant important for our heart, but prevents the brown 'age spots' on the back of our hands." As we discussed this Regis interrupted and said, "The audience is taking over our show," and everyone laughed. Regis is very warm and friendly and visits with the audience during each commercial break.

Regis Philbin was giving away 3 million dollars for a department store promotion a few blocks from our store in Torrance, CA. The McFarland girls went to see his event and when it was over, Regis came to our store and shocked all of our customers! Later, over lunch with all the McFarland family, Regis said he not only takes our vitamins, but he works out regularly to stay in shape, including weight lifting and doing cardio exercises. One of my sons said, "He's got muscles that would put men 20 years younger to shame." If you don't get a chance to win a million, at least it's within your control to get in shape, stay healthy and feel like a million, like Regis!

The Trinity Broadcasting Network—TBN

The door has been opened many times for us to be on this fabulous network. Mother and I were invited to be on the *Joy* television program with the delightful host, *Jim McClellan,* in the early '80s to discuss our book *Take Charge of Your Health.* TBN is a Christian network in Tustin, California. At that time the show was seen in many states. Mother and I did numerous programs together, and, years later, I appeared with my beautiful daughter, *Laura McFarland.*

Praise the Lord

TBN's most popular evening program, *Praise the Lord,* had both Mother and myself on several times. I could hardly believe it when response letters came from the tip of South Africa to the islands of the West Indies, and Canada.

The Doctor's Night

You will see references in this book to *The Doctor's Night,* which are prime-time, three-hour television programs on TBN. These doctor programs have gone on for years and are one of the station's most requested. They consist of several medical doctors and myself discussing all aspects of health and nutrition. I always count it an honor to be asked to participate. My part of the show is to discuss proper nutrition and how to build health and improve our sense of well-being. It always amazes me how the switchboard at their station lights up with calls from people all over the world who want to know more about good health. In this book, I've tried to answer many of the most frequently asked questions from these television programs, knowing that they are the most common and relevant to a wide variety of people.

Trinity Broadcasting Network is now seen almost all over the world. In fact, as of April 1999, *Paul Crouch* states they have 977 stations worldwide of which 551 are foreign stations. What an amazing accomplishment!

Paul and Jan Crouch, TBN owners, are also very interested in their health. Jan Crouch says that taking the Pink Pack for Women these last 15 years has kept her well. She also takes other nutritional supplements and our protein powders.

Doctor to Doctor

Laura and I were on *Dr. Helen Pensanti's Doctor to Doctor* health program for almost two years doing a television program each week (about 63 programs). This was a tremendous amount of work as we prepared food and nutritional dishes, teaching the audience how to cook, and providing recipes for those who wrote in to the program. People are in great need of information about nutrition, and they are eager to learn! I can't thank my precious Laura enough for helping me "pull it all together."

The Carol Lawrence Show

It has also been a wonderful experience being a frequent guest on Carol Lawrence's television program on TBN. Carol is a beautiful actress, singer, and dancer who is a big advocate of good nutrition, and we had wonderful discussions many times on her shows. Carol was the original Maria on Broadway in *West Side Story* and has a "Star" on the Hollywood Walk of Fame for live theater.

This Is Your Day!

I was invited to do a week of television programs with *Benny Hinn* on his daily program, *This Is Your Day*. Benny Hinn is very interested in keeping his audience and partners of his ministry healthy. He offered my original *Aging Without Growing Old* book on his show as a gift to his audience for any donation, because he wanted his people to read it and stay well. Though he has a healing ministry, he knows that many are not healed. There is so much we can do ourselves, in changing our eating habits and in taking nutritional supplements, to keep us active and well. That was our combined message to his audience!

Hope Builders

The television program, *Hope Builders,* features *Steve Brock,* a fabulous singer on TBN. Steve also travels the world with the Benny Hinn Crusades. I was invited to be his television guest for three programs in Palm Desert, California, at the Desert Falls Country Club, to discuss current health issues. According to his lovely wife, Pat, they received a tremendous amount of mail from these programs. It's a wonderful privilege to have the opportunity to share "hope" for good health to his many viewers.

New TV Series—*Doctor to Doctor*

This is a series I am on each week with Dr. Makena Marangu, and Dr. Helen Pensanti. We individually discuss an important health issue and I make my presentation from a nutritional perspective I think might interest the viewers. It has become a very popular program since so many people have been helped through a better understanding of nutrition and how to live a healthier life. I have really enjoyed being a part of these programs. In fact, one of my daughter's friends saw me on this program in BonAire, off the coast of Venezuela, in their hotel room after snorkeling! It is amazing how these programs are seen throughout the world.

Trinity Christian City International

This is a fabulous facility in Costa Mesa, California, where many of the TBN television programs are broadcast. *Jan Crouch* asked if I would give a seminar on nutrition every month. Lecturing for two hours really keeps me on my toes and reading all the latest literature. I am so grateful to my dear daughter, Laura, for helping me with this project. She usually brings along her son, Tyler, my precious grandson who also helps!

Radio talk shows

When the first edition of *Aging Without Growing Old* was released, I was, and still am, booked on many call-in talk shows, all across America. I would first discuss my book and then talk to the radio audience, answering their questions. It is always interesting to me how many speak of the numerous drugs they are taking. This makes me more convinced than ever that we need to start on an excellent nutritional program early in life and not wait until we are ill.

Following Her Example

What I know about nutrition was not necessarily gained in a classroom. I do have a Bachelor of Science degree in Foods and Nutrition from Pepperdine University, but most of what I know was learned at Mother's side.

In following her example, I began reading the classic works of early researchers. I became part of a group that started the American

Nutrition Society in the South Bay area of southern California and served as the group's Program Chairman and President for many years. I've also been involved in our industry many, many years, serving on the Board of Directors of the National Nutritional Foods Association (NNFA) and on the Golden West Regional Board of the NNFA. At the 1996 NNFA national convention in Nashville, I was honored with an award for ongoing and continued support of the nutrition and health industry. I am also a member of the American Academy of Anti-Aging Medicine. I stay current with nutritional and scientific literature, and attend lectures and seminars across the nation, even in other parts of the world.

The third generation

Our adult children have joined my husband, Don, and me in our family business. Gary is Purchasing Director and buyer for Lindberg Nutrition and our mail order company Nutrition Express. Dan is our Marketing Director for the entire organization. Our daughter, Laura, also received her Bachelor of Science degree in Foods and Nutrition from Pepperdine University. She has worked in our store, helped in the mail-order department with her dad, assists me with lectures, appears on television with me, and is by my side just as I was with Mother. Our son Douglas is a Medical Doctor specializing in Emergency Medicine. He has been involved with product development.

Though the number keeps changing, we are currently the proud grandparents of twelve grandchildren—two granddaughters and ten grandsons. How blessed we are to be "Papa Don" and "Nonnie" to these beautiful and healthy grandchildren.

There are NO "magic bullets"

When we discuss the subject of aging, we must lay the nutritional foundation for abundant health. As much as we may dream about the "magic bullet" that will prevent aging or the degenerative diseases that usually accompany growing old, there is no such pill yet. I have compiled a tremendous amount of information for you to help you along this anti-aging path. I make no claims in this book that any one nutrient, vitamin, mineral, hormone or practice will help every person. All the nutrients your body needs must be supplied in sufficient and balanced quantities in order for your body to be properly nourished. This book provides you with a complete nutrition program that will help you achieve optimal health now and for the rest of your life!

Aging
Let's Slow It Down

Holding Back the
Hands of the Biological
Time Clock

*We shouldn't think of growing older as a time of
physical degeneration, senility or becoming
cantankerous. Our goal should be to maximize our
vitality, doing what contributes to optimum health, so
we can maintain our zest for living.*

—GLADYS LINDBERG

My Mother, Gladys Lindberg, had a simple test for establishing the true age of a person. She would tell you to pick up the skin on the back of your hand and pull it up taut, hold it for a few seconds, and then let go. If your skin snapped back, Mother declared you to be young, regardless of your chronological years. If your skin "crawled" back, you were old. Truly old skin may take a minute or more to return to normal. Mother, of course, loved to show her customers how elastic her own beautiful skin was. Check yours. Compare your skin with younger and older friends. Later I will discuss how to keep your skin young and elastic.

We Each Have Two Ages

There is our *chronological age*, which involves the celebrating of birthdays and passing of years, and our *biological age*, which reflects the rate at which we are getting older. Everybody ages at the same chronological rate, but people do not age at the same biological rate. You will find the skin-test comparison interesting, especially if you smoke and drink alcohol. The goal of nearly everybody I know is to reduce the rate at which they age biologically!

My husband and I were high school sweethearts and continued dating throughout college. Don received a football scholarship to the University of Southern California, and we didn't marry until 1955, after college. We attended our 50th Manual Arts high school reunion and were looking forward to meeting our friends from long ago. When we arrived at the hotel, Don said he was going to ask directions to the ballroom, but I assured him we would find our friends without difficulty. Well…we found a ballroom with lots of celebrating, happy senior citizens. Don hesitated before going in, saying, "This can't be our class; they look too old." Of course it was our group!

We realized very quickly how fast the years had flown by. I had never thought much about our own aging until we attended that party and saw many of our long-lost friends. We were all about the same chronological age (except the "new" wives of several of the men), but we certainly had many different biological ages. Some looked great, but others I recognized only by the high school photo on their name tag. What caused the difference in the aging of our friends?

Is There an Aging Clock?

Aging is influenced by many factors, including genetics, lifestyle and what has been called an "aging clock." This aging clock regulates specific changes at various times throughout our lives. An example of this internal time clock would be when our bodies start producing hormones that control our growth and sexual development, a time called puberty. Another example of this internal time clock would relate to women and menopause. Women enter menopause at different ages, from early '40s to mid-'50s.

At the time of mid-life, for both sexes, our body starts to wind down. A signal is sent by the level of our hormones that we are past our prime. Our body is now more vulnerable to various illnesses and degenerative diseases.

An important aspect of aging is the decline of key physiological functions: vision impairment with cataracts, glaucoma, brittle bones and dowager humps (usually associated with osteoporosis or osteoarthritis), weaker muscles and loss of strength, diseases that shorten life (such as cancer, heart disease, diabetes), a weakened immune system, senility or memory loss, and the list goes on.

Many of these conditions are not necessarily true signs of aging but rather the result of combinations of long-term nutritional deficiencies and decreases in our natural hormone levels. Physical activity and our positive mental attitude also play an important part in preventing this "disease" of aging.

Holding back the hands of the biological time clock

In the mid-'60s, Dr. Leonard Hayflick published an interesting paper in which he concluded that human cells have a definite number of cell divisions built into their genetic code. In other words, our cells are capable of reproducing themselves only so many times. This conclusion, in turn, suggested that there was a limit to the human life span.[1] The idea of a biological time clock was born.

Several years later, however, at the Miami Symposium on Theoretical Aspects of Aging, a researcher reported that only in certain cell cultures did cells stop dividing, while in others they continued to divide. This researcher also noted that cells that had stopped dividing could be stimulated to divide again.[2]

Other scientists picked up on this possibility, and in 1976 a researcher reported that red blood cells in a culture with partial vitamin

E deficiency were destroyed eight to ten percent faster than cells with adequate vitamin E.[3] Another scientist enriched human cells in a test tube with vitamin E and found that he could prolong the cells' life-span for as many as 120 generations of cell division, compared to a span of 50 generations for untreated cells![4] Vitamin E was apparently acting as an antioxidant in this experiment.

Today the findings seem to point toward a two-sided truth. On the one hand, we do have a biological clock within each cell that limits its age. On the other hand, we can intervene in this cell mechanism and add time to the clock, as the researchers did with vitamin E. There is more valuable information on vitamin E in the *Antioxidant* chapter, and throughout this book.

Every human being begins life as a single cell, a fertilized egg. By the time he/she reaches adulthood, the body consists of 100 trillion cells. The cell is the fundamental component of all living things. As cells deteriorate, people age. As cells malfunction, people get sick. If we had a better understanding of cell function, people might live longer and stay healthier.[5]

Every living cell in your body is made of protein. Furthermore, every cell must have a continuous supply of protein to maintain its life. Protein foods are often referred to as the building blocks of the body, necessary for tissue repair and the construction of new tissue.

When you have unhealthy cells, cells that are missing the essential amino acids (proteins), the body will "cement" you together with scar tissue. My Mother, Gladys Lindberg, the famous pioneering nutritionist, would explain it this way:

The scar tissue appears:

- in your eyes as *cataracts;*

- in your lungs as *emphysema;*

- in your liver as *cirrhosis;*

- in your kidneys as *nephrosis;*

- in your arteries as *arteriosclerosis;*

- in your nerves as *multiple sclerosis;*

- in your brain as *senility* (when it obstructs the flow of oxygen to the brain).

"Usually vitamin and mineral deficiencies go hand in hand with protein deficiencies, but this state is preventable, and often reversible, if we give our bodies all the nutrients it needs," she would say.

Cell function is the basis of all life. As we grow older, trillions of body cells reproduce countless times and in the course of reproduction gradually change. To reduce biological aging, our goal is to maintain the reproduction of our cells with minimal deterioration or change.

Every cell has a limited life. It performs its function in the body, then reproduces itself and dies. At any given time, thousands of your cells may be dying, while thousands more are being born, some faster than others. Fat cells, for example, reproduce slowly, while skin cells reproduce approximately every ten hours.

Only one type of cell doesn't follow this pattern—the cells of your brain. You were given your lifetime supply of brain cells at the time of your birth. When these cells become worn out and die, some authorities report they are never replaced. Others are now reporting they can regenerate. Scientists tell us that by age 35, a person is losing 100,000 brain cells a day. I always wonder who is counting! Fortunately, whether they can regenerate or not, the initial supply is so great that this loss is scarcely noticeable.

DO WE HAVE CONTROL OVER AGING? Much of aging has to do with our lifestyles, choices and personal environment. The good news is that this is something over which we do have some control. A number of things cause damage to our cells, such as ultraviolet light, x-rays, smoking, alcohol, lack of exercise, chemicals in our foods, processed or oxidized fats, and many other factors. But damage to cells can be minimized in many ways, as you will see throughout this book. Scientists are increasingly focusing their research on the entire process of aging and are defining it as an instant-by-instant destruction of weakened, undefended cells that on a massive scale leads to the degeneration of the body and even the mind.

Living on this side of disease

An overwhelming number of people, young and old, simply don't feel well. They do not have an obvious illness, yet they do not feel well on a consistent basis. They are living in the twilight zone of health—without a major problem or life-threatening disease, yet with a multitude of minor problems that keep them from experiencing the full vitality and energy of health. They are, indeed, "living on the edge of disease."

It is easier to say what aging is NOT. It is not senility and poor health. These are conditions generally brought on by chronic malnutrition and inattention to what the body needs to maintain its vigor at any age. Unfortunately, senility and aging are often equated. The truth is that everybody ages, but only some become senile. Senility is not inevitable. Memory loss, inability to store new information, and certain personality quirks associated with senility can be postponed, if not prevented, as you will see.

Just as senility is not inevitable, neither are most chronic degenerative diseases. A person can age without many of the conditions we have come to assume are inescapable. Yes, we can slow down and in many cases prevent this physical and even mental degeneration. Let's understand through the information in this book that disease is not an inevitable part of aging, and it is possible for us to not only live a long life, but to be strong and healthy as we go down this path during our lifetime.

Yes, we can slow down this whole aging process and even restore our youthful zest for living and loving. So let's get started!

The Value of Scientific Research and Medical Studies

Throughout this book you are going to find numerous references to scientific research and medical studies. Some of the studies are very recent; others are classic studies. Just because a medical study is old doesn't make it invalid. Some 25 years ago I heard distinguished physicians discuss studies that linked a folic acid deficiency to gross birth defects. And yet, this finding has been reported recently as if this fact was just discovered.

I attended a conference at the National Institutes of Health in Bethesda, Maryland, in June 1996 with my daughter, Laura. I was excited to visit our government's highest scientific institute. They were sponsoring the presentation that dietary supplements can help normal, healthy, well-nourished, active people improve their performance. The conference was entitled "The Role of Dietary Supplements for Physically Active People," and it was co-sponsored by 11 divisions of the NIH.

After a few presentations, it was obvious the select audience had more information than the panel of experts. One of the speakers was a young Ph.D. from a renowned university who spoke about vitamin E.

The information presented was very basic and "surface level" as far as I was concerned. After the lecture, I asked this young lady if she had read any of the classic vitamin E studies conducted by Drs. Wilfrid and Evan Shute of Canada. She had never heard of them. How sad to miss out on their wealth of knowledge! Their research on vitamin E was presented widely in the mid-'50s, '60s and even the '70s. They worked with 38,000 cardiac patients and documented tremendous benefits of vitamin E in preventing heart disease. They also authored several excellent books such as *The Heart and Vitamin E*, revised in 1977. Their research stands as valid today as it was back then. "New research" touting that vitamin E can prevent heart disease, increase immunity, even prevent hot flashes in menopausal women, is only now gaining the attention it should have had 40 years ago.

JAMA reports adverse drug reactions kill 100,000 annually.

Information that *more than 100,000* patients die and another 2.2 million are harmed in American hospitals every year by adverse drug reactions from *properly administered pharmaceutical drugs* sent shock waves through our country. This report placed deaths from adverse drug reactions as the fourth leading cause of death overall, depending on how conservatively one analyzes the data.[6] This report was published in the April 15 *JAMA*, and was discussed only briefly on television, but reported in the *New York Times,* plus many of my nutrition newsletters. It is interesting that the annual reports from the Center for Disease Control (CDC) have shown for years that thousands of adverse reactions, including deaths, are attributed to prescription drugs.[7]

I feel that these kinds of reports are making people realize they need to learn how to take charge of their health through dietary modifications and aggressive nutritional supplementation, so they can eliminate some of their unnecessary medications. This is one of the reasons so many are turning to alternative medicine.

The November 11, 1998 issue of the *JAMA* was devoted to alternative medicine. One of the articles was entitled "Trends in Alternative Medicine Used in the United States, 1990–1997." David Eisenberg, M.D., summarized his study on the extent the public has adopted alternative medicine since 1990. Dr. Eisenberg reported that 46.3 percent of Americans visited an alternative practitioner in 1997. There were 629 million visits to alternative care practitioners, which exceeds total visits to all conventional physicians. This is really amazing when you realize most of this is paid for by the patient and not by medical insurance. This amounted to 27 billion dollars spent on alternative therapies in 1997.[8]

My son, Douglas McFarland, M.D., has shared information with me from copies of a newsletter he now receives called *Alternative Medicine Alert, A Clinician's Guide to Alternative Therapies*. The series started in January 1998 and is dedicated to educating medical doctors on alternative therapies and the scientific basis for their use. Recent information reported on how glucosamine sulfate, vitamin C, vitamin E, evening primrose oil, milk thistle, and many other supplements are now going "mainstream." How grateful I am that our medical profession is becoming educated about some of these natural therapies and that they recognize their importance in the care of their patients.[9]

Most of the natural or alternative therapies reported in my book are backed by many decades of information and hundreds and hundreds of scientific papers. You will educate yourself about this alternative medical information as you read through this book.

"Healthy people don't have that."

In my nutritional counseling when I hear most of my clients' list of symptoms and ailments, I quickly tell them, "I am not a medical doctor and do not treat disease, but healthy people don't have that; let's make you healthy."

What is it that healthy people don't have? Perhaps first and foremost, they don't have major degenerative diseases—cancer, heart trouble, crippling arthritis, osteoporosis, mental illness, senility or Alzheimer's, diabetes, emphysema, arteriosclerosis (hardening of the arteries), atherosclerosis (fatty deposits in arteries), and others.

Research statistics tell us that degenerative diseases are responsible for more than 70 percent of all deaths in this country. I once heard former Surgeon General C. Everett Koop say that "dietary imbalances" are the leading preventable contributors to premature death in the United States. This is borne out by the Center for Disease Control, which has stated that 54 percent of heart disease, 37 percent of cancer, 50 percent of cerebrovascular disease (pertaining to the blood vessels of the brain), and 49 percent of atherosclerosis is preventable through lifestyle modification. In all, some 1.6 million deaths a year may be related to poor nutrition! As startling as these figures may be, there is great hope for people willing to take charge of their health. Most people are aging too rapidly and are dying from something that can be prevented! Many are finding there is a great deal they can do to help themselves.

We need to recognize that the degenerative diseases that are rampant today were hardly known before the Industrial Revolution, which brought people from farms into the cities. People in past generations faced major killers that were more commonly associated with germs, parasites, or viruses—diseases such as smallpox, influenza, plagues, and diphtheria. These have almost all been conquered, thanks in large part to the discovery of antibiotics and modern means of refrigeration and sanitation.

The major causes of aging and degenerative diseases are associated generally with the absence or lack of some substance from our system. Stated in other terms, the person with any of these diseases is generally missing something that would otherwise keep him or her well. That "something" is nearly always associated with things people can take into their bodies, and in many cases it is something related to nutrition. In very simple terms, malnutrition is a significant cause of aging and degenerative diseases. This is often caused by a lack of certain vitamins, minerals, or trace elements.

Our goal, then, is to make sure that we take into our bodies all that we need to maintain excellent health and eliminate those things from our diet that we know damage our health. It sounds simple, and in many ways it is. Unfortunately, there is much confusion about what constitutes an "adequate diet"—a diet that promotes total health and a feeling of well-being, strength, energy, and vitality. One nutritionist says one thing, another contradicts. One book reports certain findings, and another refutes its claims.

You are unique!

No two individuals have the same genetic code, cellular structure or hormone balance. We all take individualized routes through life, encountering different environments and stressors. Despite our unique nutritional differences, our goal of optimal health is shared by all.

Good health is far more than simply the absence of disease. Your body is always trying to make you well. It is constantly in the process of making trillions of new cells. These cells have to reach into your bloodstream to obtain more than 40 chemicals: amino acids (the building blocks of protein), fatty acids, minerals, trace elements, vitamins, and enzymes. These chemicals must come from the food we eat, the water we drink, and the air we breathe. When our food is hydrogenated, homogenized, refined, microwaved, preserved, emulsified, pasteurized, chemicalized, colored, bleached, and sterilized, something is lost. In many cases, it is our health that is lost!

Each of us has a unique and individually determined biochemical heredity pattern. The exact amount of each nutrient that you need is as distinct as your fingerprint or voice print. When you experience a health problem, your body is sending you a signal that your body cells are ailing. They are not being provided with the nutrients they need to sustain and propagate healthy cells, tissues, and organs.

Your body may be able to get along without a particular nutritional substance for days, weeks, months, even years; but if the pattern continues, chances are you will eventually develop a health problem. Some people will develop problems sooner than others. Some will develop more severe problems than others. But eventually, all of us are subject to problems if we don't provide our bodies with the materials needed for rebuilding healthy cells.

Many fail to understand the role of nutrition and unknowingly deprive themselves of optimum health. Their minor abnormalities, left uncorrected, frequently lead to more serious disease. Recognizing subtle deviations from good health and taking steps to correct them early is preventive medicine at its best. And that's what this book intends to help you accomplish.

Maintaining a zest for living

I often see clients who have been customers of ours for...can you believe for 50 years! My Mother, Gladys Lindberg, placed them on her program and they have stayed with it through the decades. Why? Because it worked for them. They look great, are feeling well, and are aging with grace. They are free of disease. So they return again and again to continue doing what they know works so well for them. They often tell me amazing stories about how their health was radically transformed years ago by Mother's advice. The following is a classic example of one of those stories. You can imagine how surprised I was when Linda referred to Mother, from the podium, at a recent health convention!

The beautiful actress, Linda Evans, is forever grateful.

While at the Natural Products Expo West in Anaheim, California, I attended a lecture by the lovely *Linda Evans*. She was representing

Ostivone, a product I discuss in the *Osteoporosis* chapter.

Linda Evans is the exceptionally beautiful actress who played the beautiful blond "Krystle" on the television program *Dynasty*. This television series seemed to be everyone's favorite for years and years. At the lecture, Linda presented a compelling testimony on how sick she had been when in her 20s. She stated she had developed terrible allergies, asthma and hives that caused her face to break out and eyes to water. As she said, "I was a mess." She was allergic to everything—dust, the food she ate, and even the trees in her backyard!

Linda explained that she had the best medical specialists in the country treat her for over a year and a half. She was hospitalized at St. Johns in Santa Monica for almost a week, where she was given every test imaginable. Some of these specialists even flew in from the Mayo Clinic. The diagnosis was idiopathic (of unknown cause) allergies and edema. The prescribed treatment was to give herself daily shots for the rest of her life so she could "live" with the condition. She described how, when she was trying to give herself the first injection, that she decided then and there to find another answer.

Linda told how she heard about Gladys Lindberg, the owner and nutritionist of Lindberg Nutrition Service. She went to see Mother at our store on Wilshire Boulevard near Beverly Hills. Mother put Linda on a complete nutritional program, starting with Lactobacillus Acidophilus, to re-establish friendly bacteria in her intestinal tract. Linda took the *Lindberg Pink Pack*, which is our complete vitamin and mineral packet for women. She also drank our *serenity cocktail* (no longer available) mixture for breakfast and mid-afternoon. This powder combination was to provide her with all of the known and unknown nutrients in high enough potencies to build her up. The Hydrochloric acid and Pancrea-Lind (pancreatic enzymes) helped her digest and assimilate her food. Mother knew that we are usually not allergic to things we digest, so Linda needed help in digesting her food. (At the lecture, Linda simply told the audience what she was taking, but I am explaining to you why.)

Mother explained to Linda that her adrenals were exhausted and she needed to build them up. She had told Linda that she did not need to accept the advice that she would not get well. Mother used her favorite phrase, "Healthy people don't have 'that,' so let's make you healthy." As you can see, Mother never believed in the "magic bullet" approach. She knew Linda needed the full gamut of nutrition, and Linda was willing to do it all.

The next part of her testimony was thrilling to hear. She stated how the nutrition program worked, and she got well and was able to lead a normal life again. What a blessing; she had no more allergies!

I went backstage to meet Linda and told her I was Gladys Lindberg's daughter and that I was thrilled to hear her speak. I sent her my original *Aging Without Growing Old* book, and we later talked on the telephone and she gave me this precious statement that I want to share with you.

> I shall be forever grateful to Gladys Lindberg for her wisdom and understanding of proper nutrition. With her help, and a change in my attitude, I was able to heal myself of my allergies. This was in the early 1970s and I have blessed her a million times since.
>
> —LINDA EVANS

This is a classic example of what I have heard all my life. I don't care where I am or even what country I am in, it is always amazing how people will approach me and tell me a story similar to Linda Evans'! What a thrill to know Mother blessed Linda with newfound health, as well as many thousands more throughout the years.

"They can't kill me now."

A woman recently came into our southern California store with her darling mother who was visiting from Alabama. The mother had been a mail-order customer for more than 35 years. When she came to visit her daughter in Los Angeles, she insisted on visiting our store to meet me, because I was Gladys Lindberg's daughter.

I found this spry little woman with steel-gray hair pushing her own shopping cart through the store. She told me how she once had been so sick that her doctors had said there was no hope for her. She said, "I had everything wrong that could go wrong. They just gave up on me. I came to see Gladys Lindberg, and she saved my life." She went on to inform me that she is now 96 years old. "They can't kill me now," she said with a twinkle in her eye. "I just go on and on." And off she went, buzzing through our store and loading up her cart with the *Pink Pack* and other products that had been recommended to her "way back in the '50s."

When I meet women such as she, I know that the medical establishment would label her story as "anecdotal," but to me, it is a miracle. This woman was not part of a double-blind, crossover study. Still, she is enjoying good health at age 96. As far as I'm concerned, she is the beneficiary of the best nutritional wisdom Mother had to offer... and that

I am delighted to share with you in this anti-aging book.

Don't change a thing!

Another woman called to ask me if she should change what she had been taking, which was our special Varsity Pack 2, the athletic vitamin and mineral pack. This is the packet that was originally designed for amateur and professional athletes. In talking with her, I discovered she was driving her own car, working in her yard, and taking complete care of herself as her husband had passed away the year before. She still had all her mental faculties and had no real complaints but was just "moving a little slower." In ordering her vitamins, she wondered if she should change what she was doing. She said she had been faithful in following Gladys Lindberg's advice for more than 35 years. Her voice sounded quite young, so I finally asked, "How old are you, honey?"

She replied, "89."

I immediately responded, "Don't change a thing!"

The higher potencies in these vitamin and mineral packets worked for her. I am sure at 89 we would all love to still be driving our car and be completely independent.

Baby boomers and senior citizens alike want to age without growing old. Such people as these are enjoying great health; they have aged without growing old. Nutrition has played a major role in preventing their physical and mental deterioration. Many of the baby boomers and senior citizens I see have maintained a zest for living, loving, working, and growing. They are still striving to be the very best they can be, at whatever age.

I have always maintained that you can improve with age—that you can retain an attractive appearance and vitality while enjoying optimum health. However, health is not something that just happens.

Let's build you up! My role as a nutritional counselor is to discuss a person's eating habits and to suggest dietary changes that may help to encourage good nutritional practices. This includes supplementation of all the essential vitamins, minerals, proteins, fatty acids, herbs, the natural hormones and single amino acids when necessary. Exercise also fits into this formula. Moderate-intensity exercise, such as brisk walking 30 minutes a day, improves immune function and mood, prevents migraines, lowers blood pressure, and decreases the disability that affects inactive people as they age.

I also believe in the power of prayer. Medical research has even proved it works! We also need a positive mental attitude, continually telling ourselves how great we feel. I try to inspire my clients to "take charge of their health," and when they do so, many of their physical and emotional problems improve and even disappear.

Make a decision today that you are going to strive for optimal health—the best health you can possibly have—and that you are going to become healthy through natural and nutritional means. You can enjoy greater health at any age, so let's make you healthy! You can take charge of your health...and slow down the aging process...beginning now!

The Significance of Vitamins, Minerals and Herbs

Important Nutrients for Health and Healing

When the missionary zeal took hold of me, I was thrilled to read the works of the pioneering doctors. Their tremendous results helped chart my path and open my eyes to this whole field of nutrition.
—GLADYS LINDBERG

The late Albert Szent-Gyorgi, M.D., Ph.D., was a brilliant researcher who received the Nobel Prize for Physiology and Medicine for the isolation of vitamin C, as well as the Albert Lasker Prize for his theory of muscle contraction. One of his classic statements was that "the whole idea of a vitamin is a paradox and difficult to digest. Everybody knows that things we eat can make us sick, but it seems utterly senseless to say that something that we have *not* eaten could make us sick. And this is exactly what a vitamin is: *A substance that makes us sick and even die by not eating it.*"[1]

I believe this statement is one that truly reflects the great importance of vitamins. If we do not obtain the vitamins or minerals we need from our food supply or in supplement form, we can become sick and even die. The Scriptures tell us: "My people are destroyed for lack of knowledge" (Hos. 4:6). Classic examples of this in history are diseases that caused a tremendous amount of suffering and millions of deaths for "lack" of a certain vitamin and the knowledge that it was needed.

Today, researchers know that each of the diseases below is the result of a deficiency of an important molecule in the organs and tissues of the body.

- **Scurvy.** In the 1700s, British sailors perished for the lack of knowledge that ascorbic acid, or vitamin C, prevented scurvy. It was not until 1928 that Dr. Szent-Gyorgi was able to obtain vitamin C, and not until 1939 that it was named ascorbic acid and recognized as a possible dietary deficiency. The bioflavonoids such as grape seed and pycnogenol also help prevent scurvy.

- **Beriberi** results from an insufficient supply of the vitamin B_1 (thiamin). The word *beriberi* means "extreme weakness" in the Singhalese language. It was common in Asia where the diet was limited to white rice in which the B_1 was refined out.

- **Pellagra** was caused by an insufficient supply of vitamin B_3 (niacin) that resulted in dermatitis, diarrhea, and dementia (confusion and memory loss).

- **Pernicious anemia** results from an insufficient amount or absorption of vitamin B$_{12}$ (cobalamin). An intrinsic factor is essential for the absorption of vitamin B$_{12}$.

- **Rickets** is caused by a lack of vitamin D in the diet or insufficient exposure of the skin to sunlight.

- **Goiter** can be prevented by taking the mineral iodine and kelp.

- **Anemia** is treated and prevented by taking the mineral iron.

- **Osteoporosis** can be prevented by taking calcium, magnesium, vitamin D, boron, ipriflavone and even the use of natural progesterone hormone cream.

- **Spina Bifida** and other birth defects can be prevented if the expectant mother takes the B-vitamin, folic acid.

The causes of these diseases may be obvious to many, but we also need to be able to recognize subclinical deficiencies, or "pre-disease" symptoms, and reverse trends before they develop. The more we learn about these deficiency symptoms, the more we are equipped to take charge of our health and the health of our loved ones.

Many people are finally realizing that the average American diet is far from adequate and actually causes some of the diseases we face today. Some of the diet-induced diseases that have become major killers are heart disease, many forms of cancer, diabetes, osteoporosis, arthritis, and premature aging. Other conditions such as allergies, obesity, chronic fatigue, impotence, birth defects, and so forth can also be directly related to nutritional imbalances in our bodies.

In all, deficiencies of certain vitamins and minerals can be involved in the death of millions of Americans annually. You only need to walk into any nursing home to see outright evidence of deficiencies—especially scurvy—that have not been recognized, and therefore, are not being corrected.

Scurvy in This Day and Age?

I am sure you have seen older people who have deep red bruising (sometimes almost purple) on their hands and arms. They may even tell you they don't know why any slight bump or scrape seems to cause it. Their gums bleed easily, especially when they brush their teeth.

Wounds don't heal, their skin is rough, and their muscles waste away. In Mother's old classic medical books there were photographs of scurvy and the symptoms appear identical. We all know scurvy has been conquered ... or has it?

In these classic books the recommendation is always vitamin C. I often wonder what these older people must be doing or drugs they are taking that are either destroying their vitamin C or increasing the need for vitamin C and the bioflavonoids in their bodies.

This story is tragic to me because everyone thinks scurvy is from the old days. Information reported in the *Journal of the American Medical Association* stated, "Scurvy is a disease that can mimic other more serious disorders ... and because clinical features of scurvy are no longer well appreciated, scorbutic patients are often extensively evaluated for other disorders."[2]

Michael Rosenbaum, M.D., said, "Most physicians believe that everyone gets all the vitamin C they need, so they fail to suspect scurvy when faced with the symptoms. The symptoms of scurvy can mimic the symptoms of cardiovascular disease, arthritis, infectious disorders, and many other common illnesses usually treated by means far more expensive than vitamin C supplementation." He went on to say, "A lot of illness and unnecessary medical treatment might be prevented by making sure everyone got plenty of vitamin C in their diets."[3]

If you see your loved ones with these symptoms, recommend vitamin C with bioflavonoids and Pycnogenol or grape seed extract on a daily basis. Read more about these nutrients in the next chapter.

Vitamins

Vitamins are not the fuel, but they are like the ignition switch
that sparks the fuel and keeps the engine running.

A vitamin is a group of organic compounds that, in very small amounts, are essential for normal growth, development and metabolism. With a few exceptions, they cannot be synthesized or made in the body and must be supplied by the diet. Vitamins are produced by living material, such as plants and animals, as compared to minerals that come from the soil. Lack of sufficient quantities of any of the vitamins produces specific deficiency diseases. In fact, if a substance does not produce a deficiency symptom when it is removed from the diet, it is not considered a vitamin.

Each vitamin functions in many diverse roles and always with other essential nutrients. They participate in a variety of life-building processes, including the formation and maintenance of blood cells, hormones, all the cells and tissues of the body, and even the creation of our genetic material.

Vitamins contain NO calories.

Vitamins are not used as sources of energy as some believe. They contain no calories, and they cannot make you fat. They are used to form enzymes that are biologic catalysts in many metabolic reactions within the body. Several vitamins help convert the calories in carbohydrates, protein, and fat into usable energy for the body. In other words, vitamins are not the fuel, but they are like the ignition switch that sparks the fuel and keeps the engine running. When vitamins are not present in sufficient quantity, metabolism ceases or is impaired.

CLASSIFICATIONS OF VITAMINS

Vitamins are generally classified as water-soluble or fat-soluble.

Water-Soluble Vitamins dissolve in water and are not stored by the body to any great extent. These include vitamin C, or ascorbic acid, and all the B-vitamins:

- B_1 (Thiamin)
- B_2 (Riboflavin)
- B_3 (Niacin, which includes niacinamide and nicotinamide)
- B_6 (Pyridoxine, which includes pyridoxal and pyridoxamine)
- B_{12} (Cobalamin)
- Folic Acid
- B_5 (Pantothenic Acid)
- Biotin
- Choline*
- Inositol*
- PABA* (Para-amino-benzoic acid)

*While essential vitamins for humans, these are not officially recognized as B-vitamins, but are considered part of the "B-complex" family.

Note: *Niacin can be made in the body from the amino acid, tryptophan.*

The Fat-Soluble Vitamins dissolve in fat and in substances that dissolve fat. These vitamins are stored in the fatty parts of the liver and other tissues. The fat-soluble vitamins are:

- Vitamin A   - Vitamin E
- Vitamin D   - Vitamin K

Note: *Vitamin D is called "the sunshine vitamin" because when the ultraviolet rays from sunlight hit the skin, a form of cholesterol in the body is converted into vitamin D.*

What increases your need for vitamins?

When you perspire, take diuretic drugs (such as high blood pressure medication), or have diarrhea, you lose an abnormal amount of water-soluble vitamins. Stress and exertion also deplete the body of these valuable nutrients. Actually, our supply of these vitamins is constantly being diminished by the activity of our own bodies. Therefore, if we are to maintain even reasonably good health, these vitamins have to be replaced on a routine basis. A variety of factors can cause a person to expend, excrete, or malabsorb certain vitamins and minerals. Some of these are listed in the following chart.

FACTORS THAT CAUSE VITAMIN, MINERAL DEPLETION

tobacco	estrogen	prescription drugs
sugar	rancid fats	emotional strain
antibiotics	aspirin	mineral oil
antacids	tranquilizers	sleeping pills
surgery	sickness	accidents
diuretics	laxatives	polluted water
fluoride	pesticides	food additives
polluted air	pregnancy	extreme cold
extreme heat	lactation	oral contraceptives
cortisone	salt	chlorinated water

Any one of these factors can cause the body to need an increase in vitamins and minerals... and most people today encounter one or more of these factors on a daily basis!

Other factors that impact our lives

There are other important factors in our modern lifestyles that affect our health. These include:

- ❧ the kinds of food you eat.

- ❧ how these foods are prepared, processed, preserved, sprayed.

- ❧ the physical, mental, and emotional stress you experience.

- ❧ the environment in which you live and work, and the contaminants to which you are exposed.

- ❧ your unique, individually determined biochemical heredity pattern or genetic code.

- ❧ the type and amount of exercise you do, or do not do.

- ❧ the quality of soil in which your food was grown.

- ❧ the type of water you drink—tap water is full of impurities, distilled has had all the minerals removed.

All these factors affect your unique requirement level for any particular vitamin or mineral.

DO I REALLY NEED TO TAKE VITAMIN AND MINERAL SUPPLEMENTS? is a question I hear often. The good news is that I hear this question less today than several years ago. The general public is becoming much more informed about the need for vitamins and minerals. Many people now come to me with a list of products they have "heard about," eager for more information or advice related to their specific health concerns.

Still, a great many people seem to feel that they can get all their daily requirements for vitamins and minerals from a "well-balanced diet" without taking additional supplements.

The diet we tend to think about as being well-balanced is one that came from our nation's agricultural heritage. Our great grandparents came from the farm, where they performed hard physical labor all day and consumed between 4,000 and 5,000 calories per day. They got their milk right from the cow and their fruit and vegetables from the garden. They ground their own whole grains and ate five or six times a day. They did not need vitamin or mineral supplements because they received enough of these nutrients from the large amounts of natural and fresh foods they consumed.

Can't burn all those calories

Most of us today cannot consume those large amounts of natural and fresh foods like our ancestors. We do not do as much physical labor so we cannot burn the extra calories or we'll gain weight. The food we eat today varies considerably in the amount of nutrients it contains, the way it is grown, the chemicals sprayed on it, how it is processed, and very often, in the way we store or prepare foods in our own kitchens.

Our farm-fed ancestors did not eat the processed, man-made, chemically enriched, synthetic fast food we consume today. For the most part, they did not need to supplement their diets. The foods of today are not the foods of our ancestors.

Not getting the minimum RDAs

Furthermore, the United States Department of Agriculture has stated that as many as one out of every two Americans are not getting the minimum RDAs (Recommended Dietary Allowances) as the result of their current diet. Even though these guidelines reflect a minimal level, one half of our population falls below minimum![4]

In addition to that reported fact, government statistics have shown that fat consumption has increased by 30 percent and sugar consumption by 50 percent in the past several decades. The average American consumes approximately 170 pounds of sugar each year, which is about one half pounds a day.[5] Remember, this is per every man, woman and child. Average means that some are eating less but many Americans are eating even more.

TOP TEN ITEMS PURCHASED IN GROCERY STORES

Ranked by dollar volume as listed in the Top Ten Almanac are as follows:[6]

1. Marlboro cigarettes
2. Coca Cola Classic
3. Pepsi Cola
4. Kraft Processed Cheese
5. Diet Coke
6. Campbell's soup
7. Budweiser beer
8. Tide detergent
9. Folger's coffee
10. Winston cigarettes

You will note there's not one whole food on this list! If the most popular purchases are nicotine, sugar, caffeine and sodium-rich processed foods, what can we expect in the way of health?

Other studies

    Time magazine has reported that only about 9 percent of

Americans manage to consume five servings a day of fruit and vegetables, according to the National Center for Health Statistics.

- A USDA survey of 21,500 people showed that over a three-day period, not one of them consumed 100 percent of the RDA for ten nutrients—the RDA already being too low, in my opinion.

- Surveys have shown that on the average, an elderly person takes between six and nine prescription drugs a day. Many of these drugs rob the body of vitamins and minerals in a variety of ways such as: increasing urinary excretion, blocking absorption, binding to nutrients and deactivating them, destroying nutrients, causing nutrients to be used up more rapidly, and increasing loss of nutrients in the stool.[7]

Our most intelligent decision

It seems the most intelligent decision a person can make today is to begin to take vitamin and mineral supplements on a daily basis.

When clients tell me they cannot afford vitamins, which can cost about as much as a cup of coffee or a soft drink, I tell them *they cannot afford NOT to take them!* Vitamins and minerals are our best anti-aging insurance policy. I believe you will agree with me as you read the tremendous research in the rest of this book.

Vitamins and Minerals Are Safe and Effective

As we and others in the nutrition field fought the proposed legislation designed to require prescriptions for vitamins, the very popular radio commentator Paul Harvey joined in the fight. At stake was our right to sell, buy, and take the vitamins we want. The forces against the free access to vitamins claimed the American public was wasting its money on vitamins. The public said back, "It is my money to spend as I see fit." The tactic of the anti-access group then changed its emphasis to say that vitamins are dangerous and toxic. This has been their message for a number of years. At the core of this issue is if vitamins are turned into prescription drugs, pharmaceutical companies could charge a great deal more for them. Is it economics, far more than science, that fueled their concern?

Paul Harvey report

When it comes to the safety of vitamins, Paul Harvey wrote in one of his columns:

- A recent eight-year study at 72 poison control centers revealed that sleeping pills and tranquilizers killed 460 people.

- Analgesics led to 715 deaths.

- Anti-depressants accounted for 805 fatalities.

- Cardiovascular drugs killed another 360.

- There were 2,500 people killed by accidental or intentional overdose of drugs.

- During those same eight years the number of people killed by vitamins was zero!

- There were no reported fatalities from taking vitamins either by children or adults.

- All suggest that vitamins, whatever their benefits, are 2,500 times safer than drugs.

Meanwhile, doctors who do recognize benefits from vitamin therapy are recommending them to overcome high cholesterol, to reduce cancer risk, to prevent or relieve many chronic health problems.[8]

Within the scientific community, Dr. Linus Pauling was a great champion in proclaiming the safety of vitamins, even when they are taken in large amounts. Side effects occur very infrequently and are rarely serious, and those that do occur often relate to factors other than the vitamins themselves.

Julian Whitaker, M.D., the physician with whom I have appeared many times on the Trinity Broadcasting Network program *The Doctor's Night*, wrote recently, "*According to detailed analysis of all available data, there are over ten million adverse reactions yearly from FDA-approved, over-the-counter, and prescription drugs. We are not talking about mild nausea or headaches. Between 60,000 and 149,000 people die per year from adverse drug reactions, according to the* Journal of the American Medical Association. *Each year, more Americans die after taking prescription drugs than died in the entire Vietnam war. This constitutes a real public health issue.*"[9]

Dr. Whitaker makes a very important point. "Only a single death related to a vitamin supplement was reported in the United States by the American Association of Poison Control Centers (AAPCC) in 1990. Only one death! After investigation by Citizens for Health, there is good reason to question whether this death was attributable to the supplement, as the young man suffered paranoid schizophrenia and was also taking six major drugs at the same time, along with the vitamin niacin." Whitaker said, "I personally would wager that his death was attributable to the six drugs that caused his liver damage."[10]

Abram Hoffer, M.D., Ph.D., said in the *Journal of Orthomolecular Medicine:* "Vitamins that are safe even in large doses have not been acceptable to the medical profession, and their negative side effects have been consistently exaggerated and over-emphasized, to the point that many of these so-called toxicities have been invented, without there being any scientific evidence that these side effects are real."[11]

A Growing Acceptance of Vitamins and Minerals

I had the honor of meeting Dr. Abram Hoffer, a Canadian psychiatrist and editor-in-chief of the *Journal of Orthomolecular Medicine,* one evening at an Alternative Cancer Treatment seminar. Dr. Hoffer is one of the pioneering medical doctors in the area of nutrition. He stated that almost every modern, acceptable treatment we see in medicine today seemed to require 40 or more years of use and study before it became widely accepted. Dr. Hoffer said he started the clock in 1957 when he first published a paper describing the use of large doses of vitamin B_3 (niacin) for the treatment of acute schizophrenia. He projected that by the year 1997 this information would become recognized as the best treatment for schizophrenia and that orthomolecular medicine would be accepted by the medical profession. Well, it hasn't happened yet! Indeed, the field of orthomolecular medicine stems from this paper of Dr. Hoffer's, as well as several others like it.

Dr. Hoffer and vitamin B_6

Dr. Hoffer has also researched vitamin B_6 (pyridoxine) and first published his studies on this important vitamin in 1975. He believes that 75 percent of people who are severely ill with mental disorders also need much larger amounts of vitamin B_6.

He writes: "As well as being mentally ill, these patients may have constipation and abdominal pains, unexplained fever and chills, morning nausea (especially if pregnant), low blood sugar, impotence or lack of menstruation, and nerve symptoms such as amnesia, tremor, spasms, and seizures. About one third of all schizophrenic patients suffer from this need for very large amounts of vitamin B_6 and niacin."[12]

Orthomolecular medicine

It was actually Dr. Linus Pauling who defined the term "orthomolecular" and placed his immense scientific prestige and knowledge behind the concept. Orthomolecular medicine means using certain nutrients in much larger amounts than is customary to satisfy the excessive need for the nutrients at various sites in the body. Dr. Pauling's work on vitamin C has been one of the major factors in swaying public opinion—and the opinions of those in the scientific community—to take vitamins more seriously. Dr. Pauling first studied the impact of vitamin C on colds and flu, then in the treatment of cancer, and finally in the role vitamin C plays in preventing hardening of the arteries. I once heard Dr. Pauling say at a conference that if he had started his research with heart disease instead of cancer, he would have found the cure for heart disease. You will read more in the *Heart* chapter about Pauling's work, especially how vitamin C prevents the oxidation of fats in the arteries and is one of the main benefits of vitamins.

Minerals
*Just as with vitamins, never underestimate
the importance of minerals to your total well-being.*

People often think of minerals as relating only to teeth and bones, but minerals also preserve the vigor of the heart and brain, as well as the muscles and the entire nervous system. About 5 percent of your total body weight is mineral matter. They are found in your bones, teeth, nerve cells, muscles, soft tissues, and blood.

Minerals are important in the production of hormones and enzymes, in the creation of antibodies, and in keeping the blood and tissue fluids from becoming either too acidic or too alkaline.

Some minerals, such as sodium, potassium, and calcium, have electrical charges that act as a magnet to attract other electrically charged substances to form complex molecules, conduct electrical impulses along nerves, or transport substances in and out of the cells. In the blood and other fluids, minerals regulate the fluid pressure between cells and the blood. Minerals also bind to proteins and other organic substances and are found in red blood cells, all cell membranes, hormones, and enzymes, the catalysts of all bodily processes.[13]

Minerals are essential for human health

The essential major minerals (sometimes called macro-nutrients or nutrients needed in larger amounts) include the following:

- calcium
- phosphorous
- potassium
- sulfur

- sodium
- chloride
- magnesium

Other essential minerals (also called micro-nutrients or trace elements) are found in the body in only small amounts. The most important trace elements are:

- iron
- zinc
- selenium
- manganese
- copper
- cobalt

- iodine
- molybdenum
- chromium
- boron
- vanadium[14]

Still other essential trace elements that appear to be important for other warm-blooded animals (although not specifically studied thoroughly in human beings yet) are such minerals as fluorine and silicon. Generally we have no problem getting enough of these in our diets. Still other trace amounts of the following minerals are usually found in the body, but little is known about how they affect the maintenance of normal bodily processes at this time: arsenic, barium, bromine, cadmium, germanium, strontium, gold, silver, aluminum, tin, nickel, bismuth, and gallium. Many of these are actually known to be toxic, including lead and mercury, so their presence in the body may not reflect an element of health.

Mineral Deficiencies

Mineral or trace element deficiencies occur much more often than vitamin deficiencies. Those at increased risk for mineral deficiencies are people who eat low-calorie diets; the elderly; pregnant women; vegetarians; those who take certain drugs, including diuretics; and those living in areas where the soil has been depleted of certain minerals.

Vitamins are usually present in foods in similar amounts around the world, but this is not true for minerals. Geologic conditions make certain areas rich in minerals and trace elements, while the soil in other areas of the world is scarce in minerals and trace elements.

Minerals can work either together or against each other. Some compete for absorption. When this happens, a large intake of one mineral can actually produce a deficiency of another. This is especially true of the trace minerals iron, zinc, and copper. Some minerals can enhance the absorption and use of other minerals, as in the case of calcium, magnesium and phosphorous that all work together well. Absorption of minerals is generally dependent on the body's particular needs.

Herbs

We often refer to herbs as "God's first pharmacy."

Herbs have been valuable sources of natural medicine for thousands of years. They have had a remarkable history of curative effects, especially when used in a proper way.

Every plant on this earth is part of God's creation and has a purpose. One of the best arguments for saving the rain forest is that it may contain as yet undiscovered plants that may help to cure cancer, AIDS, and other killer diseases. Even as we must keep an eye to the future, we also know that a number of well-researched herbal products are already available today. Herbs known in various parts of the world—but that still have not been researched or accepted in our nation—may be valuable in treating various diseases. While herbal medicine is not the focus of this book, I do believe we should use the most researched herbal products when necessary.

In other chapters we will discuss a number of herbs, such as alfalfa, astragalus, cat's claw, echinacea, goldenseal, garlic, ginkgo biloba, ginseng, hawthorn berry, milk thistle, valerian root, etc.

Mother Nature's Remedies

The leaves, flowers, bark, berries, or roots of plants are fast becoming the treatment of choice for millions of Americans. In fact, more than 1.6 billion dollars worth of herbal products are sold each year in the United States alone.[15] Packaged as capsules, tablets, teas, concentrated extracts, tinctures, and salves, these botanicals, as they are also called, are a natural and safe alternative to drugs. The medicinal herbs are those valued in the treatment and prevention of illness. Herbs have been found to help in a variety of conditions, including viral infections such as influenza.

Herbs as pharmaceutical agents

Herbs contain powerful pharmaceutical agents. In fact, an estimated one third of our pharmaceutical drugs are derived from plants. For example, white willow bark led to aspirin; the opium poppy is the basis of the opiate narcotic drugs; and the foxglove herb gave rise to Digitalis, the heart drug. More recently, the Pacific Northwest yew tree has been used to make Taxol, a drug used to treat ovarian cancer. Two of the most useful chemotherapy drugs, Vincristine and Vinblastin, are derived from the common plant Madagascar periwinkle *(Vinca rosea)*.[16] French oncologist Dr. Leon Schwarzenberg has said that "28 of the 32 most commonly used modern chemotherapeutic drugs were discovered by chance and are derived from plants."[17]

A number of other drugs are extracted from plants. A danger arises, however, when these drugs no longer have the herbal components in their natural state.

Herbs as preventive measures

The medicinal herbs are valued not only for their ability to treat illness but also for their capacity to prevent illness, which is why some are recommended as a preventive measure. Herbs have great potential to improve the quality of a person's life, especially when they are combined with proper diet, nutritional supplements, rest, exercise, and a healthy mental, emotional, and spiritual approach to living. Many herbs are referenced throughout this book in connection with specific conditions.

As a general guideline, most of the bitter-tasting herbs are medicinal herbs. The pleasant-tasting herbs are potentially less toxic and can be used more often. All plant roots and bark are naturally fungicidal and bactericidal. (If they were not, pathogens would destroy them in the ground.) Some herbs should not be used for extended periods of time, so always follow the directions.

A general rule is that the active ingredients in most herbs are more potent when the herbs are freshly picked, but since this is not practical for most of us, it is wonderful to know many parts of the plant can retain their medicinal value for years, if thoroughly dried.

The parts that may be included are the fresh leaves, flowers, berries, seeds, roots, and bark. They can be used in their natural form, or they can be found in the form of tablets, capsules, liquid beverages, extracts, powders, tinctures, creams, lotions, salves, and oils. We are constantly learning so much about the value of these natural medicines that have kept many cultures and early civilizations alive and healthy. Read more about the value of herbs in chapter four.

$\mathcal{P}$romoting Longevity
with Antioxidants

Live a Long Life by
Preventing the Killer Diseases

Every minute in your body, three billion cells die and three billion cells are created! To properly replenish these cells, your blood needs 40 different chemicals, including oxygen, hormones, enzymes, vitamins, and minerals. When any of these are lacking, your body cannot make the necessary repairs, and if deficiencies are not corrected, disease will result and we age.

—GLADYS LINDBERG

very day we are bombarded with substances that can cause damage to our bodies at the cellular level. We are exposed repeatedly, and almost constantly in some cases, to unnecessary x-rays, radioactivity, the effects of a diminishing ozone layer in our atmosphere, smog, chemical products that give off volatile fumes, and even chemical dumping. Our homes are filled with toxic substances such as asbestos, vinyl chloride, glue that holds our rugs together, lead based paints, and formaldehyde (found in plywood, particle board, paints, plastics, and detergents). We use dangerous chemical "bug bombs" to rid our homes of pests, and in the process, contaminate every area of our homes and yards with toxic chemicals.

Alternative Medicine: The Definitive Guide explains how the radiant energy emitted by computer screens, television sets, microwave ovens, fluorescent lights, high voltage electric power lines over some of our homes, electric heating in the ceilings of some homes, and even the energy from electric blankets and heated waterbeds can interfere with the body's own electric field.

Perhaps the most widespread pollutant over which we have control is tobacco smoke, which has been cited repeatedly as a contributing cause of cancer...and still, people smoke.

Potential dangers

Added to these potential dangers are preservatives and chemical additives in our foods, agricultural pesticides, chemical sprays, food processing, cured and processed meats and the tremendous amount of sugars added to our food. Even mercury amalgam fillings in our teeth have been linked to a weakening of the immune system.

Then, if we add mental stress that we're subjected to every day, it's easy to understand why "living" can be hazardous to one's health!

Regardless of the arguments that might be drawn related to the impact of any pollutants or energy sources, the net effect of all these forces striking our bodies from within and without on a daily basis must be seen as staggering. At no other time in history has the human population been bombarded by so many factors on a consistent basis, all of which "run down" our battery. Is it any wonder that we are seeing such a rapid increase in cancer, tumors, leukemia, infertility and congenital birth defects?

All of these pollutants weaken the body's ability to function, and in turn, make the body more susceptible to foreign invaders. These attacks ultimately impact the health of the individual cells in our body. What does exposure to these environmental toxins do to a cell? It causes free radical damage that is one of the main theories on aging at the cellular level.

What Is a Free Radical?

A free radical is a molecule that has lost a vital piece of itself—one of its electrically charged electrons that normally orbit in pairs. To restore balance, the free radical frantically tries to steal an electron from a nearby molecule or give away its unpaired electron. In doing so, it wreaks molecular havoc, careening into protein, fat, and the genetic DNA of cells, disfiguring and corroding them. If the target is fat, the radical can set off wildly destructive chain reactions that break down membranes, leaving cells to disintegrate. If the radical hits protein, it can destroy the cell's ability to function. If it hits DNA, it can cause mutations that incite cells to aberrant behavior. Over time, free radical damage leaves the body aged and diseased.

In an analogy, Bruce N. Ames, Ph.D., University of California at Berkeley, likens the production of free radicals to the smoke and soot by-products produced by a wood-burning fireplace. To carry the analogy further, the waste of a wood-burning fire is easily channeled away from your home's interior by your fireplace chimney, but in the body, free radical by-products are not so easily eliminated. Certain free radical scavengers must help remove these harmful free radicals from the body.

Dr. Ames said, "We need free radicals to live, but they're also the bane of our existence. Through free radical reactions in our body, it is as though we are being irradiated at low levels all the time. They grind us down." He has calculated that each of our cells endures 10,000 oxidative hits every day from errant free radicals, but that most of these cells are immediately repaired.[1]

The point to be made, of course, is that even if we lived in a pure environment, our own bodies would produce free oxygen radicals. There simply is no way to avoid their presence within the body.

Many free radicals are produced in our personal environment, such as sunlight, smog, high altitude, exposure to x-ray, toxins in food and water, pollen, ozone, molds and dust, and so forth. We can't avoid free radicals. They are everywhere. What we can do is attempt to diminish their impact on the body.

Free radical damage can impair the immune system and result in various types of cellular damage. As might be expected, such cellular damage is associated with many of our degenerative diseases: Lou Gehrig's disease, arthritis, Alzheimer's disease, some types of cancer, heart attacks, hardening of the arteries, Parkinson's disease, cataracts, cerebral vascular changes that we know as senility, and many others.[2]

What can we do? Free radicals are rendered harmless by antioxidants. Antioxidants are the "saviors" in this process. An antioxidant is a substance that can donate a sought-after electron to a free radical without becoming dangerous itself. An antioxidant that comes into contact with a free radical puts an end to the rampage of cellular and bodily destruction.

Antioxidants Can Prolong Life

Antioxidant literally means "against oxidation." Antioxidants are the good guys that continually combat the harmful effects of oxidation in the body. They are constantly on duty to render wayward free radicals harmless. The net result of their work is that they prolong the life of cells, and thus, prolong life itself. Taken in sufficient amounts, antioxidants can saturate all of our cells and tissues to provide protection against free radicals.

In the laboratory, antioxidants have been shown to prolong the life of mice. Denham Harman, M.D., who developed the free radical theory of aging more than 40 years ago, discovered that sick, old mice actually seemed to get younger when given massive doses of vitamin A. Although Harman has shown that resistance to disease decreases with age, these older mice developed fewer infections and their immune systems improved dramatically.[3]

I like to think of antioxidants as the "good guys" in the war against aging. They can prevent or repair damage to the cells. They are important nutrients in detoxifying the body and cleaning up harmful wastes. Your body makes special antioxidant enzymes, but you can also get many antioxidants in foods and nutritional supplements. The following chart identifies important antioxidants.

THE MAJOR ANTIOXIDANTS

❧ Vitamin A ❧ Vitamin C ❧ Vitamin E ❧ Selenium ❧ Beta-Carotene

OTHER EXCELLENT ANTIOXIDANTS

- Bioflavonoids
- Ginseng
- Molybdenum
- Zinc
- L-Cysteine
- Melatonin
- Copper
- Ginkgo Biloba
- Pycnogenol
- B-vitamins
  (folic acid, riboflavin, B_{12})
- N-Acetyl-Cysteine
- Carotenoids (lycopene, beta-carotene, alpha-carotene, cryptoxanthin, lutein/zeaxanthin)

- Garlic
- Manganese
- Echinacea
- Milk Thistle
- Wheat and Barley Grass
- CoQ10 (Coenzyme Q_{10})
- Alpha-Lipoic Acid
- Glutathione
- Grape Seed Extract
- DHEA
- Acetyl-L-Carnitine
- Conjugated Linoleic Acid

Knowing the Value of the Antioxidants for Our Immune System

There are several thousand research articles in medical literature on the value of the antioxidants. I want you to see how we can incorporate this information into our lives.

Two antioxidants are variations of Vitamin A:

- **Vitamin A**—known as retinol or retinyl. It is always found in animal products—such as liver, milk, eggs, butter, cream, and fish liver oil.

- **Carotenoids**—which we see most commonly as beta-carotene, is converted to vitamin A once inside the body. Typically found in carrots, sweet potatoes, and many other dark green vegetables and fruit characterized generally by yellow/orange pigment. The body converts beta-carotene into vitamin A in most people, but many others have difficulty in this conversion.

Hypothyroidism and diabetes

Dr. Sheldon Hendler reported, "Note that those with *hypothyroidism* and some with *diabetes* may not be able to efficiently convert beta-carotene to vitamin A and may thus assume a yellowish pigmentation in the skin even at lower doses. This pigmentation is not harmful in itself and will fade once beta-carotene intake is stopped or reduced."

"Those who note yellowish pigmentation while taking beta-carotene in moderate dose ranges and who have not previously been diagnosed as diabetic or as having hypothyroidism should be tested for these conditions."[4] Dr. Hendler also said he has seen a number of cases where low-dose beta-carotene supplementation has unmasked these diseases. Read about the home thyroid test in Chapter 10.

Carotenoids: fruit and vegetable antioxidants

Virtually all carotenoids work as antioxidants to rid the body of potentially cell-damaging free radicals. High blood levels of carotenoids are usually associated with a lower risk of degenerative disease. Recent research suggests that carotenoids lower the risk of certain cancers such as lung, stomach, cervix, breast, oral and bladder cancer. According to cancer researcher Gladys Block, Ph.D., an extensive and unimpeachable analysis of nearly 200 studies from 17 countries showed that eating fruit and vegetables regularly slashed your chances of getting cancer in half.

In at least 21 population-based studies, there is a 20 to 50 percent reduction in risk for many, but not all, cancers among those who are in the top quarter of fruit and vegetable intake, as compared to those in the bottom quarter. The researchers found the survival rates were much higher for women with lung cancer, endometrial cancer, cervical dysplasia (a precancerous condition of the uterine cervix), and they were less likely to develop pancreatic cancer.[5]

Carotenoids also appear to enhance the immune system and protect against age-related ailments such as stroke and heart disease.[6] Although over 600 different carotenoids have been characterized, they are simply divided into two families. There are more than 4,000 chemically unique *flavonoids* that have been identified in plants. Only 40 to 50, however, are found in the American diet, and only about 14 are actually absorbed and found in the bloodstream. See the following chart for major carotenoids.[7]

Phytonutrients

Also known as *phytochemicals*, either term simply refers to plant-derived nutrients. Carotenoids are phytonutrients, the nutritional elements that occur naturally in fruit and vegetables, giving them their distinctive yellow, orange and red colors. Green leafy vegetables are also high in carotenoids, but chlorophyll hides the yellow and orange pigments. Vegetables rich in carotenoids include carrots, tomatoes, sweet potatoes, broccoli, spinach and kale.

You may have heard the recent campaign to convince Americans to eat five servings a day of fruit and vegetables. As far as I am concerned, that's a minimum! Place your emphasis on organically grown fresh fruit and vegetables for maximum benefit.

Deeply colored fruit and vegetables are a sign that flavonoids and antioxidants are present! Red grapes and red onions have much more antioxidant value than green grapes and white onions. Blueberries contain an exceptionally high concentration of antioxidant flavonoids, as do strawberries, blackberries, bing cherries and boysenberries. Look for dark, richly colored fruit and vegetables at your market!

Important Studies on the Value of Carotenoids in Relation to Cancer

The following startling facts were confirmed through scientific studies:

- Scientists found that women with lung cancer who loaded up on vegetables nearly doubled their survival time compared with those eating the least amount of vegetables. They found tomatoes, oranges, and broccoli appeared to improve survival times the most.[8]

- Deep colored fruit and vegetables were a major deterrent to endometrial cancer. Others found tomato eaters were five times less likely to develop pancreatic cancer.[9]

- A study over a 19-year period showed that a diet with low beta-carotene consumption caused a seven-fold increase in the risk of lung cancer.

- Beta-carotene reversed the progression of premalignant lesions in the mouth.

- Postmenopausal women with a high intake of vitamin C reduced their risk of breast cancer by 16 percent, and vitamin C, vitamin E, and beta-carotene were also linked to protection against cervical cancer.[10]

There are many, many other studies that have associated carotenoids with a lower rate of cancer. It sounds to me as if the nutritional advice given for the last 50 years of "eat your dark green and yellow vegetables" and "drink your carrot juice" has had more merit than some have given it!

No adverse effects have been reported in people who have taken natural forms of beta-carotene for many, many years.[11]

MORE ANTIOXIDANTS

❧ Antioxidant	❧ Potential Benefits	❧ Where to Get It
Alpha Lipoic Acid	Extends the effects of other antioxidants, including vitamins E, C, and glutathione.	Red meat, potatoes, brewer's yeast.
Selenium	Reduces the risk of some cancers; enhances the effects of vitamin E.	Brewer's yeast, fish, liver, garlic, Brazil nuts, asparagus, mushrooms.
CAROTENOIDS Lycopene	Reduces the risk of certain cancers and cardiovascular disease.	Tomatoes, guava, watermelon, apricots, pink grapefruit.
Lutein Zeaxanthin	Prevents age-related macular degeneration (an eye disease resulting in blindness).	Spinach, broccoli mustard and collard greens, kale, hot chilies.
Beta-carotene	Limits oxidation-type reactions and neutralizes free radicals inside the cell; protects lipoproteins against oxidative damage.	Carrots, spinach, kale, sweet potatoes, tomatoes, papaya, apricots, melons.
Alpha-carotene	Inhibits the production of skin, liver and lung cancer cells.	Pumpkin, cantaloupe, yellow and red peppers, carrots, corn.
Cryptoxanthin	High levels are associated with a significant reduction in cervical cancer risk.	Peaches, tangerines, oranges, papaya, nectarines.
Bioflavonoids	Decreases risk of cardiovascular disease and some cancers; enhances the effects of vitamin C.	Onions, buckwheat, most fruit, including grapes, plums, apples, cherries, white rind of citrus fruit.[12]

Valuable Protection of Vitamin A (Retinol)

Even in the early days of vitamin research, discoveries pointed to the amazing infection-fighting properties of vitamin A (retinol or retinyl), derived from fish liver oil. An early sign of vitamin A deficiency is damage to the lining of respiratory, digestive and urogenital tracts. Vitamin A helps to maintain protective barriers against infectious organisms entering the body by preserving the integrity of the skin and mucous membranes. This is why all good parents gave their children cod liver oil (a natural source of vitamin A and D). It kept their children well.[13]

A vitamin A deficiency also increases susceptibility to viral, bacterial, and protozoal infections and makes these problems worse and more often fatal. In sum, vitamin A is vital to the health of our immune system![14]

Protective against cancer

Not only does vitamin A (fish liver oil) protect against infection, it appears to be one of the most important protective nutrients against cancer. Whether it is a result of its antioxidant properties or its ability to impact the organs and cells of the immune system, vitamin A appears to be one of our strongest allies against degenerative diseases that cause aging.[15]

- Since the '20s, a deficiency in vitamin A has been linked to the development of cancerous tissues, particularly in the lining of the respiratory, gastrointestinal, and genitourinary tracts.[16]

- In a study of 16,000 men, a deficiency of vitamin A was clearly associated with an increased risk of cancer, independent of age or smoking habits. The authors of this study concluded that measures should be taken to increase serum-retinol levels in men and women as a possible means of reducing cancer.[17]

- Breast cancer patients with higher blood levels of vitamin A responded twice as well to chemotherapy as women with lower levels. Scottish researchers reported an association between improved chemotherapy response and higher vitamin A levels for patients with cancer of the breast, cancer of the bowel, and melanoma.

- Studies revealed that men with prostate cancer had low levels of vitamin A.[18]

♪ One study tested vitamin A on 370 people who underwent operations for lung cancer. Some of them took 300,000 IU of the vitamin daily for a year; the others did not. After 12 months the vitamin takers remained free of new tumors for a longer period and developed far fewer tumors than the people who did not use supplements.[19]

Extensive surgery

Similar studies have shown that vitamin A is very helpful in stimulating an immune function that is often suppressed with extensive surgery. Cancer patients received 1.5 million IUs, while surgical patients were given 300,000 to 450,000 IUs daily, just before major surgery and for seven days after surgery. These patients showed increased T-cell activity several days after surgery, while the control group showed the usual immunosuppression. They had no signs of toxicity from these mega-doses, which of course were given under medical supervision and only for a short period.[20]

Is vitamin A toxic?

The *American Journal of Clinical Nutrition* has reported that in adults, vitamin A toxicity is uncommon at doses less than 100,000 IU per day. In cases of genuine toxicity, when vitamin A is stopped, the symptoms generally are relieved within a short amount of time. In humans, five cases of birth defects have been reported in which the mother took high doses of vitamin A during pregnancy. *However, the Journal reported, there was no clear cause-and-effect relationship between the vitamin A and the birth defect in any of these cases.* The intake of high vitamin A may have been coincidental to other factors.[21]

According to the *American Academy of Pediatrics, vitamin A toxicity generally does not occur unless someone consumes more than 1,000,000 IUs in a two- to three-week period.*[22]

Furthermore, you may find it interesting to know that the liver stores up to 1,000,000 IUs of vitamin A, so it is clear to see that this vitamin is vital to the body's health. Cod Liver oil is one of the best forms of natural vitamins A and D for children and teens.

Symptoms of overdose

It is important to recognize the symptoms of a vitamin A overdose, which include chronic headache, vomiting, loss of hair, dryness of the mucous membranes, and liver damage. When the vitamin A is stopped, the condition clears up.

"There has never been a vitamin-caused fatality."

Biochemist Richard Passwater, Ph.D., says, "In 50 years of vitamin supplementation, there has never been a vitamin-caused fatality reported in an adult in the U.S., nor has there been a reported death of a child due to the accidental consumption of a jar of vitamins."[23]

Vitamin A saved 300,000 children's lives

Vitamin A supplements saved the lives of at least 300,000 children in developing countries in 1997, according to the United Nations Children's Fund (UNICEF) report *The State of the World's Children, 1998.*

Vitamin A deficiency, which affects about 100 million children worldwide according to the report, has long been known to cause blindness. It is now known to also impair the immune system and cause maternal mortality, a distinct problem among women in impoverished regions.

"There's mounting evidence that improved nutrition, such as an adequate intake of vitamin A and iodine, can bring profound benefits to entire populations," says Kofi A. Annan, secretary-general of the United Nations.

A dozen field studies, conducted in Brazil, Ghana, India, Nepal and elsewhere, indicate that supplementing the diets of children at risk of vitamin A deficiency, in particular, saved lives that would otherwise be taken by diarrhea, measles and malaria. Supplementing also reduced the incidence of pregnancy-related deaths among women—and even the incidence of children born with HIV/AIDS.

Deaths from diarrhea, which currently kills 2.2 million children a year, were reduced by 35 to 50 percent with vitamin A supplementation.

The number of deaths due to measles, which kills nearly one million annually, were reduced by half, an effect believed to stem from vitamin A's crucial effect on immune system functioning.

Pregnancy-related deaths were reduced by an average of 44 percent among pregnant Nepalese mothers who received low-dose vitamin A supplements. Nearly 600,000 women die worldwide each year from pregnancy-related causes.

This fascinating report in *Nutrition Science News,* March 1998, even described more evidence on the importance of vitamin A for malaria and other infections such as cough and diarrhea. Giving vitamin A to third world countries has actually been the mission statement of several companies in our industry.

Caution urged with vitamin A in pregnancy

The New England Journal of Medicine reported in November 1995 that women who take large doses of vitamin A around the time of conception or early in their pregnancy run a higher than average risk of delivering infants with birth defects. This study was widely reported on all the television newscasts.

My two pregnant daughters-in-law called me in a panic, thinking they may have damaged their unborn babies since they were taking vitamin A. I reassured them that the vitamins they were taking only contained 7,500 IU of vitamin A in the form of fish oil, and the rest was from beta-carotene. I realized that a great many pregnant women must have felt fear about this also.

During the time of conception or during the first several months of pregnancy is the period considered the greatest risk. Taking excessive vitamin A at these times did not mean that a baby would definitely suffer defects; it only meant the risk was slightly higher.[24] *This study was based on women questioned from memory on what they ate during their pregnancy from 1984 to 1987, so I question why it took over ten years for the information to be reported.*

Vitamin A is essential for normal cellular differentiation and in regulating organ development in the fetus. The medical literature has also shown that a deficiency in vitamin A causes the same type of birth defect that excessive amounts may cause.[25]

According to one major survey, one half of Americans consume 19 percent or less of the RDA for vitamin A, and one fourth of the population consumes no more than 11 percent of the RDA.[26]

So, the conclusion drawn from the vitamin A and pregnancy study is, yes, there is a risk of taking too much vitamin A if you're pregnant, but the risk is generally overstated.[27]

The researchers recommended that pregnant women either limit their vitamin A consumption to 4,000 to 8,000 IU daily, or alternatively, take beta-carotene.[28] Beta-carotene is only converted into vitamin A when the body needs it; therefore, you do not have potential toxicity problems with this precursor to vitamin A.

Antioxidant Value of Vitamin C for Mature Adults

Vitamin C is one of the most widely heralded antioxidants. The proper use of ascorbic acid (vitamin C) throughout life may provide the long-awaited breakthrough in geriatrics. Vitamin C can prolong the period of "vigorous and healthy maturity," not just the life span, according to Irwin Stone, M.D.[29]

Symptoms of old age

Years ago, Dr. Walter H. Eddy of Columbia University pointed out that many typical signs of old age are actually symptoms of subclinical scurvy! These include wrinkles or loss of skin elasticity, loss of teeth, and brittleness of bones. He theorized that the scurvy-preventing properties of vitamin C are required even more as a person ages, because absorption is often poorer with advancing years and much of this vitamin is destroyed by the intestine when the stomach fails to produce normal amounts of hydrochloric acid.[30]

Vitamin C infections and intracellular cement

Vitamin C is easily destroyed by light and air, and is absent from most cooked or canned foods. Many of the blood-thinning drugs that older people take may interfere with vitamin C. Research has pointed toward the need to increase the vitamin C dosage as the years pass. You see, although you may be getting enough vitamin C to prevent scurvy in its grossest forms, because of the interference from drugs and medications, you may lack sufficient vitamin C to ward off colds; to minimize aging; and to prevent cancer, infections, and other diseases.

Consider for a moment that most animals produce between 10,000 and 20,000 mg of vitamin C every day in their bodies, and they do not have heart attacks and strokes. (Humans do not manufacture vitamin C in their bodies and must obtain it from outside sources.)

The best for life extension

Vitamin C may well be one of the best life-extending and anti-aging products available to us, yet because it is so inexpensive and completely non-toxic, many people ignore its value.

Vitamin C is a potent broad-spectrum, non-toxic virus fighter when used in large doses. One of vitamin C's most important functions is the synthesis, formation, and maintenance of a protein-like substance called collagen. Collagen is the "cement" that supports and holds tissues and organs together, much like steel rods in reinforced concrete.

The late Fred Klenner, M.D., one of the pioneering authorities on the clinical application of vitamin C, regularly gave large amounts of vitamin C by injection to his patients with meningitis, encephalitis (inflammation of the brain), polio, viral pneumonia, pesticide contamination, and many other serious diseases. Many of Dr. Klenner's patients were not expected to live at the time he began giving them vitamin C therapy. However, with vitamin C given in massive amounts, sometimes around the clock, a good percentage of them recovered quickly and were discharged from the hospital in three or four days! Antibiotics had been given previously to these same patients without success.[31]

Virus fighter

Dr. Irwin Stone has written about Dr. Klenner's work: "The main value of his work is in showing that any active viral disease can be successfully brought under control with ascorbic acid (vitamin C) if the proper large doses are used. It is inconceivable, but true, that Klenner's pioneering work has been almost completely ignored; no large-scale tests have been made to explore the exciting possibilities of his provocative clinical results."

Dr. Stone continued, "Millions of dollars of research money have been spent in unsuccessful attempts to find a non-toxic, effective virus fighter, and all sorts of exotic chemicals have been tried. All the while, harmless, inexpensive, and non-toxic ascorbic acid has been within easy reach of these investigators. More than 10,000 studies over the past four or five decades have shown vitamin C to be effective in battling a long list of human ailments. It might prove to be the 'magic bullet' for the control of viral diseases."[32]

The role vitamin C plays

Through the years, a number of people have said that vitamin C is excreted in the urine and those taking large amounts of supplements are wasting their money. The gentleman who won the Nobel Prize for Medicine in 1937 for his isolation of vitamin C and flavonoids, Albert Szent-Gyorgi, M.D., Ph.D., was one of the most respected and honored biochemists of the 20th century. He contended that his research showed that vitamin C transduces protein into a living state and enables it to perform in our bodies. He wrote, *"The more ascorbic acid is available, the better the protein will work...The ascorbic acid ingested by man is excreted only partly with his urine. Its greatest part simply disappears! What happened to it is a mystery. My studies indicate that it is incorporated into the living machinery!"*[33]

This wise and honored scientist, who died at the age of 93, also discovered the *flavonoids*. He gave a friend with bleeding gums crude vitamin C from lemon and his condition cleared up. When the problem reappeared, he gave an even purer form of vitamin C and expected even better results. But the purer vitamin C did not work. Dr. Szent-Gyorgi then isolated the flavonoid portion, the white part on an orange or grapefruit rind, gave it to his friend, and the problem cleared up. He named the flavonoids vitamin P, but it was not considered a true vitamin and was abandoned.

Dr. Szent-Gyorgi saw vitamin C as a cohesive force that holds living structure together. He said, "One should not wait for the application of this vitamin until one gets ill, trying to put the situation right by taking big doses. We should take it all the time." He also commented: *"I strongly believe that a proper use of ascorbic acid can profoundly change our vital statistics, including those for cancer."*[34]

Vitamin C and cancer

Some significant studies have been done that show large doses of vitamin C have a life-extending effect for patients with advanced cancer, as well as a preventive effect. Gladys Block, Ph.D., epidemiologist at the University of California, summarized more than 140 large-scale population studies on the relationship between vitamin C or vitamin C-rich foods and cancer. With possibly fewer than five exceptions, every study pointed toward a positive benefit from vitamin C, with more than 110 studies finding statistically significant reduction in the risk of virtually all kinds of cancer with a high intake of vitamin C.[35]

Cancer patients seem to have a much greater requirement for vitamin C than normal healthy individuals, apparently because all available vitamin C is mobilized by the body in its effort to boost natural resistance and repel invasive malignant growth.[36]

Vitamin C dosage

The older we become, the less we are able to store and use vitamin C. Therefore we need to increase our intake of vitamin C. Dr. Pauling recommended 10 grams (10,000 mg) of vitamin C to be taken daily for cancer patients. Most animals manufacture about this amount, calculated to the body weight of a human being. Dr. Pauling believed that if animals naturally make this amount, it is because they need it in these quantities to keep them in strong health.

Timed release vitamin C is not recommended in these high doses. The preferred way to take high doses (10 grams per day), would be to divide the vitamin C throughout the day. Make sure to take it with food. I prefer you take capsules, not tablets. You may also use the buffered form in which minerals are combined with vitamin C to make it non-acidic. A healthy individual would do well with 3 to 6 grams (3,000 mg to 6,000 mg) of vitamin C a day.

Pycnogenol and Grapeseed Extract
Contain Free Radical Scavengers

A group of plant *flavonols* exert many health promoting effects. Dr. Albert Szent-Gyorgi isolated them in the white part of an orange and grapefruit rind. Grapeseed extract is also part of the flavonoids. These are nutrients produced in many plants and when they are used by the body, they are often referred to as *bioflavonoids*. More than 4,000 chemically unique flavonoids have been identified in plants. This is only a small fraction of the total number that are likely to be present in nature, since only a few plants have been systematically examined for their flavonoid constituents.[37]

The early French explorer, *Jacques Cartier*, had just discovered Canada's Gulf of St. Lawrence, around 1534, when he and his crew were trapped by the winter ice. Trying to survive on salted meats and biscuits, his crew began dying of scurvy—a severe lack of vitamin C. Some friendly natives showed Cartier how to prepare a tea containing the bark of the Maritime pine and its needles. Soon the men not only got rid of their scurvy, but their appetites returned and they were able to gain weight, their chronic pain vanished, and their inflamed joints became normal.

Jacques Cartier's personal journal explaining these amazing results was discovered some 400 years later, and *Professor Masquelier* of the University of Bordeaux, France, was intrigued by Cartier's story. The French researchers set out to find more about this special pine tree, its bark and needles. Masquelier later termed the active components of the pine bark, "Pycnogenols."[38]

European physicians have known since 1950 that Pycnogenol strengthened capillaries and reduced swelling in the legs and ankles. They have used Pycnogenol with great success against hay fever and allergies since 1960. In the '70s, enthusiastic users called Pycnogenol "the skin vitamin" and the "skin cosmetic in a pill." However, it was not until 1986 that the great antioxidant power of Pycnogenol was fully realized.[39]

Professor Masquelier researched the flavonoids in pine bark, grape skins, and various nut shells. He found the richest source of the most bioavailable and bioactive flavonoids were in the bark of the Maritime (Landes) pine bark that he later trademarked as Pycnogenol by Horphag Overseas, Ltd.

Desirable effects

Pycnogenol and grapeseed complexes are potent antioxidants and free radical scavengers that help prevent "oxidative" damage that has been linked to the aging process. Because of their antioxidant activity, they have been used in Europe to treat a number of ailments: vein and capillary disorders including venous insufficiency, varicose veins, capillary fragility, and vascular disorders of the retina. Perhaps the most significant use will be in the prevention of atherosclerosis (hardening of the arteries from cholesterol deposits) and the resulting complications of heart disease and strokes.

In vitro (in a test tube or other equipment) studies measured the antioxidant activity of Pycnogenol as 20 to 50 times stronger than that of vitamin C and vitamin E, respectively. It should not replace vitamin C or vitamin E, but it is considered a helper and intensifies the vitamins' actions.

From a cellular perspective, Pycnogenol has the unique ability to cling to cellular proteins, strengthening and protecting them. This physical characteristic, along with Pycnogenol's ability to protect against both water and fat-soluble free radicals, provides incredible protection to the cells against free radical damage, according to Dr. Michael Murray and Dr. Richard Passwater.[40]

Lowers cholesterol in animals

In addition to preventing damage to the lining of the artery caused by cholesterol, Pycnogenol extracts have actually been shown to lower blood cholesterol levels and to shrink the size of cholesterol deposits in the arteries of animals. They also prevent destructive enzymes (elastase and collagenase) from eroding arterial walls, according to Dr. Passwater. Presumably they may exert similar benefits in humans.

The value of pycnogenol is that it protects us

Dr. Richard Passwater has said that it "can help protect you from approximately 80 diseases, including heart disease, cancer, arthritis, and most other non-germ diseases that are linked to the deleterious chemical action of free radicals...In addition to its antioxidant protection that slows the damage associated with aging, Pycnogenol restores elasticity and smoothness to skin via its influence on skin protein formation. What is even more exciting is that Pycnogenol is more than a powerful antioxidant; it nourishes blood cells, blood vessels, and the skin."[41]

Pycnogenol is unique because it may help alleviate hay fever and other allergies by reducing histamine production, providing relief for allergy sufferers. It strengthens capillaries, prevents bruising, improves peripheral circulation, reduces varicose veins, and improves capillary resistance and permeability. These flavonols are also metal chelators.[42]

This valuable nutrient also enhances immune response, reduces diabetic retinopathy, fights inflammation and improves joint flexibility. It acts against stomach ulcers and inflammation, treats chronic venous insufficiency, reduces capillary fragility and much more.[43]

Recommended dosage

You will find several Pycnogenol and grape seed extracts in your nutrition store. The Horphag Research Ltd., in the UK has done most of the scientific research with Pycnogenol, and they continue to support international research. These are both excellent products you may want to add to your nutritional program, along with your complete vitamin and mineral formulas. The current suggested dosage for both is one milligram (mg) per pound of body weight, so a 130-pound woman would take three 50 mg tablets or capsules.[44] For therapeutic purposes, the effective dose would be about 1.5 mg for one pound of body weight. A 150-pound person would take 225 mg for the first seven to ten days and half that dose thereafter for maintenance.[45]

Dr. Robert Atkins feels for all practical purposes, the difference between Pycnogenol and grape seed extract is slight, but grape seed is much less expensive and the dosage remains about the same. Dr. Atkins says, "To limit a heavy menstrual flow or stop bleeding gums, I'll tell a patient to take 1,000 mg of grapeseed extract three times per day. At that dosage a therapeutic change can come about in as little as a month. For instance, by the time of her cycle, a woman accustomed to a heavy seven-day menstrual flow might finish within three or four days."[46]

The Amazing Benefits of Vitamin E on Immunity

Vitamin E (d-alpha tocopherol) is a powerful antioxidant that seems to have a number of immune-protective and immune-stimulating effects. It protects against free radicals and blocks some of the negative prostaglandins (a group of hormone-like fatty acids produced in small amounts in the body) that slow down the immune system. Vitamin E also protects cell membranes, thereby making them more difficult for viruses to attack.[47]

Read your labels—Use natural vitamin E

Even though the label implies natural, it may not be. Natural vitamin E is designated by "d" (not dl) alpha-tocopherol. The "d" means it is from a natural source, usually from soy oil; the "dl" means it is synthetic and made from petrochemicals, and of course much cheaper. Most of the nutrition-oriented doctors agree that the natural d-alpha is the effective form of vitamin E. There is not just alpha, which is the most researched and effective, but also beta, gamma, and delta tocopherols, which are also important.

Aging and immune response

Aging is associated with changes in the immune response, which can contribute to increased incidence of infectious disease and tumors in the elderly. Although all aspects of the immune system are affected, the main alterations occur in the cellular area of the immune system.[48]

It recharged their immunity

Nutritional manipulation of the immune system is the most practical way of delaying or reversing the age-associated changes in the immune system. A study reported at a seminar conducted by the N.Y. Academy of Science showed even though the immune response declined with age, it reverted almost to the level of young people after administering 400 to 800 IUs of vitamin E. A level of vitamin E greater than the RDA has been shown to enhance the immune system and reduce the incidence of age-associated diseases. For most of the healthy elderly subjects studied, it "recharged" their immunity, giving their bodies the ability to produce higher white cell counts when faced with infection. The proliferation of white blood cells that fight infection increased by ten to 50 percent within 30 days. Some functions improved as much as 80 to 90 percent.[49]

Vitamin E and cancer protection

Hundreds of studies have shown that the higher the intake of vitamin E, the less likely the risk of cancer.[50] *In an eight-year study of more than 36,000 adults, the people with the lowest levels of vitamin E had the greatest risk of developing cancers of all kinds.*[51]

Vitamin E has been shown to lower the risk of breast cancer, epithelial cancer and cancer due to carcinogens. In fact, one study in the *British Journal of Cancer* found that the group of *5,000 women with the lowest blood serum levels of vitamin E had four to five times the risk of developing breast cancer, stomach cancer, cancer of the pancreas, and cancer of the urinary tract.*[52]

Another study showed that vitamin E levels in the blood were lower in the patients that developed lung and colorectal cancers than in the group that did not.[53]

Vitamin E's role is preventive

It cannot reverse already existing damage. The presence of other antioxidants magnifies vitamin E's potency. Vitamin C, the carotenoids and selenium are partners that enhance the anti-cancer shield.

Vitamin E dosage

Many authorities agree that a person should take 400 IUs to 1,200 IUs of vitamin E from natural d-alpha tocopherol daily. Wilfrid Shute, M.D., one of the early researchers using vitamin E in his clinic in Canada used up to 3,200 IU a day.

NOTE: *If you have high blood pressure, you should consult your physician before increasing your intake beyond 800 IUs, due to its blood thinning properties. If you are using anti-coagulation drugs, or have a pre-existing hypertension condition, or any other medical problem, you should first consult your physician before taking larger doses of vitamin E supplements.*

High intensity exercise and free radicals

While we were attending a meeting of the National Nutritional Foods Association, my husband Don and I had the opportunity to meet Kenneth Cooper, M.D., founder of the Cooper Aerobics Center in Dallas, Texas, and the author of *Antioxidant Revolution*. Dr. Cooper is the father of the worldwide aerobics movement that started America running. He has found in recent years that high-intensity exercise, the type of training that athletes undertake, may actually produce an excess of free radicals, which leads to disease. Many veteran distance runners have died of cancer, heart attacks, and other chronic diseases.

Dr. Cooper acknowledges that strenuous exercising generates large numbers of free radicals as a by-product of deep or "heavy" breathing. He strongly recommends that those who exercise aerobically take the three major antioxidants—vitamins C, E, and beta-carotene—as the most effective way to combat or reduce the production of free radicals throughout the body. He has reported that vitamin E supplements prevent much of the free radical damage, particularly to the DNA (deoxyribonucleic acid) where mutations can lead to cancer.[54]

Vitamin E prevented DNA damage

In a series of experiments at the University of Ulm, Germany, Gunter Speit, M.D., has found that only the consistent daily consumption of 1,200 IUs of vitamin E daily prevented DNA damage from exercise.[55] What valuable information for athletes or those of us involved in heavy aerobic activity!

Dr. Cooper's extensive research has also shown that 30 minutes of low-intensity exercise three to four times a week is more healthy than strenuous exercise, and it can help reduce mortality from all causes. This amount of exercise sounds "livable" to me. More information on Dr. Cooper's program will be found in chapter 8.

Tremendous Benefits of Selenium

Selenium is a powerful antioxidant and a valuable protective agent against cancer, coronary artery disease, strokes, and heart attacks. It also plays a very important role in helping to reduce the incidence of many diseases associated with aging.[56]

Selenium can stimulate increased antibody response to germ infections when combined with vitamin E. In research conducted by Soviet scientists, this antibody response increased as much as 30-fold in some studies.[57]

Selenium and vitamin E work together synergistically. Most researchers study the effects of only one nutrient at a time and can easily miss the value of the combined effects. Generally speaking, vitamin E and selenium do not replace each other, but work best when taken together.

Many of these studies have found that people with low selenium levels also tended to have low vitamin E levels.

Protective against cancer

A substance that can cut cancer occurrences by almost 40 percent and decrease the cancer death rate by 50 percent should be heralded as our greatest medical breakthrough and dispensed to every person in the world. I cannot understand why this valuable information isn't broadcast everywhere.

More than 400 research and scholarly articles have documented the role of selenium in cancer prevention.

Studies in the early 1970s revealed that selenium was protective against cancer in laboratory animals. Dr. Gerhard Schrauzer of the University of California at San Diego and Dr. Richard Passwater conducted a series of experiments that showed an optimal selenium intake reduced the incidence of spontaneous breast cancer in susceptible female mice from 82 percent to 10 percent merely by adding selenium to their drinking water.

Dr. Schrauzer said, *"If every woman in America started taking selenium (supplements) today, or had a high-selenium diet, within a few years the breast cancer rate would decline drastically."*[58]

Dr. Schrauzer also remarked that if a breast cancer patient has low selenium levels in her blood, her tendency to develop metastases (other tumors spreading from the first tumor) is increased, her possibility for survival is diminished, and her prognosis in general is poorer than if she had normal blood selenium levels.

I had the honor of meeting Dr. Schrauzer at an Alternative Cancer Treatment Seminar. His research results and recommendations should be shouted from the housetops! I try to spread the word every time I have an opportunity to discuss nutrition on a television or radio program or even during my lectures. Everyone should be taking selenium as a preventive measure.

Fifty percent of cancer deaths could be prevented

A spectacular study was reported in December 1996 *Journal of the American Medical Association (JAMA)*. Researcher Larry Clark, Ph.D., of the University of Arizona, demonstrated perhaps the most successful cancer prevention study ever executed. He showed that taking 200 micrograms of selenium daily, for about seven years reduced the occurrence of all cancers in a group of 1,300 older people by 42 percent and cancer deaths by nearly 50 percent compared with those on a placebo (sugar pill).

This study was the culmination of more than 40 years of research, supporting unequivocally the cancer-preventing aspects of this unique trace mineral. Selenium had the greatest impact on prostate cancer. The study showed the following information in the death rate from the three most prevalent cancers:

63 percent reduction in prostate cancer

❧ 58 percent reduction in colon or rectal cancer
❧ 45 percent reduction in lung cancer.[59]

In fact, the results of the study were so astounding that the study was ended early. The doctors and researchers conducting the study felt that, given the dramatic reduction in cancer, it was unfair to wait any longer to release the news to anyone wanting to start protecting themselves against cancer.

Mitchell L. Gaynor said: "the relatively large size of the study and the deeply significant cuts in death and incidence rates makes it very likely that this piece of work will be one of a number of classic studies in the 1990s that permanently alter the conventional wisdom of medicine," as reported in *Dr. Gaynor's Cancer Prevention Program.*

Again, it really upsets me that there have been over 400 research and scholarly articles on selenium, and this cancer cure and preventive information has been available for 40 years and still this information has not been reported.

Selenium dosage

A general recommendation is that people take 200 to 400 mcg (micrograms, not milligrams) daily as a supplement. Dr. Passwater has recommended giving 600 mcg per day to patients with cancer. Even after taking this dose for years, patients had no toxic side effects. If you have cancer, suggest that your physician read the *JAMA* article and check your blood level to determine if you should increase your selenium to 600 mcg. This is one trace mineral that you should not take more than is recommended, as high doses may be toxic. More is not necessarily better.

Alpha Lipoic Acid
Prevents Oxidative Damage

It has taken a long time for the concept of free radicals to be accepted as a disease-causing agent. However, it was also a long time before Louis Pasteur's germ theory was widely accepted. A free radical is just as deadly as a germ, but in a different way. Of course, neither one germ nor one free radical presents a grave danger by itself. It is when these free radicals multiply and create chain reactions that they cause damage over time, altering bodily functions and causing degenerative diseases that impact aging.

Free radicals damage capillary and nerve endings, damage proteins that may create cataracts or damage elastin and collagen that are associated with aging and wrinkles. Free radicals also damage tissues where inflammation is present, such as with arthritis and asthma. Free radicals are a major cause of many of the complications associated with diabetes. Antioxidants neutralize free radicals, preventing them from causing harm, and alpha lipoic acid is a valuable antioxidant.

Your body's chemistry is dependent upon oxygen, and yet normal body processes—metabolism, respiration, and so forth—create harmful oxygen-containing molecules as by-products. Fortunately, we now have many antioxidants, including alpha lipoic acid, to protect us against these by-products of normal metabolism. In fact, antioxidants may eventually play a significant role in the treatment of arthritis, AIDS, diabetic retinopathy, and other conditions.[60]

Alpha lipoic acid, or lipoic acid, protects the liver and detoxifies tissues of heavy metals such as excessive iron and copper, and the toxic metals cadmium, lead, and mercury.

Alpha lipoic acid also has the unique ability to enhance the antioxidant power of vitamins C, E, and glutathione (an amino acid) in the body, creating an antioxidant network that gives you more complete protection against damaging free radicals. Unlike other valuable antioxidants, alpha lipoic acid is the only fat and water-soluble free radical antioxidant; therefore, it is easily absorbed and transported across cell membranes, protecting us against free radicals both inside and outside our cells.

An exciting antioxidant

Alpha lipoic acid is an important link in the vital antioxidant network, and it is multifunctional. There are hundreds of studies over 40 years revealing how alpha lipoic acid performs many functions in the body, but it has only recently been noticed by the public. It has been shown to energize metabolism, to be a key compound for producing energy in the muscles, and it is important for everything we do, from physical activity to thinking. Alpha lipoic acid unlocks energy from food calories and directs these calories away from fat production and into energy production.

The excitement about this nutrient can be seen in the many recent studies focusing on how alpha lipoic acid improves the physique, combats free radicals, protects our genetic material, slows aging, helps protect against heart disease, cancer, cataracts, diabetes, and many other diseases. It is also being studied in the treatment of Parkinson's disease and Alzheimer's disease. Alpha lipoic acid is especially suited to protect nerve tissues against oxidative damage.[61]

Diabetes link

Diabetics (both insulin and non-insulin dependent) will be excited to learn that *alpha lipoic acid* has been used successfully for nearly 30 years in Germany, not only to normalize blood sugar levels, but to protect against the damage caused by diabetes. According to Dr. Richard Passwater, *it has reduced the secondary effects of diabetes, including damage to the retina, cataract formation, nerve and heart damage, and it also increases energy levels. These patients were given levels as high as 600 mg per day with great results.* Study after study reported that alpha lipoic acid safely regenerates damaged nerves. It protects through its antioxidant and antiglycemic actions. It is the agent of choice for the prevention of diabetic complications, including neuropathy (damage to the peripheral nerves that connect the central nervous system), cardiomyopathy (any disease of the heart muscle), and retinopathy (disorder of the retina).[62]

Alpha lipoic acid improves the blood flow in nerve tissues, improves glucose utilization in the brain, and improves basal ganglia function. The researchers observed no adverse effects from the high dosage of 600 mg per day of alpha lipoic acid for diabetes.[63]

It is imperative that diabetics monitor their blood sugar levels closely and make appropriate adjustments to their medication.

Natural sources

It is interesting that the richest source of naturally occurring alpha lipoic acid is found in red meat. It is also present in certain plants, such as potatoes. Under normal conditions, our bodies contain small amounts of alpha lipoic acid, but it may not be a sufficient level to provide optimal protection from free radicals.

Alpha lipoic acid dosage

It is difficult to obtain enough alpha lipoic acid through the diet to obtain this wonderful protection, so supplementation is suggested. The typical preventive, daily supplementation range for healthy adults appears to be 100 to 200 mg, depending on your weight. Higher amounts may also be taken, depending on your condition. There are no clinical, toxicological, or other studies that have shown a serious adverse effect from alpha lipoic acid supplementation. It has been used for more than three decades at high dosages (300 to 600 mg a day) to treat diabetic neuropathy. A toxic dose, in animals of several species, has been noted but this dose translated to 30,000 to 37,500 mg (30–37.5 grams) for a 165-pound human.[64]

Alpha lipoic acid supplementation is not recommended for pregnant women, until further studies are completed. Alpha lipoic acid supplements are available without prescription in nutrition stores.

Zinc Promotes T-Cell Immunity

Zinc is an extremely important antioxidant mineral that is an immune stimulant, specifically promoting T-cell immunity. Individuals with low zinc levels have been found to have lowered resistance, atrophied thymus glands, and a reduced number of mature T-cells. Under these conditions, many immune functions are likely to be impaired, including antibacterial activity of your T-cells (from the thymus) and B-cells (from the bone marrow).

More than 200 enzymes or "biologic catalysts" require zinc for their activity, including the enzymes involved in the production of nucleic acids DNA and RNA. In addition, zinc lends its hand to form the so-called zinc fingers, which allow proteins to bind specifically to nucleic acids. Zinc also plays a role in the structure and function of cell membranes.[65] Upon the first sign of cold and sore throat symptoms, zinc has the ability to shorten and decrease the severity of colds when taken in the form of zinc lozenges. Also it is known as the "clear skin" mineral.

Benefits of Coenzyme Q$_{10}$

Coenzyme Q$_{10}$, more commonly referred to as CoQ$_{10}$, appears to be a vital catalyst in the creation of the energy that cells need for life. Dr. Karl Folkers has shown that CoQ$_{10}$ fights aging by stimulating immunity. Immunoglobulin or antibody G (IgG), the major antibody in the blood, rose significantly in patients receiving oral doses of 60 milligrams of CoQ$_{10}$ daily. The rise of antibodies usually happened between one and three months after the treatment began.[66]

Breast Cancer

The treatment of breast cancer with CoQ$_{10}$ was reported at the Eighth International Symposium on Biomedical and Clinical Aspects of Coenzyme Q$_{10}$, November 1993, held in Stockholm, Sweden.

Knud Lockwood, M.D., and Karl Folkers, Ph.D., treated 32 "high risk" breast cancer patients with these supplements:

- 2,850 mg of vitamin C
- 2,500 IU of vitamin E
- 96,667 IU (58 mg) of beta-carotene
- 387 mcg of selenium
- 1.2 grams of linolenic acid, omega-6 (GLA)
- 3.5 grams of omega-3 fatty acids (EPA)
- 90 mg of CoQ10

"No patient died and all expressed a feeling of well-being," wrote the researchers. "These clinical results are remarkable since about four deaths would have been expected. Now, after 24 months, all still survive; about six deaths would have been expected." Six of the 32 patients showed partial tumor remission.

One astonishing case

The dosage of CoQ10 was increased from 90 mg to 390 mg daily. The doctors said it was astonishing that in 30 days the tumor could no longer be felt, and 60 days later the cancer had disappeared from the mammogram and there were no traces of the mass on the x-ray. The cancer was in complete regression. Dr. Lockwood said that in his 35 years of practice with over 200 patients a year, he had never witnessed a spontaneous complete regression of a breast tumor measuring as much as 1.5 to 2 centimeters.

Dr. Lockwood was not using CoQ10 as a magic bullet, but it was given with the other nutrients I just reported. CoQ10 was used as an adjunct to conventional cancer therapy.[67]

Dr. Folkers summarized the case histories of ten diverse cancer patients who were treated with CoQ10 and survived for periods of five to 15 years. For some of these patients, evidence of cancer was no longer present.[68]

Another high-risk case was treated with 300 mg of CoQ10 after undergoing non-radical breast surgery. Three months later, no cancerous tissue could be detected.[69]

The summary from Drs. Folkers and Lockwood was, "The relationships of nutrition and vitamins to the genesis and prevention of cancer are increasingly evident...The bioenergetic activity of CoQ10, expressed in hematological or immunological activity, may be the dominant but not the sole molecular mechanism causing the regression of breast cancer."

Protects the brain

CoQ10 has also been linked to protection of the brain. Researchers believe it is important in protecting the cells' mitochondria, which may result in helping prevent degenerative brain diseases like Alzheimer's disease, Lou Gehrig's disease, and gradual loss of memory and brain function usually associated with aging. CoQ10 is thought to be one of the few substances that can actually penetrate and restore vitality to the mitochondria, according to Dr. Denham Harman, a leading free radical researcher.[70]

Unfortunately, the body's production of CoQ10 begins to decline around age 20, often leaving people seriously deficient by middle age, when the body needs to fight off aging diseases. CoQ10 is valuable in protecting the heart. Read all the details in the *Heart* chapter.

CoQ10 dosage

The recommendation is usually 60 to 90 mg a day for generally healthy people. Some suggest 120 to 390 mg for those who want to prevent signs of aging or who have cancer or heart problems. It should be taken with a fat-containing food or with a meal, in divided doses.

One of the best aspects of CoQ10 appears to be that the substance has virtually no side effects. It is one of the safest substances ever tested, even at very high doses. No significant toxicity in animal or long-term human studies has been recorded.[71]

Glutathione Is a Major Enemy of Free Radicals

Glutathione is manufactured in the liver by three naturally occurring amino acids—*cysteine, glutamic acid,* and *glycine.* Glutathione is a powerhouse antioxidant. A lack of it in the cells is considered by some researchers to be the foremost cause of premature aging. It protects every cell, tissue, and organ in the body. In one study, those with 20 percent higher blood levels of glutathione had only one third the rate of arthritis, high blood pressure, heart disease, circulatory symptoms, diabetes, stomach symptoms, and urinary tract infections when compared to those with lower glutathione levels. Dr. Mara Julius, the author of this finding at the University of Michigan, said, "Even in very old age, people with the highest levels of glutathione bounce back from diseases and accidents the same way much younger people do. They are just more vigorous."[72]

The Anti-Aging Benefits of Glutathione

Jean Carper reports that glutathione:

- protects from cancer
- rejuvenates immunity
- blocks damage to the cells by breaking down free radicals
- rejuvenates old and weak immune systems
- prevents lung injury from free radicals
- fights against the free radicals produced by rancid fat
- keeps blood cholesterol from oxidizing and becoming toxic
- cures some forms of Type II diabetes
- helps prevent macular degeneration
- maintains healthy immune function.[73]

John T. Pinto of Memorial Sloan Kettering Cancer Center in New York calls glutathione the "master antioxidant" because it protects every cell, tissue, and organ in the body. He says, "If you deplete glutathione, the cell disintegrates and loses its immune activity. If you add glutathione to that ailing cell, it regenerates and becomes immuno-efficient."[74]

Glutathione protects the body against powerful natural and man-made oxidants. It helps the liver detoxify poisonous chemicals and even helps protect the integrity of red blood cells. It helps prevent macular degeneration and age-related eye disease.[75]

Another researcher has noted that glutathione can deactivate at least 30 cancer-causing substances.[76] Glutathione works synergistically with vitamin C and selenium.

L-glutamine (an amino acid) also helps boost blood levels of glutathione. Digestive juices can break down supplemental glutathione into other substances, so we must make certain to consume the chemical building blocks that form glutathione in the body. In fact, taking the amino acid supplement L-glutamine is apt to boost your blood levels of glutathione much better than taking glutathione directly.

Douglas Wilmore, M.D., a professor of surgery at Harvard Medical School, has researched L-glutamine, the amino acid that can boost glutathione levels, and says, "It's an awesome anti-aging agent, essential for anyone who is ill or under stress. It strengthens immunity, hastens recovery, and actually rejuvenates muscles weakened by wasting illnesses." He said to make sure you take it with vitamin C and selenium.[77]

L-Glutamine dosage

L-glutamine is relatively inexpensive and readily available, and it greatly enhances the body's production of glutathione. L-glutamine appears safe even in high doses. Daily doses of up to 40,000 mg have been taken under the supervision of a physician with no noticeable adverse effects, says Dr. Wilmore. A typical dosage among researchers who have studied this substance is 2,000 to 8,000 mg daily in tasteless powder form and more if fighting an infection.[78]

L-glutamine can be found in your nutrition store in 500 or 1,000 mg capsules or powder form. After learning the value of glutathione, I now add one scoop (1 teaspoon) of powdered L-glutamine (equals 5,000 mg) to my protein shake in the morning. A study at Louisiana State University Medical College showed that as little as two grams of L-glutamine increased growth hormone levels by 430 percent.[79] Increasing growth hormone levels has been directly correlated with increased lean body mass, increased fat burning, and improved strength. I vote for all of these!

Glutathione is found in whole fruit and vegetables, walnuts, orange juice, and fresh meat. Especially rich sources are raw avocado, watermelon, fresh asparagus, grapefruit, and baked acorn squash.

Soybeans—Nature's Own Antioxidant

The soybean is another food you can add to your diet. Soybeans and soy-based products have been shown to fight chronic illnesses including heart disease and cancer, lower blood cholesterol levels, help with digestive problems, and provide a valuable source of protein for a healthier diet.

Soybeans are the only vegetable food source known to be a complete protein that contains all of the essential amino acids. They are called "essential" because they must come from our food supply; our body cannot manufacture them. They are also essential to humans in order to survive and maintain good health. Soybeans are higher in protein than other legumes, but soy's value is diminished slightly because of their short supply of the essential amino acids methionine and tryptophane.

Soy isoflavones and cancer

Isoflavones are valuable plant estrogens that are chemically structured like estrogen, and when they link to receptors awaiting estrogen bonds, they block the human estrogen from making its connection.

Therefore, they are a weaker estrogen that functions as an anti-estrogen. The two primary isoflavones in soybeans are genistein and daidzein.[80]

The *International Journal of Anti-Aging Medicine* 1998 reports that genistein prevents estrogen from causing malignant changes in breast tissue. This phenomenon is seen in both perimenopausal and post-menopausal women. Some of genistein's potent anti-cancer effects are:

- Interfering with cancer activity at every stage, including breast, colon, lung, prostate, skin, and blood (leukemia) cancers.
- Acting as anti-estrogen by competing with human estrogen for binding to estrogen receptors.
- Reducing plaque buildup in artery walls and reducing risk of heart attack, stroke, and atherosclerosis.
- Interfering with activity of enzymes, which are involved in controlling cell growth and regulation.
- Inhibiting angiogenesis (new blood vessel growth) that would, in turn, interfere with tumor growth.[81]

Genistein is attracting interest because it has been shown to block the process by which new blood vessels grow and feed malignant tumors. The U.S. National Institute of Health is now funding the testing of genistein on patients with breast and prostate cancers, melanomas, leukemia, and Kaposi's sarcoma (an otherwise rare cancer that is common in AIDS sufferers).[82]

Recommendations

Soy sauce or soybean oil *are not* good sources of protein or genistein. The best sources of soy foods are soybean protein powder, soy milk, tofu, soy nuts, miso, and tempeh. Studies have shown that isoflavones like genistein only remain in the human body for 24 to 36 hours at most. Therefore, daily servings are needed to keep the cells fully stocked with the power of soy foods.

Herbs and Other Nutrients to Build Immunity

Herbs Are God's First Pharmacy

When I was a child, the old Indian squaws taught my Mother how to make many Indian remedies, including a spring tonic using bark, roots and herbs. It was a black and bitter substance, but it gave our family a pick up after the hard South Dakota winters.

—GLADYS LINDBERG

*Y*our body is equipped with a wonderful healing system capable of handling almost any condition of infection or ill-health—provided it is given the nutritional support it needs. This health restoring mechanism is known as the immune system. There are many harmful microorganisms like viruses, fungi and bacteria that suppress the immune function. This can leave you more vulnerable to getting sick and make you susceptible to many diseases.

One essential fact must be understood if you are to maintain health: the state of your nutrition directly influences your biochemistry and your immunological system. Researchers believe that the nation-wide prevalence of chronic bronchitis, cancer, yeast infections, chronic fatigue, Epstein-Barr syndromes, and even colds and flu, reflect wide-spread immunity difficulties.

Along with all the vitamins and minerals discussed in the previous chapter, there are a number of herbs and nutrients that appear to build immunity. A few important ones you may want to consider are these:

- Astragalus
- Echinacea
- Goldenseal
- Cat's Claw
- Garlic
- Milk Thistle
- Green Tea
- Maitake Mushroom
- Shiitake & Reishi
- Beta-Glucan
- CLA
- DIM
- Indole-3-Carbinol
- Colostrum
- IP6

Astragalus Is an Immune Stimulant

Astragalus *(Astragalus membranaceus)* is a commonly used traditional herb in Chinese medicine. It has been used for 3000 years for its properties that produce resistance to disease. It is an immune system stimulant, and Chinese researchers have reported success in using it with cancer patients to offset some of the immune-suppressing effects of radiation and Western cancer drugs.[1]

American researchers at M.D. Anderson Hospital and Tumor Institute in Houston, Texas, have been working with crude extracts and a specific active component of astragalus. The compound, a polysac-charide, has been shown to be highly effective in restoring immune function to normal levels in test animals whose immune systems were suppressed by modern drugs.[2]

Astragalus is called an "adaptogen" and has been credited with producing long life for cells. It seems to protect the cells even when chemotherapy is used. When added to a cancer program, the survival time reportedly doubled among patients who received herbal therapy that included astragalus, as compared with those who received only standard chemotherapy and radiation.[3]

This herb also reportedly boosts the numbers, strength and activity of T-cells, the roving white blood cells that eliminate bacteria and viruses. It is particularly effective in warding off flu and some respiratory infections.[4]

It is also used to increase resistance to disease, but not while you are sick. It is considered the best herb in Chinese medicine to strengthen resistance. Master herbalist Janet Zand recommends an echinacea and goldenseal combination for one week, then switching to astragalus for the next week, alternating back and forth for increased resistance to infection, especially during the cold and flu season.

Echinacea: A Significant Immune Stimulant

Echinacea *(Echinacea angustifolia and purpurea)* is also known as Purple Coneflower. Researchers in Europe and the Far East have studied these two varieties of this plant extensively and have found significant immune-stimulating properties. Echinacea is one of the most potent herbs that support the immune system, and is useful for treating colds and flu.

Echinacea works like penicillin in the body with no side effects. It has been called the "King of Blood Purifiers" because it improves lymphatic filtration and drainage. It is known by herbalists as one of the best alternatives for detoxifying the blood, and is an excellent blood cleanser.[5]

Macrophages are the cells that kill and destroy bacteria, viruses, other infectious agents and cancer cells.[6] Echinacea increases natural killer cell activity, antibody binding, and levels of circulating white blood cells primarily responsible for defending against bacteria. It also exhibits interferon-like properties, and is used in the treatment of influenza and herpes, strep throat and infected lymph glands.[7]

It is among the most powerful and effective remedies against all kinds of bacteria and viral infections. It has antibiotic, antiviral, and anti-inflammatory-like properties without any reported cases of toxicity. Some have found it to be good for the enlargement of the prostate gland.[8]

Add echinacea to your list of herbal products to keep on hand. Herbalists advise not to use echinacea for a long period of time; otherwise it loses it effectiveness. It is better to alternate one or two weeks on, then one or two weeks off. Capsules and tinctures (concentrated herbal extracts) of echinacea are available in your nutrition store. Follow the instructions on the label.

Goldenseal Has Antibacterial Properties

Another herb native to North America, goldenseal *(Hydrastis canadensis)*, has been used medicinally to soothe mucous membranes that line the respiratory, digestive, and genitourinary tracts. Its major compound, *berberine*, exhibits a broad spectrum of antibiotic activity. Berberine finds its use in mouth and gum problems.[9] Goldenseal strengthens the immune system through its antibiotic and antibacterial properties. It also helps against bacteria, protozoa, and various fungi. Plus, it has been shown to activate macrophages (the cells that destroy bacteria, viruses, and tumor cells).[10]

Goldenseal has been used in the treatment of infections involving the mucous membranes, such as strep throat, sinusitis, bronchitis and urinary tract infections. It helps in inflammation of the gallbladder and stimulates the secretion of bile.[11]

The *British Pharmaceutical Codex*, 1934 states that goldenseal is useful in controlling uterine hemorrhage. It has been considered useful for arresting bleeding from the uterus and for profuse menstruation. It is an effective treatment, specific in female applications for uterine contractions and menstrual disorders.[12]

Generally speaking, goldenseal is non-toxic, but it should not be used by pregnant women or for long periods of time. Many herbal products will combine echinacea and goldenseal for their synergistic effect.

Cat's Claw May Be a "Wonder Herb"

Much is presently being written about cat's claw *(Uncaria tomentosa)*. It is also known as *una de gato*. This unique herb is actually a high climbing vine found in the highlands of the Peruvian rain forest. It has been used for hundreds, perhaps thousands, of years by the Ashanica Indians for a wide range of health problems. According to research conducted in many nations, evidence suggests that cat's claw is beneficial in the treatment of cancer, arthritis, bursitis, rheumatism, genital herpes, herpes zoster, allergies, ulcers, systemic candidiasis, PMS, irregularities of the female cycle, environmental toxic poisoning, numerous bowel and intestinal disorders, and organic depression.[13]

Brent W. David, D.C., has been working with cat's claw in the United States and has reported its remarkable ability to cleanse the entire intestinal tract and help patients who suffer from many stomach and bowel disorders, including Crohn's disease, diverticulitis, leaky bowel syndrome, colitis, hemorrhoids, gastritis, ulcers, parasites, and intestinal flora imbalance. In its healing ability and benefits to the immune system, cat's claw appears to have so many therapeutic applications that it has far surpassed many well-known herbs.[14]

Garlic Dates Back to the Bible!

Our ancestors used roots and herbs in abundance. Garlic and onions, particularly, were staples. Germs do not like garlic; in fact, they cannot live in its presence. Ancient civilizations, especially during Bible times, relied heavily on this bulb as a medication for indigestion, diarrhea, worms, skin diseases, dizziness, headaches, bronchitis, pneumonia, influenza, tuberculosis, infections, wound healing, heart problems, arthritis, aging, and even cancer.

In recent years, people have rediscovered the medicinal merits of garlic in warding off colds and in the treatment of high blood pressure, strokes, and cardiovascular disease. Interestingly, countries where garlic is consumed in large quantities—Italy and Spain, for example—have a lower death rate from heart disease than America does.[15]

A longtime friend in our industry, Charlie Fox, is the spokesperson for Kyolic Garlic, Wakunaga of America. I asked him for some scientific information on their Aged Garlic and I was amazed when I received the *Aged Garlic Extract Research Excerpts from Peer Reviewed Scientific Journals & Scientific Meetings*. The research studies are from Loma Linda University, Memorial Sloan Kettering Cancer Center, University of Tokyo, and various other universities around the world. If you read all of this literature, I am sure you would feel as I do. We must take our garlic.

Milk Thistle to Detoxify the Liver

Milk thistle *(Silybum marianum)* has been used for centuries for the treatment of liver problems. The active ingredient is a bioflavonoid mixture called *silymarin*. Research has demonstrated that milk thistle protects the liver against damaging toxins.[16] Milk thistle has been helpful in alcohol-induced fatty liver disorders, chronic hepatitis (inflammation of the liver), chemically induced fatty liver disorders, cirrhosis or hardening of the liver, hepatic organ damage, and psoriasis, according to *The Little Herb Encyclopedia.*[17]

The liver is one of the most important organs for filtering out toxins. Everyone of us are exposed to environmental chemicals, air pollutants, ozone, smog, pesticides, bacteria from food poisoning, cigarette smoke, preservatives, auto exhaust, prescription and nonprescription drugs, and alcohol, all of which can inflict severe unexpected liver injury.

Alcohol causes 80 percent of all liver disease in Western countries. Many people who are simply moderate drinkers have a fatty liver, indicating liver damage, and milk thistle would be a valuable supplement for them.

The great news is that milk thistle has been shown—in more than 200 experimental and clinical studies—to prevent and reverse liver damage and to neutralize free radicals. It also has the ability to stimulate the growth of new liver cells and to replace old damaged cells in large areas of liver tissue. Interestingly, silymarin does not have a stimulatory effect on malignant liver tissue.[18] Most of the research has been done in Germany, as that government endorses a supportive treatment for chronic inflammatory liver conditions and cirrhosis.[19]

Milk thistle helped heal hepatitis B

Considerable evidence shows that milk thistle helps in the treatment of chronic viral hepatitis. According to German research, milk thistle helped heal hepatitis B, the most common form of hepatitis usually resulting from a virus. It may also be successful in treating hepatitis C; studies to confirm it are under way. In German studies, doctors gave patients with hepatitis 420 milligrams of milk thistle extract *(silymarin)* daily for an average of nine months. It reversed liver injury, as measured by biopsy and decreased blood *transaminase* levels (transaminase is a liver enzyme that is elevated in hepatitis and is a primary marker of the intensity of the disease).[20]

Milk thistle dosage

The standardized milk thistle extract widely tested in Europe, and approved in Germany for liver disease and liver impairment, contains 70 percent to 80 percent silymarin. The recommended dose is 140 milligrams of silymarin to be taken three times a day (total 420 mg). After improvement, determined by liver function blood tests, you can cut back to a daily dose of 280 mg of silymarin, which is also the recommendation for those who just want to help prevent liver dysfunction and damage.[21]

There is no evidence that milk thistle is toxic or interacts with other medications. Surprisingly, in Germany they consider milk thistle so safe that there are no government warnings against using it, even during pregnancy and lactation.

I personally experienced excellent results with several of my clients that have taken high levels of milk thistle, well above the recommended potency. They took three capsules of the 175 mg (standardized 80 percent for 140 mg silymarin), twice a day (total of six capsules). This was actually a misunderstanding of the amount I had suggested, but the results were amazing and they experienced tremendous liver regeneration. It is an excellent addition to any complete nutrition program. Make sure the product you purchase is an extract and contains 70 to 80 percent silymarin.

Green Tea Enhances the Body's Natural Antioxidant Systems

The *International Journal of Anti-Aging Medicine* in 1998 reported that the evidence for green tea's potent antioxidant effects continues to accumulate. In a recent study researchers found that green tea compounds not only directly scavenge free radicals but enhance the effectiveness of the body's natural antioxidant systems. Green tea contains numerous cancer-fighting polyphenol compounds, including the antioxidant flavonoid *catechin*.

Studies indicate that green tea may help protect against cancers of the lungs, skin, liver, pancreas, and stomach. It also may work as a weight-loss agent by increasing fat metabolism and regulating blood sugar and insulin levels.

Green tea also boosts heart health by lowering cholesterol levels and reducing the tendency of blood platelets to stick together.[22]

Green tea contains caffeine, which occurs in small amounts (average of 20 to 30 mg per cup, if brewed for two to three minutes). This is much less caffeine than in coffee, however; an eight-ounce cup of coffee typically contains more than 100 mg of caffeine.

How to use it

There are many brands of green tea in bags and bulk form (regular and decaffeinated). Enjoy several cups a day. Green tea is also available in extract capsules that is more potent than the loose tea. The average dose is 200 mg of an extract standardized for 25 percent polyphenols.

Maitake Mushrooms

Maitake (my-tah-keh) mushrooms are highly prized both as food, as they have a good taste, and also as medicine. They are indigenous to the northeastern part of Japan. Maitake *(Grifola frondosa)* is huge, often reaching 20 inches in diameter at the base. A single cluster can weigh as much as 100 pounds; that's why it has been called the "King of mushrooms."[23]

People with serious degenerative illnesses travel long distances in search of the Maitake mushroom. Recently, Western medicine has received increased clinical and research attention.

While I was attending the American Academy of Anti-Aging Medicine convention, I had the opportunity to hear our friend Shari Lieberman, Ph.D., discuss Maitake D-fraction as an adjunct cancer treatment. She explained that the Maitake D-fraction is a protein-bound extract developed by Professor Hiroaki Nanba, Ph.D., and colleagues from the department of microbial chemistry at Kobe Pharmaceutical University in Japan.

Dr. Nanba observed: "Though it cannot be said that Maitake D-fraction and tablets are the cancer cure, one can safely say that they do maintain the quality of life of patients and improve the immune system, resulting in the possible remission of cancer cells with no side effects."[24]

Maitake contains the polysaccharides of beta-1,6-glucan with beta-1,3-glucan side chains, which results in a more complex branching structure.

The chemical structure of Maitake's polysaccharide compound is slightly different from beta-glucans found in other medical mushrooms. Known as beta-1,6-glucan, it is recognized by researchers as the most effective active agent stimulating cellular immune responses.[25]

Not only does maitake stimulate the production of immune cells, it improves their efficiency and effectiveness by increasing the chemicals that your body normally produces to stimulate these responses and target foreign substances in the body.

BENEFIT FOR CANCER AND TUMORS

Maitake D-fraction has been confirmed to have a multi-faceted benefit for cancer and tumors:

ஐ   It helps prevent the spread of cancer (metastasis).

 ♨ It activates natural killer (NK) cells, macrophages, and memory
   T cells.

 ♨ It slows or stops the growth of tumors.

 ♨ It works in conjunction with chemotherapy by lessening their
   negative side effects.

 ♨ One study reported 90 percent lessening of side effects from
   chemotherapy, including hair loss, pain, and nausea.

Other benefits of maitake D-fraction

Researchers have been working with diabetes, HIV and AIDS, high blood
pressure, high cholesterol and triglycerides, weight control, constipation,
and many other clinical cases.[26]

Maitake dosage

Look for Maitake D-fraction supplements in capsule, caplet, liquid
extract, or tincture form. The usual recommendation is one to two
grams daily for general purposes. Be sure to read the label directions.

Shiitake and Reishi Mushrooms

Mushrooms have been working their herbal magic for over 3,000 years
in traditional Oriental medicine. In China, the history of the shiitake
(shi-TAH-kay) mushroom dates back to the Ming Dynasty (1368-1644
A.D.). It has been prized both for its culinary use and as an immune-
potentiating agent. It was a remedy for upper respiratory diseases, poor
blood circulation, liver trouble, exhaustion and weakness, and to boost
"chi," or what they call the life energy. It was also believed to prevent
premature aging.[27]

Shiitake's most studied active principal, *lentinan*, is a polysaccharide
composed of beta-1,3-glucans with beta-1,6-glucan side chains.[28]
Shiitake's antiviral substance, lentinan, stimulates the immune system, as
well as activating the T-helper cells and the macrophages. Japanese experiments have found lentinan to be more powerful than the prescription
antiviral drug Amantaine hydrochloride. I am reporting this now because
you will see immune enhancing articles discussing beta-1,3-glucans and
beta-1,6-glucan, and you will be familiar with its origin.

Reishi mushroom

The reishi mushroom has also been used for 3,000 years and is considered by some to to be a medicinal mushroom. Most of these mushrooms also have the active constituent beta-glucan that supports the body's immune system in fighting cancer cells and countering the effects of aging. According to *The Little Herb Encyclopedia*, new research is showing success against chronic fatigue syndrome by the noticeable increase of vitality after its administration. In addition, it has been found that the Reishi helps regenerate the liver; reduces excessive levels of cholesterol in the blood, thus improving circulation; lowers triglycerides; reduces coronary symptoms and normalized blood pressure; and alleviates allergy symptoms. It is a powerful immune stimulating agent, with particular effectiveness against wasting and degenerative diseases. Reishi stimulates T-cell activity and inhibits replication of the HIV virus.[29]

Beta-Glucan and Immunity

Thanks to impressive scientific research and innovative manufacturing techniques there is now a product called beta-glucan (1,3-glucan) that has demonstrated significant benefits for immune function. It has now been confirmed that beta-glucan profoundly and positively activates a powerful immune-system response.

Beta-glucan is a simple polysaccharide (a carbohydrate/sugar molecule` that is found in small amounts in baker's yeast, oats, barley, and the Maitake and Shiitake mushrooms I just discussed. The beta 1,3-glucan, extracted from the cell walls of baker's yeast has also been clinically shown to stimulate a specific immune receptor site.[30]

The first research projects establishing its effectiveness was back in 1950's. A report in the journal of *Cancer*, showed that a single low dose of beta-glucan in animals revved up immunity. Low doses of this substance can help macrophages overcome tumors and infections linked to viruses and yeast or fungal conditions such as Candida albicans.[31]

It has been confirmed that when the macrophage encounters the beta-glucan molecule, the macrophage becomes activated and triggers its powerful immune stimulating capabilities.

Macrophages (literally means "big eater") are actually large white immune cells that clean up the body. They have taken up residence in specific tissues like the liver, spleen and lymph nodes, and engulf (eat) foreign particles including bacteria, dead or damaged cells. Macrophages are essential in protecting against invasion by microorganisms, as well as against damage to the lymphatic system. These immune cells can then recognize and destroy toxins, bacteria, viruses, fungi and parasites. Beta-glucan may aid the body in fighting cancer, and may help protect the body from negative effects of chemotherapy and radiation.

Macrophages stimulated by beta-glucan require extra amounts of vitamin C to function more effectively. So, if you take beta-glucan make sure you also take extra amounts of vitamin C to ensure a more effective immune response. You will find several brands of beta-glucan in your nutrition store.

Conjugated Linoleic Acid—CLA

We have known that CLA can help speed up the body's fat metabolism so more fat gets flushed out of the system, instead of getting deposited in our cells. CLA also helps the body to metabolize existing fat deposits—a key to losing weight.

But, the exciting news is that CLA has shown both in vitro and in animal models to have strong anti-tumor activity. Investigators at Roswell Park Cancer Institute in Buffalo, New York, conducted rat studies and reported CLA inhibits proliferation and induces cell death (apoptosis) of normal rat breast cells in primary culture. In other words it protected the rats against breast cancer using CLA.

Another study reported in *Life Extension, Disease Prevention and Treatment*, investigated the effect of dietary CLA on the growth of human breast cancer cells in immuno-deficient mice. Similarly, it was found that CLA inhibited the development and growth of mammary tumors. Moreover, CLA completely stopped the spread of breast cancer cells to lungs, peripheral blood, and bone marrow. These results indicate the ability of dietary CLA to block both the local growth and systemic spread of human breast cancer via mechanisms independent of the host immune system. CLA is a natural substance we need to investigate for immune support, as more information becomes available. You can find CLA in your nutrition store.

DIM & Indole-3-Carbinol

DIM (Diindolylmethane) is a very concentrated form of the phytochemical indole-3-carbinol, a compound found in cruciferous vegetables such as broccoli, cauliflower, brussel sprouts, etc. DIM is many times more potent than regular indole-3-carbinol and it has an effect on hormonal balance and estrogen metabolism. There are many references in the medical journals on the value of indole-3-carbinol and its protective effect against cancer.

The value of cruciferous phytonutrients

In 1997, researchers at Strang Cancer Research Laboratory at Rockefeller University discovered that when indole-3-carbinol changes "strong" estrogen to "weak" estrogen, it stops human cancer cells from growing (54–61 percent) and provokes the cancer cells to self destruct. Subsequent studies from the University of California at Berkeley, showed that indole-3-carbinol inhibits human breast cancer cells from growing by as much as 90 percent in culture. Growth arrest does not depend on estrogen receptors.[32]

It has been shown that indole-3-carbinol goes right to the cause of cancer and stops the mechanism that makes cells mutate and form tumors. A few of the scientific papers were titled:

- Selective responsiveness of human breast cancer cells to indole-3-carbinol, a chemopreventative agent.
- Indole-3-carbinol. A novel approach to breast cancer prevention.
- Multifunctional aspects of the action of indole-3-carbinol as an anti-tumor agent.
- Anti-estrogenic activities of indole-3-carbinol in cervical cells; implication for prevention of cervical cancer.[33]

We have always known that eating cruciferous vegetables are valuable for our health, and now we know it may even lower the risk of all kinds of cancer. Watch for more information on these natural products. They should be available in your nutrition store. Follow the recommended dosage.

Colostrum—The Immune Enhancer

I have become very excited about bovine colostrum after finding it during one of our national conventions. I even ordered a case of capsules and powder so all of my grandchildren could benefit from this wonderful product, as it is considered "life's first food".

Daniel G. Clark, M.D., wrote "When a mother gives birth to her offspring, her mammary glands provide life supporting factors that she has acquired in her lifetime. Her body concentrates these factors into a special (non-milk) immune and growth-supporting fluid called colostrum. A mother produces true colostrum for only the first 24–48 hours after giving birth."[34] This is also true for a newborn calf, as the dairy cow also produces colostrum after birth.

Dairy cows are the only animals that meet all of the essential criteria needed, as cows are accepted by virtually all other mammals, including man. For example, in the US and Japan, researchers verified, in laboratory analysis that the key immunoglobulins (the body's most important immune, growth, healing and anti-aging factors) in cows are identical in molecular combination to humans, and are not species specific but transferable from one species to another.[35]

In 1987 the International Institute of Nutritional Research reported that, "Bovine colostrum offered tremendous possibilities for providing unparalleled support for the immune system that may be the deciding factor in the body's war against illness and aging." It also reported, "Bovine colostrum is found to be safe, effective via oral administration, with no known contradictions or overdoses."[36]

Historically, bovine colostrum has played a significant role in natural healing. Hundreds of years of human use, thousands of scientific studies and human clinical trials worldwide have shown bovine colostrum to be safe and effective. The presence of such a wide spectrum of immunoglobulins, antibodies and accessory immune factors, found in colostrum, offer tremendous possibilities in the prevention of and recovery from illness. Colostrum's rediscovery and supporting research show that we had one of the most important supplements for immune enhancement and tissue repair all along.

IP6—The Anti-Tumor Substance

IP6 is an ubiquitous substance, which means it is found everywhere at the same time. It is virtually found in all fiber from whole grains and legumes. IP6 is composed of inositol with six phosphate groups attached, therefore, it is called inositol hexaphosphate or IP6. It is present in almost every cell of the body, and is essential for key body functions. The brain, the nervous system, and reproductive organs all depend on a constant supply of inositol (a B vitamin).

AbulKalam Shamsuddin, M.D., Ph.D., has been performing ground-breaking experiments on inositol and its derivative IP6, for the last 15 years. He has discovered that IP6 can effectively prevent cancer formation and shrink preexisting cancers in experimental systems, with virtually no toxicity. When he gave IP6 by mouth, or by injection directly into the tumors or intra-muscular injection, it consistently had the same effects. Whether it was tested on a colon-cancer, a breast-cancer, smooth-muscle cells, skeletal muscle tumors, or liver cancer, regardless of how IP6 was given, it showed that it inhibits the growth of cancer.

The combination of IP6 and inositol has also been shown to be an effective antioxidant and immune function booster. The combination is especially helpful in stimulating the activity of white blood cells known as natural killer (NK) cells, so called because they literally kill cancer cells, viruses, and other infecting organisms. Adding IP6 and inositol enhances the NK cells' killer instincts, according to Michael Murray, N.D., in his book, *How to Prevent and Treat Cancer with Natural Medicine*.

What forms of cancer can be treated with IP6?

Lab studies show that the combination of IP6 and inositol exerts anti-cancer effects against virtually all types of cancers, including cancers of the breast, prostate, lung, skin, and brain, as well as lymphomas and leukemia. Unfortunately at this time there are few results available from human studies.

The exciting news is that these scientists have observed that cancer cells can revert back to normal cells in the presence of IP6. Research studies have also shown that IP6 inhibits growth of human prostate cancer cells.

Take Charge of Your Health

As you read this research about these herbs and other nutrients that stimulate the immune system, I hope you are convinced that it is time to *Take Charge of Your Health* (the title of my previous book). New information about herbs and various essential nutrients are constantly reported in the news. It is one of the most exciting and rapidly growing fields of research. I encourage you to stay abreast of the information about these substances, and add them to your nutritional program. They may very well be the foremost keys to your staying in excellent health, along with all of the antioxidants we discussed in the previous chapter.

Mirror, Mirror on the Wall

Beauty Secrets for Your Hair, Skin and Nails

*No one wants to get old as we generally think of it—
the muscles becoming soft, the bones brittle, a cantankerous personality, and a senile mind. While others
have searched for the legendary "fountain of youth,"
I have been searching for something else—a way to help
people stay healthy, energetic, and attractive. My search
led to nutrition.*

—GLADYS LINDBERG

hen you look in the mirror, what do you see? Do you see soft, supple, radiant, glowing, blemish-free skin? Or do you see age spots and new wrinkles?

The skin is the first "aging" sign we tend to see in ourselves. We all want to find ways to keep our skin beautiful, soft, and we hope, wrinkle free. We will each get some wrinkles, but nobody wants them prematurely!

My Mother, Gladys Lindberg, had the most beautiful skin for her age of any woman I have ever seen. She far surpassed the "beauty experts" and "movie stars" in her beauty and grace. At age 85 she had a clear, peachy complexion and was virtually wrinkle free! She had no patchy "age" spots or blemished skin. She never smoked and avoided the sun whenever possible. This was natural beauty. Mother started her quest for health when she was 43 years old. She said her skin was blotchy and never radiant, but her program drastically changed the quality of her skin.

Important Advice for Skin Health

A woman recently came into our store looking for a "magic formula" for her deeply wrinkled skin. She was only in her mid-40s, but said her skin had changed drastically over the past months. Being quite disturbed about the situation, she came to me wanting "that miracle cream."

I talked to her for a few minutes and discovered that she had been on a severe reducing diet for several months. She had followed a diet low in protein, and over the course of those months had lost her skin tone. It had started to sag and wrinkle way beyond what would be normal for her chronological age. Most women want to be slim, but if you saw her, I'm sure you would agree, "not at that price!" Here are some things I told her that are important for healthy skin regardless of whether you're trying to lose weight or not.

Collagen—the Skin's "Cement"

Elastic skin is a sign that a person has ample collagen, the strong cement-like material that binds together the cells of your body.

Collagen is a structural tissue and it is replaced very slowly. It is made of fibrous protein. In fact, collagen comprises 30 percent of the total body protein. Its strong white fibers, stronger than steel wire of the same size, and yellow elastic networks, called elastin, form the connective tissue that holds our body together. Collagen strengthens the skin, blood vessels, bones, and teeth. It is the intracellular cement that holds together the cells in various organs and tissues. Collagen is one of the most valuable proteins in the human body. A person who has been sick, or who has been on an extremely low-protein diet, very often sees the muscles in his or her arms and legs begin to sag, which is a sign that they have probably lost collagen.

Let's Start With Protein

The building blocks of protein are amino acids. When protein is eaten, your digestive processes break it down into amino acids, which pass into the blood and are carried throughout the body. Your cells can then select the amino acids they need for the construction of new body tissue, antibodies, hormones, enzymes, and blood cells.

There are 22 different amino acids, each of which has its own characteristics, and are like the letters of the alphabet. The eight essential amino acids are like the vowels. Just as you cannot make words without vowels, so you cannot build proteins without these essential amino acids. Protein is not one substance, but literally tens of thousands of different substances. The essential amino acids must be consumed in the diet because the body does not make them.

The complete proteins that contain the eight essential amino acids come from meat, poultry, fish, eggs, milk—all dairy, cheese and soy. They are basically anything that comes from the animal. Nuts and legumes (peas and beans) contain some but not all of the essential amino acids; these are known as incomplete proteins.

In various combinations, all of these amino acids are capable of forming an almost limitless variety of proteins, each serving its own purpose.

Proteins are necessary for tissue repair and for the construction of new tissue. Every cell needs protein to maintain its life. Protein is also the primary substance used to "replace" worn-out or dead cells:

- Most white blood cells are replaced every ten days.
- The cells in the lining of the gastrointestinal tract and blood platelets are replaced every four days.

- Skin cells are replaced every 24 days.
- More than 98 percent of the molecules in the body are completely replaced each year![1]

Your muscles, hair, nails, skin, and eyes are made of protein. So are the cells that make up the liver, kidneys, heart, lungs, nerves, brain, and your sex glands. The body's most active protein users are the hormones secreted from the various glands—thyroxin from the thyroid, insulin from the pancreas, and a variety of hormones from the pituitary—as well as the soft tissues, hard-working major organs and muscles. They all require the richest stores of protein.

Next to water, protein is the most plentiful substance in your body. In fact, if all the water was squeezed out of you, about half of your dry weight would be protein.

- One third of this protein would be in your muscles,
- One fifth in your bones and cartilage,
- One tenth in your skin,
- and the rest in your other tissues and body fluids.
- Even hemoglobin is 95 percent protein. Hemoglobin is the protein in the red cells of the blood that carries oxygen from the lungs to the other parts of the body where it is used to burn molecules of food and produce energy.

How much protein a day?

Many "experts" differ on the amount of protein needed in the diet. Some suggest very low amounts; some suggest much higher amounts, especially if body building. I have found with my nutritional counseling that most people consume a very low protein diet, especially if they tell me they are tired all the time. When I have them increase their protein during the day, usually with protein shakes, it is amazing how much better they start to feel.

The following protein requirement chart is to be used only as a guideline for determining your protein requirement. You may need more, or you might be able to get by with slightly less. Your requirement depends on your percent of body fat, your weight and the physical activity you do. The higher your activity level, the more you will need to increase your dietary protein intake to repair and rebuild muscle.

If you are undergoing any type of severe stress (including the stresses of cancer, burns, radiation exposure, or pregnancy), you need more. If you are susceptible to infections you may need more.

Remember that antibodies, white blood cells, lymph cells, and every-thing our body uses to fight infections is made out of protein. I feel it is very important we look to the high side of these requirements.

DAILY PROTEIN REQUIREMENTS
FOR MEN AND WOMEN OVER 20*

IDEAL WEIGHT	PROTEIN NEEDED	SAFETY MARGIN
80 lbs	40 grams	60 grams
111 lbs	50 grams	70 grams
133 lbs	60 grams	80 grams
156 lbs	70 grams	90 grams
178 lbs	80 grams	100 grams
200 lbs	90 grams	110 grams
222 lbs	100 grams	120 grams
244 lbs	110 grams	130 grams

*Our calculations for this age group are based on the usual recom-mendation of one gram of protein per kilogram (2.2 lbs) of ideal body weight, for sedentary individuals. However, adding 20 grams of protein to the above recommendation as a safety margin will ensure getting enough protein.

Pregnant women should add an additional 20 grams, and nursing mothers should add 40 grams of protein to the above recommendation.

If you are physically active, exercising every day, figure one gram of protein per pound of lean (your ideal) weight.[2]

Three ounces of chicken yields approximately 20 grams of protein; one half cup of water-packed tuna contains 28 grams; eight ounces of low fat, plain yogurt has 12 grams. One egg provides six grams. An eight-ounce glass of low-fat milk has eight grams. Remember, there are excellent protein powders that are alternatives to traditional protein foods. There are tips in the *Let's Put It All Together* chapter for getting all the protein you need for optimal health and beautiful skin. There are also suggestions for making delicious Lindberg Super Energy Protein Shakes.

We need to remember there needs to be a balance of protein, fats and carbohydrates that Mother and I have basically taught. It is important to eat five times a day and include some form of protein at each meal or feeding. We have found this program has helped more people look and feel their best. This may be ideal for most people, but remember, we are "biologically different."

In our nutritional program I recommend a variety of complete protein foods including fish, chicken, low-fat dairy, eggs, some red meat, quality protein powders, and nutritional yeast. Also consume an ample supply of various fresh fruits and vegetables, legumes which are complex carbohydrates and include the essential fatty acids. A strict fat-free diet is not healthy for your skin. My approach is this: *You are not made of lettuce leaves. Your body is made of protein that is essential for almost every cell in your body, especially your hair, skin and nails.*

Protecting Your Skin

As we discussed more thoroughly in chapter 3 on the value of the antioxidants, we can protect our skin from free radical damage—the damage created when cells oxidize—by consuming antioxidants. Go back and read that important chapter. Beta-carotene, vitamin C, vitamin E, Pycnogenol, grape seed extract, alpha lipoic acid, CoQ10, and the trace mineral selenium are all antioxidants that have been researched the most in their advantages to the cells. Other nutrients that are good for our hair, skin and nails are listed below.

Vitamin B complex

Most of the B-vitamins are related to healthy skin. If you read the deficiency symptoms related to B-vitamins, you quickly come to the conclusion: "Take vitamin B-complex!" Roger Williams, Ph.D., discovered pantothenic acid (vitamin B5) more than 50 years ago.[3] He found that chickens suffering from "chick dermatitis" were cured quickly with pantothenic acid. Their unhealthy skin and feathers were restored to health almost miraculously. He suggested that people who had trouble with their hair and skin might enjoy the same results from pantothenic acid. Dr. Williams noted that, of all the organs of the body, the skin is the first organ that suffers from malnutrition. Other early indicators of malnutrition are found in the mouth, tongue, lips, and gums.[4]

Grape seed extract or Pycnogenol

An antioxidant that comes from Pycnogenol and grape seed extract has been shown to be important in skin health. Dr. R. Kuttan and colleagues have shown that Pycnogenol binds tightly to skin collagen and increases its resistance to enzyme degradation. It also helps repair collagen.[5] For more valuable information read the *Antioxidants* chapter 3.

Gamma-Linolenic Acid (GLA)

GLA acts as an anti-inflammatory agent with none of the side effects of anti-inflammatory drugs. It promotes growth of skin, hair, and nails. Evening primrose oil, borage oil, and black currant seed oil are natural sources of GLA in capsule form. There have been numerous studies showing the benefits of evening primrose oil in treating skin conditions. Other important fatty acids are called omega-3 fish oils (EPA) that are found in cod liver oil and cold water fish such as salmon and sardines. Flaxseed oil is also an excellent way to obtain a blend of omega-3, omega-6 and omega-9 fatty acids.

Alpha Lipoic Acid

Is an exciting natural substance and works double duty as it prevents free radical damage in every area of our body. It prevents this damage, regardless of whether it is in the brain fluids, the heart, the blood, stored fat, the pancreas, cartilage, the kidneys, the bones, the liver or the connective tissue of our skin. For that matter every cell, in every organ of our bodies needs alpha lipoic acid. It is one of the most powerful antioxidants. With all the literature I have read, the best part of the story is that it is also anti-aging.

I was excited when I discovered the book *The Alpha Lipoic Acid Breakthrough* by Burt Berkson, M.D., Ph.D. He has been working more than twenty years with this substance, and feels that alpha lipoic acid is an amazing, vitamin like antioxidant and one of biochemistry's most important findings. Ignored by the American scientific medical communities for so long, today its benefits are finally coming into light. He feels it has so many beneficial and incontestable influences on cellular function, that we should all take it.[6] This product is available at your nutrition store.

Silica

Silica or silicon is a trace mineral, and next to oxygen it is the second most abundant element in the earth's crust. It is present in connective tissue, bone, skin, and fingernails. Silicon appears to be involved in the building and metabolism of these structures.[7]

Dietary sources of silicon include vegetables, whole grains, and seafood. The herb horsetail *(Equisetum arvense)* contains a large amount of silica. It has many uses in the body, such as preventing the hair from split ends and strengthening fingernails. Horsetail also helps facilitate the use of and retention of calcium in the body.[8]

My favorite is a high-quality German liquid silica, derived from quartz crystals, that is a colloidal preparation of silica in a highly dispersible form available at your nutrition store.

L-Cysteine

The sulfur-containing amino acids (methionine, cysteine, and taurine) will provide sulfur in concentrated and easily assimilated forms. Of these three amino acids, experts find that cysteine is the most effective in relieving skin problems. Robert Erdmann, Ph.D., said this is not surprising, as a quarter of all the amino acids contained in collagen (the skin protein) are cysteine molecules. Without them, collagen would simply fall apart.[9]

All horny layers of the skin, including hair and fingernails, are high in cysteine. There is evidence that the high-sulfur proteins, cysteine being one of them, are missing in the hair of humans who have experienced abnormal hair loss. Preliminary findings indicate that daily supplementation of cysteine increases hair shaft diameter and hair growth density in certain cases of human baldness and hair loss.[10]

Carl C. Pfeiffer, Ph.D., M.D., said that egg yolks are rich sources of the sulfur amino acids, methionine and cysteine. Dr. Pfeiffer tells of the other minerals and vitamins in eggs and says, "The egg can thus be considered the ideal model of the exact nutrients to take with you to a desert island! The protein is complete, with all the essential amino acids, and the ratio of minerals is perfect for the purpose of growth. Eggs are the perfect food."[11]

Sulfur

As a component of cysteine discussed above, sulfur is necessary for healing and repair of most tissues in the body, especially our skin. It also protects us from internal injury of free radical damage, aging, cross linkages, scar tissue, and even recovery from burn and surgical incisions. Because of its ability to protect against the harmful effects of radiation and pollution, sulfur slows down the aging process. Sulfur is found in hemoglobin and all body tissues.[12]

It is called nature's "beauty mineral" because sulfur keeps the hair glossy and smooth, the complexion clear and youthful, and the nails strong. Sulfur is also important for producing collagen and keratin, important protein substances that prevent dryness and maintain elastin in the skin.

MSM (Methyl-Sulfonyl-Methane)

MSM (Methyl-Sulfonyl-Methane) is an organic sulfur, a nonmetallic element that occurs widely in nature. Sulfur is the fourth most plentiful mineral found in your body. MSM is an excellent supplement to add additional sulfur to your nutrition program. It is available in both capsules and white, odorless, crystals, and is important for your joints, hair, skin and nails. Because of all this wonderful new information, I am now adding MSM to my morning protein shake. The literature shows there is no toxic dose of MSM. The only side effect is fuller, thicker hair, less wrinkles and longer nails.

MSM is also available in a cream used topically to aid skin disorders. MSM cream is helpful in treating acne, psoriasis, eczema, dermatitis, dandruff, scabies, diaper rash and certain fungal infections.[13] More information on MSM is found in the *Arthritis* chapter 11.

Water

Water is essential for beautiful, soft, supple skin. Your daily diet should include the equivalent of eight to ten glasses of pure water. This keeps enough moisture in your body and hydrates your cells. Caffeine and alcoholic drinks pull moisture out of your system.

The Skin's Two Biggest Enemies

Most of us know that the skin's biggest enemy is the *sun*. Regular exposure to ultraviolet rays erodes the elastic tissues in the skin, causing a person to wrinkle prematurely. The ultraviolet energy from the sun produces free radicals in the fats stored in the skin cell membranes. Years of sun exposure may lead to malignant melanoma, the most serious form of skin cancer—which has risen five- to six-fold around the world in recent decades! The second most common type of skin cancer is squamous cell carcinoma. It, too, is on the rise.

The next biggest enemy of the skin—smoking cigarettes. If you don't smoke, minimize your exposure to people who do. People who smoke a pack-and-a-half a day wrinkle about ten years sooner than a non-smoker. I am sure you can bring to mind several acquaintances who smoke—and generally, you will find that their skin is prematurely wrinkled, especially around the mouth and lips.

One cigarette destroys about 25 mg of vitamin C, the important nutrient for building collagen.[14] If you do smoke and can't quit, learn that you must take high antioxidants to protect yourself from this damage. Most experts would suggest at least 4,000 mg to 8,000 mg of

vitamin C divided through the day, 800 IU of v[...]
mcg of selenium to help protect you. Free rac[...]
time a person is exposed to sun, smoke, er[...]
alcohol, and drugs. If you live in an area with l[...]
drink alcohol, or if you are taking drugs of ar[...]
antioxidant protection. Go back and read the /[...]

Special Help for Skin Conditions

To help with various skin or hair conditions, we recommend a complete nutrition program that you will find in the last chapter, *Let's Put It All Together.* In addition to the nutrients that are a part of that plan, some people need "extra" nutrients for specific areas of concern.

Live with Regis!

I had written Regis Philbin for tickets to his show, *Live With Regis and Kathie Lee,* prior to visiting New York with my daughter-in-law, Gabrielle, for a wedding. Regis has taken my Lindberg Varsity 2 Vitamin & Mineral Packs for about 20 years. Graciously, he provided us with VIP tickets.

During the program, Regis introduced me, and Kathie Lee Gifford asked, "If you had one vitamin to choose above all others, which would it be?" Relative to all of the important research I reported about in this book, I replied, "Vitamin E." I proceeded to explain about the age spots we may develop on our hands and face. As we discussed this, Regis finally said, "the audience is taking over this show," and everyone laughed. He then told the audience how he has taken our Lindberg Varsity Pack 2 vitamins for many years.

Age spots or liver spots

When you are deficient in vitamin E, fatty substances may turn into brown spots usually called "age spots." Some refer to these as "liver spots." We are most familiar with them when they appear on the face, arms, and back of the hands. Such deposits are not just on the surface skin, however. According to Roger J. Williams, Ph.D., the author of *Nutrition Against Disease,* these deposits can also be found in the brain, heart, adrenal glands, and other parts of the body. They are directly linked to a lack of vitamin E.[15] Dr. Williams recommends you not only increase your intake of vitamin E, but all of the antioxidants. It is especially important to take vitamin E before these "liver spots" begin to appear on your skin.

Note: *You must make sure, of course, that these "age spots" are not pre-cancerous lesions. If one of these brown spots pops up "out of the blue," or an* *ne suddenly changes shape, becomes raised, or bleeds, be sure to have a matologist take a look at it. You need to be certain it is not an early form of skin cancer.*

Deep red bruising

I am sure you have seen older people with deep red bruises on their hands or arms. Usually, this age group will tell you that they do not know why any slight bump or scrape seems to cause it. Could it be that these bruises are a result of a classic vitamin C deficiency? If you see your loved ones with these red bruises, recommend vitamin C with bioflavonoids and Pycnogenol, or grape seed extract, in large enough amounts, on a daily basis. This will help to clear their skin up and prevent it from happening again. Go back and read the signs and symptoms of scurvy (the old time sailor's disease) in chapter 2.

Wrinkles

Hans Selye, M.D., the original stress doctor, experimented with premature aging and found that wrinkles could be prevented with large amounts of vitamin E. It may be that the multiple stresses that induce aging cause cells in the lower layers of the skin to be destroyed. Bits of scar tissue then take their place, and wrinkles result as the scar tissue contracts.

If wrinkles come from cells being damaged, the best prevention is to take all the antioxidants (especially A, E, C, selenium, CoQ10 and grape seed extract or Pycnogenol) and other nutrients to prevent healthy tissue from damage. MSM (organic sulfur) has also been shown to help prevent wrinkles.

Eczema

Eczema is also called *atopic dermatitis* since the symptoms and therapies are similar to dermatitis. It may be caused by low adrenal function, irritants, allergies, or nutritional deficiencies. Symptoms usually consist of blisters, red bumps, swelling, oozing, crusting, scaling, and itching. Melvyn Werbach, M.D., in *Nutritional Influences on Illness*, reported several research studies in which patients took three to nine grams of MaxEPA (omega-3 fish oil) daily in divided doses, along with vitamin E. Other researchers used two grams, twice daily, of evening primrose oil after meals, while continuing on their regular medication. Results were noticeable in about 12 weeks, and after 11 months more than half were rated improved. If you add the mineral zinc to your diet, improvements could even be more dramatic. In one study, taking 50 mg of chelated zinc twice a day along with other nutrients resulted in full remission in all except one severe case.[16]

The other nutritional supplements that have been shown to help are EPA/DHA from cod liver oil and cold water fish, flaxseed oil, a "stress" B-complex, vitamins B₆, C, E, and the minerals magnesium and zinc. I would also recommend adding vitamin A from fish oil at 25,000 IUs a day. If you are not pregnant, that amount can even be increased. Many people cannot convert beta-carotene to true vitamin A (retinol). Go back and read about the value of vitamin A in chapter 3.

Note: *According to several researchers, if you have eczema, dermatitis or psoriasis, you may be low in stomach acidity and need to take hydrochloric acid tablets or capsules discussed in chapter 17.*

Dermatitis

Symptoms of dermatitis are similar to eczema and include itching, flaking, oozing, crusting, scaling, and thickening of the skin. It may be caused by an allergic reaction to certain foods or substances. The nutritional supplements recommended would be basically the same as for eczema with the addition of digestive enzymes, especially hydrochloric acid.[17]

Psoriasis

Psoriasis looks like patches of skin that are thickened and reddened and covered with scales. It usually does not itch and shows up most often on the arms, elbows, behind the ears, scalp, back, legs, and knees. Authorities suggest taking the essential fatty acids, evening primrose oil, vitamin A (fish oil), folic acid, B-complex, B₆, vitamin C with bioflavonoids, zinc, lecithin and digestive enzymes.[18]

According to an article in the *Journal of the American Academy of Dermatology*, researchers found that the active ingredient in cayenne pepper (capsaicin), "topically applied, effectively treats pruritic psoriasis." This ointment reduced the severity of psoriasis, including less scaling, thickness, and redness.[19] You can find this ointment at most nutrition stores. I would also suggest MSM, the organic sulfur cream for your skin.

Sunburns

A sunburn can be very damaging to the skin. Over exposure of the skin to the ultraviolet radiation in sunlight causes inflammation and burns. First-degree burns are when the skin reddens, affecting only the top layer. Second-degree burns create blisters and usually heal without scarring. Third-degree burns result in more severe damage to the skin. These burns are susceptible to infections and must be treated by a doctor. Secondary infections may follow once the skin has peeled.

Repeated over exposure to the sun and sunburns increases aging and the risk of skin cancer. Prevention is your best defense.

According to Drs. Evan and Wilfrid Shute, vitamin E should be taken to aid in the healing process. Vitamin E may even be applied topically to the burn or scar.[20] Another popular topical remedy is to apply cool aloe vera gel liberally to the burned area. You may also mix the gel with vitamins A and E.

Vitamin C with bioflavonoids and zinc are also important for wound healing. Also try to consume high protein foods and be sure to supplement your diet with vitamin B-complex, especially pantothenic acid to help regenerate the body.

Note: *With any serious burn, seek medical attention before applying anything to the skin.*

Acne

Acne is inflammation of the skin generally due to clogged pores. It may be worse at adolescence, just prior to menstruation as hormones change, when a person is under stress, or when the diet is poor. If you have this problem, add extra vitamin A (water-soluble from fish oil), beta-carotene, zinc, a "stress" vitamin B-complex, vitamin B_6 (especially for acne associated with menstruation), essential fatty acids such as evening primrose oil, flaxseed oil, brewer's yeast, vitamin C, and digestive enzymes (pancreatin and betaine hydrochloric acid with pepsin).

Jonathan V. Wright, M.D., says, "In my experience, the use of hydrochloric acid supplements in adequate doses is extremely effective in reducing the severity of acne, and, in some cases, nearly eliminating it..."[21] Adding lactobacillus acidophilus appears even more helpful than using hydrochloric acid and pepsin supplements alone. Acne rosacea is often associated with low stomach acidity. Make sure there is no constipation (you need at least two movements a day), as this can be a major cause of breakouts. MSM cream, a form of sulfur, may also be helpful. Also add several MSM capsules or powder to your nutritional program.

Tea tree oil is a natural, topical antibiotic and antiseptic. Use the product full-strength on blemishes two to three times a day. A study conducted by the Department of Dermatology of the Royal Prince Alfred Hospital in New South Wales, Australia, found that a 5 percent solution of tea tree oil was as effective as benzoyl peroxide for most cases of acne, without the irritation. Benzoyl peroxide is the active ingredient in many over-the-counter acne products, but is extremely drying.

Dandruff

We all know about those little white flakes that appear on the hair that causes itching, scaling, and redness of scalp. The only symptom that has been tied absolutely to a selenium deficiency is dandruff.[22] So take the trace mineral, selenium, and a variety of nutrients, such as extra vitamin B_6, vitamin A, vitamin B-complex, vitamins C and E, zinc, plus the essential fatty acids.

Shingles

Shingles, a type of herpes, comes from the chicken pox virus, a virus that never leaves the body. Shingles often start after a period of major stress or illness. According to Adelle Davis, the diet for anyone with boils, abscesses, carbuncles, impetigo, or viral infection such as shingles should be the same as for other infections. Vitamin A and E should be particularly emphasized while infection symptoms persist, and for three or four months afterward. Be sure to take a complete vitamin and mineral formula to rebuild your entire system, especially the adrenals.[23]

The amino acid L-lysine has been effective in some studies. A Mayo Clinic double-blind and placebo-controlled study, used 1,248 mg of L-lysine daily. This dose was consistently and significantly effective in reducing the recurrence rate of herpes outbreaks. Administering L-lysine did not, however, reduce the duration or severity of attacks once underway. Given L-lysine's low toxicity there is little to lose and potentially much to gain in taking lysine according to Sheldon Saul Hendler, M.D., Ph.D.[24]

Lendon Smith, M.D., says to "try a daily dose of B_{12} (1,000 mcg) intramuscularly for five to ten days. Use vitamin C, perhaps up to bowel tolerance—somewhere at 1,000 mg level every waking hour or two. Continue for two weeks, then taper off. Vitamin E locally and orally is soothing and might cut down the chance of scarring."[25]

If you are suffering from distressing skin pain from shingles, there is also a natural, safe product for you to use. It is from the red-hot cayenne pepper, the same hot pepper you use to spice up your chili. According to *Alternative Medicine*, the active ingredient in this pepper is *capsaicin*, and when used properly, it may relieve skin pain. When this natural capsaicin cream or ointment is applied to the skin, it creates a sensation of warmth. Generally you can expect to experience pain relief after about two weeks of therapy, or a little longer. Many doctors prefer to use capsaicin for skin pain relief rather than drugs as it has fewer drug interaction problems.[26]

Recognizing Deficiencies Related to Hair, Skin and Nails

Recognizing minor abnormalities to good health and taking steps to correct them is preventive medicine at its best. On the following pages I have described just a few deficiency symptoms that many people experience.

I want to restate my long-standing belief that all vitamins and minerals work together. For example, if you are deficient in riboflavin (vitamin B2), you can almost bet that you also are deficient in vitamins B6, B3, and so forth. The B vitamins work together, and a deficiency in one nearly always signals deficiencies in the others. That is why we recommend complete vitamin and mineral formulas in sufficient potencies that contain all the vitamins and minerals you need in doses to do you some good and prevent these deficiencies.

Other deficiencies are described in the appendix, *Vitamin and Mineral Summary Chart,* located at the end of the book.

Protein Deficiencies

- Puffy bags under the eyes, especially in the morning, may indicate a lack of protein.

- Water retention. General puffiness around the eyes, as well as swollen ankles, face, and hands, can result from a protein deficiency.

- Nails are made of protein, not calcium as some think. A protein deficiency can be marked by split, extremely thin nails. Nails that fail to grow quickly lack protein.

- The structure of the hair follicle is protein. There are eight amino acids that the body does not produce and that therefore must come from complete protein foods such as eggs, dairy (milk, cheese, yogurt, cottage cheese), soy, meat, fish, and fowl. Quality protein powders can fill this nutritional requirement for complete protein foods. It's a great reason to use protein powders. Eat small meals often with protein at each meal.

L-Cysteine and L-Methionine are the sulfur amino acids that form "keratin," which is the protein structure of hair. Studies have shown that supplementing with L-cysteine may prevent hair from falling out, as well as increase the diameter of the hair shaft. These amino acids have been found to increase hair growth by as much as 100 percent.[27] Egg yolk contains the highest amount of these two amino acids. You may also purchase L-cysteine and L-methionine individually at your nutrition store. Another easy way to add sulfur to your diet is to take MSM.[28]

Vitamin Deficiencies

These deficiency symptoms are related to the hair, skin, eyes, nose and mouth. The following covers deficiencies that you can see when you look into a mirror. There are other *mental* and *emotional* symptoms found in chapter 7.

Vitamin A—Retinol

- The ideal source of vitamin A is fish oil-based. Some individuals cannot convert beta-carotene to true vitamin A, so when I discuss the value of vitamin A, I do not mean beta-carotene in these cases.

- An emulsified (water soluble) vitamin A is available as some people may not be able to absorb the oil form.

- Drying out of the skin may signal deficiency—also rough, horny skin especially on upper arms and thighs. The skin starts to look like goose bumps that don't go away.

- The skin has four layers of cells. Lack of vitamin A on the bottom layer causes the cells to die too quickly. The body sends white blood cells to bring these dead cells to the surface; the manifestation may be a pimple, sty in the eye, a carbuncle, or a boil. Dead cells behind the ear drum create a fertile environment for infection and may be a primary cause of ear infection.

2. A vitamin A deficiency may result in bits of mucous accumulating on the eyelashes at night and the eyelids may feel stuck together in the morning. It also results in a sensitivity to bright lights and glare.

2. Vitamin A helps prevent and cure night blindness and day blindness, because it restores visual purple to the eye.

2. Vitamin A supplementation is helpful with dry eye disease, in which the tear ducts dry up. It is also helpful to those whose eyes become "tired" quickly and those who experience red "rims" around their eyelids.

2. A severe deficiency can cause retinitis pigmentosa, a slow but eventual degeneration of the retina. This condition causes blindness in thousands of Americans each year and is usually preceded by years of night blindness and other symptoms of vitamin A deficiency.

2. This vitamin is essential to the normal structure and behavior of the tissues lining the mouth, nasal, sinus, and respiratory tract.

Vitamin B2 (Riboflavin)

2. This is a widespread deficiency in America. It may take a long time to correct.

2. Deficiency can cause sensitivity to light, so that you feel you must wear dark sunglasses. It can also cause faulty vision in dim illumination, burning or itching eyelids, and eyes that water easily and become bloodshot when they are strained.

2. Cracks in the corners of the mouth.

2. Deficiency is often marked by magenta or purplish tongue, and lips that tend to crack and become rough, often feeling chapped. Tiny flakes of skin may peel from lips, and whistle lines or wrinkles from the lips toward the nose may appear.

❧ The nose, chin, and forehead take on an oily appearance, and fatty deposits accumulate under the skin, when vitamin B2 is deficient.

❧ A severe deficiency can cause the skin at the corners of the eye to split, and the eyes burn and become fiery red.

❧ B2 is helpful in preventing cataracts and glaucoma.

Vitamin B3 (Niacin or Niacinamide)

❧ Deficiency is marked by a brilliant red, coated tongue; mouth, throat, and esophagus may become inflamed. It may be difficult for older people to eat.

❧ Canker sores may indicate a vitamin B3 deficiency.

❧ Mental disturbances may also be a sign of deficiency, especially schizophrenia.

Pantothenic Acid (Vitamin B5)

❧ Pantothenic acid has been found to be a factor in restoring gray hair to its normal color in experimental animals, although this finding has not as yet been confirmed in humans. Rats deficient in pantothenic acid had hair that turned coarse and gray prematurely, and they seemed to age faster.

❧ Helpful with dermatitis and eczema. It supports the adrenal glands.

❧ An enlarged, "beefy," furrowed tongue may signal a pantothenic acid deficiency.

Vitamin B6 (Pyridoxine)

❧ Most recognized deficiency is greasy, scaly dermatitis—even between eyebrows, sides of nose, around mouth, and behind the ears. The skin may be red and inflamed and scaly with dandruff.

❧ Babies get "cradle cap" and colic when their mothers are deficient in B6 during pregnancy.

❧ Slight B6 deficiency is dry skin with oily T-zone (forehead, nose, and chin).

    ♨ Outbreaks of acne just before menstrual period may also be a B_6 deficiency. In one experiment, 72 percent of women taking 50 mg of B_6 daily for one week before and during their periods had no more acne.

Vitamin B₁₂ (Cobalamin)

    ♨ A deficiency can result in pernicious anemia, which is characterized by extreme pallor (paleness), weakness, sore and inflamed tongue that may appear smooth and shiny, numbness and tingling in the extremities, weak pulse, stiffness, drowsiness, irritability, depression, and diarrhea, poor appetite, growth failure in children, and tingling sensation (a feeling of "pins and needles" in the hands and feet). Vitamin B_{12} injections may be necessary to clear up an extreme deficiency. Mental disturbances may also be a sign of a deficiency and include change in mood, mental slowness, and even severe psychotic symptoms.[29]

PABA (Para-Amino-Benzoic Acid)

    ♨ PABA has been shown to help the skin condition "vitiligo," in which the skin loses its pigment and turns white. This condition may also be linked to low adrenal and low thyroid function.

    ♨ Supplementation can help block the harmful effects of ultraviolet light that cause sunburn and skin cancer.

    ♨ PABA has helped reverse gray hair in rats. Deficiencies in pantothenic acid, biotin, and folic acid are also related to gray hair.

Folic Acid (Folacin or Folate)

    ♨ Folic acid restores gray hair to natural color.

    ♨ The deficiencies are much the same as for vitamin B12. An inflamed and sore tongue may occur.

Biotin

    ♨ Helps with hair growth.

    ♨ The first symptom of deficiency is usually scaly dermatitis.

2 A deficiency can result in an increased sensitivity of the skin, even burning or a prickling sensation. Pallor, or an extreme or unnatural paleness, may also occur.

Choline and Inositol

2 May help prevent thinning hair and baldness. It is also a lipotropic factor (a fat emulsifier), which helps fats to move normally, without getting deposited in the lining of the arteries. Its highest concentration is found in the heart and brain. Also used for weight loss. Soy lecithin granules are an excellent source of choline and inositol.

Vitamin C (Ascorbic Acid)

2 Deficiency marked by bruising (hemorrhaging under the skin). Older people are most susceptible because the medication they often take destroys vitamin C in their body.

2 Vitamin C forms collagen in the skin, which is the "cement" that supports and holds the tissues and organs together. It keeps the youthful skin tissues soft, firm, supple, and wrinkle-free. Collagen helps keep your skin from sagging.

Bioflavonoids

2 Help prevent bruising, which results from broken or damaged capillaries.

2 Bioflavonoids have been shown to relieve the painful throbbing and swelling of mild cases of varicose veins, and to help eliminate the small veins that can appear on the face.

Vitamin D

2 When ultraviolet rays from sunlight hit the skin, a form of cholesterol in the body is converted into vitamin D. Dark skinned people do not produce their own vitamin D as efficiently, since their dark pigment screens out much of the ultraviolet rays. If you are indoors for several months of the year, be sure to supplement with extra vitamin D.

Vitamin E

- Experiments with premature aging found that wrinkles could be prevented by giving large amounts of vitamin E.

- Pregnancy mask—the brown pigmentation that appears on the face of some pregnant women may be caused by a vitamin E deficiency, or may indicate low adrenal function. A woman with this condition may also need extra pantothenic acid.

- Liver spots or age spots—brown pigmentation on the back of the hands caused by oxidation of fats—are linked to a lack of vitamin E. It is essential that a person take all the antioxidants—beta-carotene, vitamin C, selenium—for healthy skin.

Mineral Deficiencies

These deficiency symptoms are mostly related to what you can visually see in the mirror.

Calcium

- In many cases, a calcium deficiency is responsible for dark circles under the eyes. Allergies may also cause this.

- Vertical ridges in the nails.

Iodine

- A deficiency may cause goiter, which is characterized by an enlarged thyroid gland that can cause bulging of the eyes plus other symptoms. If your eyes seem too large and protruding, read more about the thyroid gland in chapter 10.

Iron

- An iron deficiency results in nails being concave or spoonlike in shape—both fingernails and toenails. The nails may also lack their normal half-moon shape at the base of the nail.

- Vertical ridges in the nail may be a sign that anemia is present. This may also be a sign of a deficiency in zinc or calcium.

◊ Skin lesions such as pimples, boils, and the like are far more likely to occur in individuals low in iron.

Potassium

◊ A deficiency in young people may result in acne, while in adults a deficiency can cause dry skin.

Sulfur

◊ Sulfur is found in every cell of the body and is particularly necessary for beautiful hair, skin, and nails.

◊ Protein foods, such as egg yolks, are the richest food source of sulfur, including the supplement MSM.

Selenium

◊ The only symptom tied to a selenium deficiency is dandruff. This trace mineral is sometimes added to shampoos to treat seborrhea dermatitis (dandruff).

Silica or Silicon

◊ Has been found to help with hair, skin, and nails. It helps build connective tissues in the body.

Zinc

◊ White spots on the nails or nails with an opaquely white appearance can signal a zinc deficiency.

Other Considerations

Low Thyroid

◊ A low thyroid output can cause hair to become coarse, dry, and brittle. Hair loss can be quite severe.

◊ The nails become thin and brittle and typically show transverse grooves in those with low thyroid production.

◊ Edema (swelling) of eyelids and face may be an indication of low thyroid.

◊ Skin cold to the touch, especially hands and feet.[29]

What Should You Apply to Your Skin?

Your skin is the largest organ of your body. It breathes and releases toxins if necessary through perspiration. What most people don't realize is that *whatever you put on your skin absorbs into your bloodstream!* So read the labels and be aware of the chemicals in your make-ups, creams, and cleansers that you use daily.

Your nutrition store has a wide variety of natural skin and hair-care products, most of which do not have the high price tag of cosmetic counters. These natural cosmetics use the least toxic preservatives and substances to preserve their product.

Along with suggesting that a person eat a healthy diet and take vitamins, especially the antioxidants, the minerals, and fatty acids, most leading nutritionists frequently recommend certain skin-care products that have a long history of documented beneficial effects. Some of these substances have been used successfully for thousands of years.

Replenishing antioxidants directly on your skin is a wonderful way to keep your skin healthy and youthful. The antioxidants, especially vitamin A, vitamin E, and vitamin C, work together to boost the entire antioxidant network within the skin, providing wonderful protection against free radicals. Optimal skin care requires these antioxidants be taken orally and applied directly to the skin.

Vitamin E oil is a cellular healer

Vitamin E is a fantastic antioxidant and cellular healer that the skin can absorb. The pure oil is wonderful for treating scars, burns, and other skin rashes, as it both moisturizes and heals wounds. Dr. Evan Shute did this original research using vitamin E for scars and burns.

There are various potencies of vitamin E oil available, some with 5,000 IU per one-ounce container, others with as much as 32,000 IU—a very heavy and sticky consistency.

My Special Formula

Into a small cream pitcher, I pour 1 ounce of "Jason's Cosmetics" 32,000 IU vitamin E oil into four ounces of "Desert Essence," 100 percent pure cold-pressed Jojoba Oil. Then I squeeze 30 or more 10,000 IU vitamin A capsules into the mixture. I stir it up and pour it back into the original bottles. There are many brands in your nutrition store, but these are the ones I have been using.

In the evening I cleanse my face with this oil, using a warm, wet washcloth to wipe off the oil and my makeup. Then I spread this oil combination again over my entire face, neck, and arms. It will absorb quickly. If you use this again in the morning, your face will be soft and moist. Ladies, apply this mixture to your legs after you have shaved. My husband uses this instead of aftershave lotion. This is also a great massage oil.

Vitamins A and E: One of Mother's Beauty Secrets

Natural vitamin A from fish oil is the form I use with the mixture above. Vitamin A is a key vitamin related to skin health and is a potent free radical scavenger. I don't use cod liver oil as it smells too fishy.

Vitamins A and E were one of Mother's beauty secrets, although she freely told everyone about them. She always squeezed 10–20 vitamin A softgels (25,000 IU each—available at that time) into her night-time moisturizing cream, along with 10 to 20 softgels of vitamin E (400 IU) to really feed her skin. She knew the moisturizing cream helped her skin assimilate the oil vitamins. You will not believe how great your skin will look and feel!

Jojoba Oil: A Pure Natural Plant Extract

Jojoba oil is another fantastic oil for skin and hair, but it is only for external, topical use. This oil is a pure and natural plant extract that penetrates and moisturizes the skin without leaving an oily residue. It can be used to remove makeup and cleanse clogged pores, leaving the skin clean and blemish free. It is excellent for inflamed skin, psoriasis, eczema, acne, and as an aftershave moisturizer.

Use this luxurious oil to soften your hands and feet. Rub the oil into your skin after bathing. It is very similar to human sebum, which oils the hair and skin, and it helps your body retain body heat and prevent sweat evaporation.

Jojoba oil rarely goes rancid because of its natural antioxidant properties. The vitamins A and E can be added to this natural oil, as I discussed.

Every few weeks, use jojoba oil for moisturizing the scalp to prevent dandruff. It is also good for split ends. After the oil is massaged into your scalp and hair, wrap your hair in a scarf and go to sleep. In the morning when you wash your hair, you will find it vital again, with lots of body and shine.

Vitamin C Is Now Added to Lotions

Information has been in the news lately about vitamin C in various skin products, and how it helps with wrinkles and fine lines. Recent studies suggest that vitamin C applied externally to the skin may do what was once considered impossible—stimulate the growth of new collagen.

Vitamin C is essential for the production of new collagen. As we age, there is a decline in the amount of available vitamin C in the skin. When taken orally, most of the antioxidant supplements are used within the cells of the body and do not get delivered to skin cells.

Dr. Lester Packer in his book, *The Antioxidant Miracle*, reported several studies showing that high-potency vitamin C creams (with over ten percent concentration of vitamin C) can increase the level of this important vitamin in the skin. According to animal studies conducted at Duke University Medical Center, skin cells treated with vitamin C actually become thicker, which is a sign of collagen regeneration.[30]

Dr. Packer reported, "Applying vitamin C directly to the skin will help to restore skin tone, plump up wrinkles, and fill in small lines, giving skin a more youthful look. Topically applied vitamin C improves blood supply to the skin, giving the skin a more youthful glow. In addition, vitamin C serums can minimize fine lines, reduce light wrinkles, and improve skin color and tone."[31]

Vitamin C can effectively stimulate collagen and elastin tissue in the dermis layer, making it appear smoother and plumper. Therefore, the appearance of wrinkles and sagging is reduced. Vitamin C creams are particularly effective at hiding the light wrinkles around the eyes.[32] I use "Jason's Cosmetics" Hyper-C Serum.

Suggestions

After you wash your face, apply vitamin C serum directly on the clean surface. Do not apply any moisturizers underneath; they will interfere with the absorption of the vitamin C. The skin soaks in these nutrients and benefits from them both internally and externally! I use this several times a week.

Aloe vera has been used since Biblical times

Aloe vera is a plant that everyone should have in the home for skin emergencies. Aloe vera has remarkable healing abilities. It has properties for promoting the removal of dead skin and stimulating the normal growth of living cells. Its enzymes dissolve dead surface-layer cells, tighten pores, and have antibacterial qualities that fight infection. Aloe can also stop pain and reduce the chances of scarring while helping the healing process. It is valuable for minor cuts, itching, and first- and second-degree thermal burns.[33]

Interestingly, aloe has a composition similar to that of human blood plasma and seawater. Its pH is the same as human skin.[34]

To use fresh aloe, simply cut off part of an aloe vera leaf, split it open, and spread the gel over a burn, cut, scrape, or infection. Aloe can also be used as an aftershave lotion or moisturizer. There are many aloe vera products, from cosmetics to pure juice and gels, in your nutrition store.

Royal jelly softens skin and reduces wrinkles

A number of products on the market contain the ingredient royal jelly. In a paper titled *Royal Jelly in Dermatological Cosmetics*, Hans Weitgasser, M.D., a German dermatologist, has written, "Through local application as an ingredient in face masks, creams, and lotions, royal jelly has tremendous effects at the cellular level. With regular use, the skin becomes soft and wrinkles disappear."[35]

Royal jelly apparently works by stimulating the circulatory system, delivering more food and oxygen-laden blood to nourish the skin and remove waste from it, according to Elfried Kirschbaumer, M.D., also a German dermatologist. Ninety percent of his patients showed a tightening of sagging skin in the face, muscles, and breasts.[36]

Alpha hydroxy acids are a natural "peel"

Everyone who is interested in skin care has no doubt heard about the Alpha Hydroxy Acid (AHA) products that have flooded the market in recent years. They appear to work as "natural" chemical peels.

Strong chemical peels, which many dermatologists use, destroy the upper layer of skin cells and trigger new collagen production at a deeper level. The new collagen helps preserve the skin's elasticity and makes it look more youthful. Fruit acids work in a similar way, but they are more natural and gentler. There is also less irritation, and they do not result in extreme sun sensitivity, which often occurs with the use of standard chemical peels and certain skin drugs.

The fruit acids are a gentle, effective way to treat wrinkles and fine lines. Alpha hydroxy acids remove dead skin by loosening the intracellular cement between the old and new epidermal cells and dissolving the dead surface cells. This improves the skin's texture and causes discolored patches to slough off and disappear.

There are several kinds of AHA's available: glycolic acid from sugar cane; malic acid from apples; citric acid from oranges, lemons and limes; tartaric acid from wine grapes; and lactic acid from milk. Glycolic acid has the smallest molecules and is more effective at exfoliating (sloughing off dead cells to renew skin) while those made with lactic acid are more moisturizing.[37]

If you have sensitive or fair skin, take special care. AHAs may irritate your skin. Start with a product that has a lower percentage of AHAs (two to four percent), and work up to higher, more effective percentage levels.

Chamomile is more than tea

Chamomile is an anti-inflammatory herb that is finding increased application for topical treatments of skin disorders such as psoriasis and eczema. Chamomile's primary active component, levomenol, may help reduce lines and wrinkles caused by the sun and environmental factors. This key therapeutic component in chamomile promotes the skin's ability to heal itself.

Doctors at the Dermatological Clinic in Bonn-Venusberg, Germany, found that levomenol can inhibit the release of histamines, which are a major contributing factor in psoriasis, eczema and contact dermatitis.

According to Rob McCaleb, President of Herb Research Foundation in Boulder, Colorado, levomenol supports skin metabolism and contributes to the acceleration of cell and tissue regeneration, at the same time inhibiting inflammation. By stimulating the skin to repair itself, levomenol reestablishes "normal structure to damaged skin." CamoCare is a cosmetic company that uses levomenol in their CamoCare Gold line of fine cosmetics found at your nutrition store.

Tea tree oil (Oil of Melaleuca)

Tea tree oil is a topical oil known as "Oil of Melaleuca." This is an incredible germicide, bactericide, and fungicide that doesn't damage healthy skin. It cleans an affected area and lets the body heal itself. For centuries, the aborigines of Australia have used the leaves as poultices for infected wounds and skin problems.

Tea tree is effective in treating all sorts of skin conditions, including psoriasis, without irritating the skin. It also relieves a variety of skin conditions such as burns, acne, cuts, insect bites, stings, rashes, athlete's foot, sores, and can be used as a flea repellent, and as a product to combat nail fungus. Some medical journals recommend Oil of Melaleuca as a vaginal douche for yeast problems (candida albicans).[38]

This is one product everyone should have in their medicine cabinets. It is a totally safe and natural product, but again, only for external use.

Wild Yam Versus Natural Progesterone Cream

The Mexican yam (Dioscorea villosa) was first chronicled for its miraculous healing properties in 25 B.C. by the Chinese, who highly valued the herb. It has played a prominent role in folk medicine for several centuries, but it was not until 1936 that Japanese researchers extracted a chemical called diosgenin from the dioscorea yam and discovered that the extract was remarkably similar to some of the adrenal hormones in the human body, including progesterone.

Most evidence shows wild yam extract does not raise progesterone blood levels as originally thought. Women with menopausal symptoms who want to naturally balance their hormones must make sure that natural progesterone has been added to the wild yam cream. Dr. John Lee recommends 450 to 500 mg of USP progesterone per one ounce, topically. In both the Young Women's and Menopause chapters I discuss how and why you use the progesterone creams.

Special Suggestions

Avoid strong soaps

When you bathe, avoid using strong detergent soaps. These soaps strip away natural oils and moisture from your skin. Instead, try mild, unperfumed soaps. Excessive bathing or showering robs your body of natural moisturizing oils, as the water is usually very alkaline.

Oil baths: A great home remedy for people with itchy skin, eczema, or very dry, flaky skin

Put about six inches of warm water in your bathtub. Then add one to two cups of inexpensive white vinegar to help turn the alkaline water into a more neutral ph. Your skin has a slight acid mantel to it and city tap water is very alkaline.

To this, add three to four tablespoons of oil (almond, soy, safflower oil—the type of oil you normally would use in cooking). Stir it up in the water. Extra virgin olive oil is great but it smells too strong for my liking. Soak in this water for about ten minutes. This allows your skin to pull in the oil, much like a sponge. Blot your skin dry with a soft towel; you do not want to wipe off all the oil.

This is an excellent treatment for children who have eczema and itch all over. Just let them play in the water for a while.

You may want to apply a thin layer of my special formula of Jojoba oil mixed with vitamins A and E to your body before you go to bed. This will really feel great!

May you always be blessed with beautiful, healthy hair, skin, and nails!

Eyes—Our Windows to the World

Preventing Glaucoma, Cataracts and Other Eye Conditions

The health of the eye is largely dependent on a variety of nutrients, especially oxygen. The amount of blood that flows through the eye highlights the essential need of proper nutrition for optimal eye health and function.

—GLADYS LINDBERG

*S*ight is our richest sense, our link to the world and its wealth of imagery. It's always amazing to me when I study the eye to think of all the processes that must take place in order for us to be able to see. Each waking second the eyes send about a billion pieces of fresh information to the brain. The eye can sense about ten million gradations of light and seven million gradations of color. We see in such detail because the eye is almost an extension of our brain.[1]

The health of the eye is largely dependent on a variety of nutrients, the foremost of which is oxygen. When the normal functions that deliver nutrition and oxygen to the eye begin to fail, many disorders soon follow. Most of these disorders are associated with aging— cataracts, glaucoma, and macular degeneration. But are they truly linked to aging? They may not be!

Signs of Aging?

Although cataracts, glaucoma, and macular degeneration have been called "signs of aging" for years, these health problems may also be averted or lessened with proper diet and nutritional supplements. In both human and animal studies, antioxidants seem to offer the greatest protection against age-related degeneration of the eyes.

Cataracts

The lens of the eye is the only transparent organ in the body. A cataract is a loss of this transparency, which eventually interferes with vision. It never causes complete blindness, because even a densely opalescent lens will still transmit light. However, with increasing loss of transparency, the clarity and detail of the image is progressively lost. Even at a fairly advanced stage, a cataract may not be apparent to a casual observer. Cataracts usually occur in both eyes, but in most cases, one eye is more severely affected than the other.

Worldwide, some 50 million people are afflicted with cataracts, including about half of the worldwide population over the age of 75. At present, about 30 percent of all Americans age 75 and older have cataracts. In fact, almost everyone over the age of 65 has some degree of cataract, but usually to a minor degree and often confined to the edge of the lens where it does not interfere with vision. More than 1.2 million cataract surgeries are performed each year in America. The condition is so common that cataracts are almost considered "normal" in the elderly.[2]

CATARACT PATIENTS DEFICIENT IN VITAMIN C. Many investigators, beginning as early as 1935, have reported that cataract patients have very little vitamin C in the aqueous humor (the fluid held between the lens and the tissue at the front of the eye). According to the late Linus Pauling, Ph.D., in a normal person there is 25 times more vitamin C in the aqueous humor of the eye than in blood plasma.[3]

Supplementation with vitamin C has caused early cataracts to regress or even disappear. The vision of 60 to 90 percent of patients with early cataracts improved in one study, with some cases of improvement labeled "dramatic."[4]

Low vitamin C has actually been labeled by researchers as the cause, not the consequence, of cataract formation. What I want to know is why, after 60 years of research, this information hasn't been told to every senior citizen as part of their health care program? Now you know!

CATARACTS CAN REGRESS, REVERSE, OR DISAPPEAR. Dr. Morgan Raiforth, a pioneering ophthalmologist, showed in a series of published photos that arteriosclerotic damage in the retinal vessels could be reversed by using 1,200 IU of vitamin E and three to five grams (3,000 to 5,000 mg) of vitamin C. The vessels in the retina of the eye are readily visible through the dilated pupil since they are covered by only a single layer of cells. As a result, all the pathological changes—such as hemorrhages, exudates (oozing of fluid from vessels), scars, and other types of damage in the arteries, veins, and capillaries—can be seen and photographed. The changes with vitamin E and vitamin C therapy are visible and dramatic in his report.[5]

An extensive review of nutrition and eye disorders appeared in the February 1994 issue of the Journal of Nutritional Biochemistry. In one U.S. study, high blood levels of vitamin E and iron were linked to a reduced risk of developing cataracts. High levels of glycine and aspartic acid, two amino acids, also decreased cataract risk, according to researcher G. E. Bunce.[6]

In another large-scale study, researchers reported that volunteers who had high levels of vitamin E in their blood had only half the risk of developing nuclear cataracts, which involve the central part of the lens of the eye, compared to those with low levels of vitamin E in their plasma. Vitamin E also offered protection against cortical cataracts, which involve the periphery of the lens.[7]

Researchers have estimated that if a person is able to delay cataract formation by only ten years, they lower their need for an operation by 50 percent. Just think of the impact in savings on our national health-care cost![8]

VITAMINS E AND C ARE BOTH VALUABLE. Many other studies have concluded that vitamins C and E are important for the prevention of senile cataracts.[9] In one study, individuals who took only moderate amounts of vitamin E (400 IU) and vitamin C (500 mg) for five years were cataract free.[10]

Ophthalmologist Robert Azar used a combined nutritional plan to reverse cataracts in his clinic, which treats 25,000 patients annually. He places cataract patients on a low fat, complex carbohydrate diet that stresses fish, fowl, and fresh produce. Patients are supplemented with vitamin C, water-soluble vitamin E, and zinc for two months. If improvement is noted, surgery is delayed. He reports that many people on the program improve enough to make surgery unnecessary.[11]

Other nutrients that are important are vitamin A (from fish oil), the bioflavonoids (extract and pine bark extract—Pycnogenol), bilberry and the complete vitamin B-complex. Research indicates that the elderly should also consider taking a complete mineral complex that includes: selenium, zinc, calcium, magnesium, and manganese—all of which have been linked in the scientific research journals to eye health.

Glaucoma

Glaucoma is a painful affliction in which there is increased pressure within the eyeball, often resulting in blindness. Glaucoma sometimes has a hereditary cause, or it may result from an eye infection, injury, or emotional stress. It can often be controlled by medication. If you have glaucoma, I suggest you follow your physician's advice, as well as the nutritional plan for cataracts described above.

Dr. Cheraskin studied 60 glaucoma patients, ages 26 to 74, and found that when vitamin C intake was increased to 1,200 mg, the pressure on the eyes was decreased.[12] Other investigators have reported similar results.

Perhaps most striking was a report in which glaucoma patients were given very high doses of vitamin C (30 to 40 grams a day, which was .5 grams per kilogram of body weight) for a period of seven months. I am sure this was a buffered powder (neutral pH) so it would not upset the stomach. The pressure in the eye decreased to about one half! This high dosage controlled the glaucoma for some patients, while others had a decrease in the amount of medication they needed to control the condition.[13]

Macular Degeneration

While cataracts are thought by many to be the primary cause of vision loss in the elderly, a little-known eye condition called age-related macular degeneration actually ranks as the leading cause of irreversible blindness among older Americans. Macular degeneration is very common; 65 percent of all 65-year-olds have clinical evidence for this disease.

Researcher Lester Packer, Ph.D., in his book *The Antioxidant Miracle* reports, "The cause of macular degeneration is unknown, although it is suspected that free radical damage due to long-term exposure to visible light and UV radiation may be responsible. Several animal studies have shown that when deprived of antioxidants, many different species, including primates, our closest relatives in the animal kingdom, are likely to develop retinal degeneration. Studies also show that exposure to bright light also accelerates retinal degeneration in animals."[14]

Macular degeneration is a progressive but painless disorder that affects the central part of the retina, causing gradual loss of vision. The retina is responsible for central vision, which is required for writing, sewing, driving, and distinguishing color. It usually affects both eyes, either simultaneously or one shortly after the other.

Degeneration begins with partial breakdown of an insulating layer between the retina and the choroid (layer of blood vessels behind the retina). Fluid leakage occurs, and new blood vessels growing from the choroid destroy the retinal nerve tissue and replace it with scar tissue. The effect is roughly a circular area of blindness, increasing in size until it is large enough to obliterate two or three words at normal reading distance.

With early diagnosis, it sometimes is possible to seal off the leakage with laser surgery. The disorder is untreatable once it has resulted in blindness.[15] The condition, however, can be helped in both early and late stages to stop or slow the degeneration, and much can be done to help prevent it. All the nutritional supplements for cataracts and glaucoma are also important for macular degeneration, especially for the preventive stage and early diagnosis. Make sure you read the rest of this chapter for various nutrients you should include in your program.

Investigators feel that a zinc deficiency may play a role in preventing macular degeneration. Zinc affects parts of the eye in which zinc is known to have an important impact on the metabolic function of enzymes crucial in vision.

Dr. Packard said that recently, researchers have offered one ray of hope. *It appears that two carotenoids, lutein and zeaxanthin, may help to prevent this disease.* They are also found in capsules at your nutrition store. The richest natural sources of these two are dark green leafy vegetables like spinach, broccoli, collard greens and hot chilies. Food is one of the most effective ways to boost the antioxidant network and to maximize health and minimize illness.

Retinopathy

This is a disease or visual disorder of the retina, characterized by hemorrhages of the retinal blood vessels. It is usually associated with either hypertension or diabetes, and it is a major cause of blindness among diabetics.

Dr. Melvyn Werbach, M.D., explains that platelets are small disk-shaped particles in the blood that are the building blocks of blood clots. Diabetics' platelets are prone to clump together. This is believed to contribute to the tendency for diabetics to develop diseases of both small and large blood vessels. Supplementation with vitamin E has been shown to reduce this abnormal clumping tendency and to reduce elevated blood fats. Vitamin E may therefore help to prevent the development of such complications.[16]

Of course, all the antioxidants I have mentioned should be added to a diabetics program, especially alpha lipoic acid that is essential for the diabetic. Chromium and selenium would also be valuable in addition to the complete vitamin and mineral formula.

PHARMACEUTICAL DRUGS. Leonard Levine, Ph.D., reports certain prescription drugs can "impair the biological health of the visual system."[17] People who experience unexpected visual disturbances when they are taking medications can't determine for themselves whether the drugs are the cause. The best course is to consult your physician.[18] The *Physician's Desk Reference* lists 94 medications that can cause glaucoma, including steroids, antihypertensives, and antidepressants. Be sure to check the side effects of the medications you are taking if you are having problems with your eyes.

Nutritional Suggestions for Various Eye Conditions

Natural herbs and supplements can help to heal your eye conditions. The following have been researched and used to help improve various conditions.

Bilberry

Interest in bilberry (Vaccinium myrtillus) was first aroused when the British Royal Air Force pilots reported improved night vision on bombing raids during World War II after they were given bilberries and bilberry jam. Subsequent studies showed that giving bilberry extract to healthy subjects resulted in improved nighttime visual acuity, especially after exposure to glare. "It helped against fatigue, reduced eye irritation, nearsightedness and nightblindness, extended the range and sharpness of vision, aided in the adaptation to darkness by accelerating regeneration of the retina and helped to restrain the development of conditions such as glaucoma and cataracts."[19]

Ginkgo Biloba

Ginkgo biloba extract has antioxidant activity, improves arterial blood flow and enhances cellular metabolism. It is known for its anti-aging properties and has been used in some cultures for centuries to help prevent degenerative changes in the eye. Ginkgo improves blood circulation in the eye and related eye structures such as the retina that helps prevent macular degeneration.[20]

BILBERRY AND GINKGO. Clinical studies in humans have demonstrated that bilberry extract (25 percent anthocyanidins), ginkgo biloba extract (24 percent ginkgo flavone glycosides), and zinc sulfate are capable of halting progressive vision loss. Bilberry and ginkgo are potent in their antioxidant and free radical scavenging activity and appear to have some degree of specificity for the eye.[21]

Importance of Carotenoids

A study reports that a higher intake of carotenoids was associated with a lower risk for macular degeneration. Writing in the *Journal of the American Medical Association*, Johanna M. Seddon, M.D., evaluated 356 cases of advanced stage macular degeneration for one year, with ages from 55 to 80 years against 520 control subjects. After adjusting for variables, she found that the highest intake of carotenoids, for example beta-carotene, was associated with 43 percent lower risk of macular degeneration compared to the lowest one fifth. "A regular intake of spinach and collard greens was especially protective," she said.[22]

LUTEIN AND ZEAXANTHIN. Two particular compounds contained in green leafy vegetables—lutein and zeaxanthin—are carotenoids. They are also members of the family of red and yellow pigments that include beta-carotene. Scientists speculate that by accumulating in the retina and filtering out certain types of light rays that may cause damage, these compounds may leave both the retina and the macula less vulnerable to degeneration.[23] Many eye care products contain these two carotenoids.

Flavonoids from grapeseed and pine bark

A group of compounds found in plants, like grape seeds and pine bark (pycnogenols), contain flavonoids that have antioxidant and anti-inflammatory effects for the eye. They are also found in high concentrations in blueberries, grapes, and other dark berries. These flavonoids improve night vision and adaptation to the dark. They help regenerate collagen and shield it from free radical attack.[24] They help strengthen and restore permeability of capillaries to allow more oxygen, nutrients, enzymes, and hormones to pass through cell membranes to replenish all the trillions of cells in the body.[25] This promotes smoothness and elasticity of the skin, improving circulation in the eyes and limbs. They also increase memory capacity since these compounds pass the blood-brain barrier.[26] They also improve visual acuity and improve capillary integrity to reduce hemorrhage in diabetic retinopathy.[27]

All the antioxidants

The Journal of Nutritional Biochemistry has also reported that antioxidants, such as vitamins E, C, and the carotenoids, can directly intercept and reduce the free radicals that damage the eyes.

G. E. Bunce, Ph.D., of the Virginia Polytechnic Institute in Blacksburg, has suggested that these substances are able to diminish, but not necessarily prevent, oxidant and photochemical damage to the lens and retina. He also recommends vitamin E, vitamin C and beta-carotene as supplements to reduce the oxidant burden. He also adds that the oxycarotenoids (lutein and zeaxanthin) are important antioxidants and serve as light-absorbing pigments in the retina.[28]

Wolfgang Schalch in *Free-Radicals in Aging* explains that of the approximately 600 naturally occurring carotenoids, lutein and zeaxanthin are crucial constituents of the macula lutea (the yellow spot in the macula). Researchers believe they may prevent damage to the eye by filtering out visible blue light.

Most of the researchers are in agreement that if you are concerned about eye health, you need to have a high daily intake of all the antioxidants to prevent free radical damage. This includes vitamins A, E, C, alpha lipoic acid, B-complex, plus the minerals zinc, selenium and lutein and zeaxanthin. Prevention is the best solution!

Addition of selenium and increased vitamin C

Wolfgang Schalch recommends a similar vitamin program like Dr. Bunce's but adds the additional antioxidant selenium in a dose of 250 mcg a day, and increases the vitamin C dose to 500 mg a day. In one study of 102 patients having acute macular degeneration for seven to 12 years, some 60 percent of those patients treated with this program reported improved or halted degenerative macular changes.[29] I personally feel if the study was conducted with a higher potency of C, would the results be even more impressive? If I had these deficiency problems I would really increase my intake of vitamins C and vitamin E. I feel Schalch's recommended doses are considered average. More is required when you are trying to overcome these deficiency conditions.

Several of the new products especially formulated for the eyes contain a variety of antioxidant vitamins, minerals and lutein. These special "eye" formulas are available in nutrition stores.

Vitamin B₂ (Riboflavin)

This vitamin is one of the most widespread deficiencies in America. It can make the eye highly sensitive to light, so that a person must wear dark sunglasses much of the time. A deficiency is also marked by faulty vision in dim light; eyelids that burn and itch; eyes that water easily and become bloodshot if strained; and a feeling of sand or grit inside the eyelid, resulting in a person constantly rubbing or wiping his or her eyes.

A person who has an increased twitching of the eyelids may have a B₂ deficiency (as well as a magnesium and B₆ deficiency). A severe deficiency is often manifested by the skin at the corners of the eye splitting and the eyes burning and becoming fiery red.[30]

Vitamin B₂ helps with the prevention of both cataracts and glaucoma, according to numerous research reports. It is a necessary cofactor for the antioxidant enzyme, glutathione reductase. A deficiency in animals leads to cataracts.

Vitamin B₆ (Pyridoxine)

If you wear contact lenses and have a problem with "dry eye disease," take note. A number of cases in Canada reported that daily supplementation with 500 mg of vitamin B6 increased tearing sufficiently to allow the wearing of contact lenses. Other supplements needed were niacinamide, vitamin C, zinc, and magnesium.[31]

Vitamin A

Vitamin A deficiency has been linked to night blindness, a quick tiring of the eyes, sensitivity to bright lights and glare, less accurate day vision, dry eye disease (the tear duct dries up), red rims around the eyelids, and mucous on the eyes at night (sometimes to the point where the eye and eyelids feel stuck together in the morning).[32]

A severe deficiency results in retinitis pigmentosa, a slow but eventual degeneration of the retina. This causes blindness in thousands of Americans each year. It is usually preceded by years of night blindness and other vitamin A deficiencies. Those with diabetes or hypothyroidism may have trouble converting beta-carotene into vitamin A, so they should take the retinol form of vitamin A found in fish oil.

The *Medical Tribune*, August 22, 1991, reported that lack of just this one vitamin leads to blindness in India and says that vitamin A deficiency affects ten to 40 million children worldwide, about half of whom live in India. In addition to blindness, such children are more likely to have respiratory or gastrointestinal problems.

Zinc

Investigators feel that a zinc deficiency may play a role in preventing macular degeneration. Zinc affects parts of the eye in which zinc is known to have an important impact on the metabolic function of enzymes crucial in vision. A double-blind, placebo-controlled trial was set up to explore this possibility. In a 12- to 24-month follow-up, they found that patients given zinc supplements had significantly less visual loss than the group that received placebos. The zinc was given in 100 mg tablet form, twice a day with meals. The side effects were minimal.[33] Just a note: some researchers feel that 100 mg of zinc should be as high as you should go.

The *Tufts University Diet & Nutrition Letter* reports that it now appears as though simply eating a diet rich in spinach, collards, kale, and other dark greens may help stave off macular degeneration. The connection, judging by new research, seems to be that certain substances in leafy vegetables and other produce are found in the portion of the eye subject to damage from age-related macular degeneration. Let's eat our vegetables and take zinc.

The essential amino acids

PROTEIN. As cells deteriorate, people age. As cells malfunction, people get sick. When you have cells that are missing the essential amino acids, the body will "cement" you together with scar tissue. When that scar tissue appears in your eyes, you have cataracts. Protein is what every living cell of your body is made of. So, get enough protein![34] I discuss the value of protein in more detail in chapter 5.

L-GLUTATHIONE. The main function of L-glutathione is to break down and dispose of potentially dangerous toxins that invade the body. L-glutathione is an antioxidant that protects every cell, tissue, and organ in the body. In addition to rejuvenating old and weak immune systems, it may also help prevent macular degeneration.

TAURINE. Taurine is a sulfur-containing amino acid, which may protect cells from the harmful effects of ultraviolet light. Some taurine is made in the body from methionine and cysteine, but eventually these sources may prove inadequate and retinal degeneration is one of the consequences. Very large quantities of taurine are found in the retina of the eye of many mammals. Taurine is present in meats and animal products but not in plant products.[35] Taurine may also be purchased as a single tablet or capsule from your nutrition store.

Exercise for the eye

Eye exercises are important for visual health. Dr. W. H. Bates developed "The Bates Method," which is a set of eye exercises to reduce eye stress and correct eye and vision related disorders. He said, "Perfect sight is a product of perfectly relaxed organs, unconsciously controlled," and that "vision improves naturally when people stop interfering with it. Under relaxed conditions, refractive errors tend to be self-correcting." Check into this method for some exercise and you may want to read his classic book, *Better Eyesight Without Glasses*.[36]

Anti-Aging Nutrients for Our Brain

What We Can Do to Enhance Thinking, Elevate Mood, Boost Memory and Prevent Alzheimer's Disease

The health of our brain and body go hand in hand. One cannot proceed without the other. Like the other organs of our body, the brain requires fuel, special nutrients, and even exercise to keep it functioning properly.
—GLADYS LINDBERG

$\mathscr{S}$cientists have been trying to unravel the complexities of the brain for centuries, but they still do not fully understand the mysteries of our body's most complex organ. Since we are all unique, I doubt that researchers will ever learn all the answers.

Still, there is now evidence that age-related changes in the brain physiology are influenced by the biochemical environment of the brain. There are numerous compounds in common foods and natural substances that can have a favorable impact on that biochemical environment. I hope to bring you some of the scientific research on these nutrients and natural products in relation to brain function.

Of all the organs in the body, the brain may be the most sensitive. In addition to the healthful benefits of thinking, learning, and reasoning, the brain is subject to many life-threatening disorders such as stroke, meningitis (an inflammation of the membranes covering the brain), senile dementia, Alzheimer's disease, and others.

Basic Brain Function

Weighing less than three pounds, the brain is one of the busiest, most metabolically active organs in the body. Although it represents less than two percent of the body's total weight, the brain is involved in 15 percent of the body's total blood flow, 25 percent of its oxygen utilization, and at least 70 percent of its glucose (sugar) consumption.[1]

Unlike other organs, the brain—which is composed of a compact network of more than ten billion nerve cells—is not capable of storing its own supply of energy. It depends, rather, on a constant flow of blood to keep it supplied with nutrients. While other organs in the body can metabolize fat and protein for energy, the brain must depend primarily on glucose from the blood for energy. Without the proper nutrients, proteins used by nerve cells in the brain cannot be manufactured, which can lead to impairment of mental functions such as memory. Finally, unlike other tissues in the body that can heal after an injury, brain cells are incapable of regenerating themselves.[2] This makes the brain especially vulnerable to illness and injury. In sum, the brain is highly dependent upon the nutrients carried to it in the bloodstream. It must have a continual supply of glucose, oxygen, and other essential nutrients.

Blood-brain barrier

Since the brain depends primarily on glucose for most of its metabolic activities, it has a special apparatus to pump glucose from the blood into the brain cells across a special blood-brain barrier. This barrier also prevents most large molecules and toxins in the blood from migrating into brain tissue, keeping many potentially damaging substances out of the brain. The barrier allows small molecules—such as oxygen, glutamine, anesthetics, alcohol, and certain toxins—to cross the barrier easily. This protective mechanism, of course, can be compromised by disease, such as infection.[3]

The quality of nutrients fed to each of these areas of the brain directly impacts a person's ability to think and remember, as well as the person's mood.

Both Physical and Emotional Involvement

Age-related decline in brain function is extremely common and sometimes is a serious problem. The condition is often referred to as senile dementia, mental deterioration, memory impairment, and cognitive decline.

Elderly individuals often are taking a wide variety of prescription and over-the-counter medications, which can adversely affect mental function. These medications can also cause mood swings and depression.

People come to me with many types of nutritional problems, and some are related to emotional ones. When a person is physically stronger and in better health, he or she very often is better equipped to cope with emotional problems or to face the difficult circumstances of their lives.

Loss of cognitive capacities

Cognition is our ability to think, reason, recognize, remember, and perceive. The progressive loss of mental agility with age has become a major focus of clinical research efforts. Beginning around midlife, the brain's higher functions of memory, learning, and concentration begin to fade. According to Parris Kidd, Ph.D., "Over the adult life span, individuals who are otherwise healthy can lose as much as half (50 percent) of their cognitive capacities, as measured from tests related to everyday tasks that rely on cognitive skills. Such progressive and insidious loss of the brain's higher functions can have a telling effect on personal productivity, can damage self-esteem, and bring considerable distress to many aging adults."[4]

Aging is stress

Aging itself is a form of stress, which we will all inevitably encounter. Stress increases our need for many nutrients, and when these needs are not met, deficiencies develop. These deficiencies, in effect, rob the brain of vitamins and minerals necessary to help brain enzymes produce enough brain chemicals to keep a person functioning at a normal level. A downward spiral can result. The greater the impact of stress, the greater the deficiency and the lower the brain function.

Positive mental attitude

I want to mention here the importance of a strong will and mental attitude of "I am going to make it," or "I am going to get well," or "Thank you, Lord, for my healing." Researchers have finally proven there is a link between the immune system and the brain.

Of course, the Bible refers to this several times. The Book of Proverbs says, "For as he thinketh in his heart, so is he" (Prov. 23:7). There is another scripture that says, "Finally, brethren, whatsoever things are true, whatsoever things are honest, whatsoever things are just…pure…lovely, are of good report; if there be any virtue, and if there be any praise, think on these things" (Phil. 4:8).

We also need to program our mind and see ourselves living a healthy, active life, free of disease, into a ripe old age. This is anti-aging at its best!

Hypoglycemia: Major Emotional Symptoms

Mood swings may be directly associated with an inadequate diet. Some of the major symptoms of hypoglycemia or low blood sugar are irritability, depression, constant worrying, unprovoked anxieties, insomnia, antisocial behavior, crying spells, lack of concentration, phobias (fears), mental confusion, and even suicidal intent. If you are experiencing depression, anxiety, panic attacks, and other emotional problems, eliminate the possibility that your problem may be the result of low blood sugar. We need to eat small feedings often, and eliminate sugar and refined carbohydrates from the diet. Include a vitamin and mineral formula to your own health-building program. Read more on hypoglycemia and a complete nutrition program in the *Let's Put It All Together* chapter.

Ruling out food factors

Foods have been known to induce depression through a variety of mechanisms, including cerebral allergy, food addiction, hypersensitivity to chemical food additives, reactions to molds, and so forth. Sugar, refined and processed foods, and alcohol have also been related to mood swings. Watch a child have an allergic response to a chocolate dessert and you will see their personality change before your eyes. Allergic disorders are common among those who are depressed.

Depression may also be associated with levels of caffeine consumption greater than four cups of coffee a day. Eliminating caffeine and sugar has been shown to lift depression within a week![5]

Vitamin and mineral deficiencies and depression

A number of vitamin deficiencies have been linked to depression, especially deficiencies in biotin, folic acid, pyridoxine (B6), riboflavin (B2), thiamin (B1), vitamin B12, and vitamin C. Folic acid, in particular, has been associated with depression. The worse the depression, the lower the level of folic acid in the blood, a fact that is often a consequence of poor diet or the use of alcohol and drugs.[6]

Mineral deficiencies of calcium, iron, magnesium, and potassium have been associated with depression. Excess or toxic amounts of vanadium have also been linked to it.

Be sure to check thyroid function

A person who is suffering from depression should also check his or her thyroid function. If you have a history of cold hands and feet, weight gain, and generalized fatigue, thyroid malfunction may be the root cause of your depression. The work of Dr. Broda Barnes has documented this connection. Read more about the thyroid in chapter 10, and take the temperature test since the blood test is not accurate.

Physical exercise helps in depression

We all feel better after taking a brisk walk or engaging in vigorous activity. Exercise increases dopamine levels in the brain and also the level of endorphins. We now know that endorphins create a sense of well-being and even relieve pain.

Physical activity tends to decrease anxiety, hostility, and other stress-related disorders. Aerobic exercises, slow jogging, stationary bike riding, or any physical exercise undertaken for at least 30 minutes to an hour is excellent. Ideally, such exercise should be part of a fitness program for everyone at least four times a week. Many authorities feel one of the main causes of depression in the elderly may be a lack of physical exercise.

Understanding Neurotransmitters

Communication within the brain, and between the brain and the rest of the nervous system, occurs through many different chemicals and electrical impulses. We think of nerve impulses throughout the body as being electrical, but the transmission of these impulses from one neuron to the next is achieved both chemically and electrically. Different parts of the brain contain different concentrations of these brain chemicals, and when these balances are disrupted, a variety of neurologic and psychiatric diseases may occur. The majority of these chemicals, known as neurotransmitters, are made up of amino acids.[7] Eight essential amino acids are found together in adequate amounts in all animal products such as cheese, milk, chicken, beef, and certain vegetable proteins such as soy.

While some neurotransmitters have an excitatory effect on the nervous system, others such as serotonin produce an inhibitory effect that soothes, calms and produces feelings of contentment.

Serotonin deficiency

The newest antidepressant medications attempt to change the serotonin balance in the brain to elevate a person's mood, but they have many side effects. Researchers at the Massachusetts Institute of Technology discovered that the serotonin concentration in the brain is directly proportional to the concentration of brain and plasma tryptophan. This was the first accepted demonstration of the direct dietary control of a brain neurotransmitter by tryptophan, a single amino acid.[8]

Serotonin has been implicated in depression, uncontrollable appetite, obsessive-compulsive disorder, autism, bulimia, social phobias, premenstrual syndrome, anxiety and panic attacks, migraines, schizophrenia and extreme violence.[9]

Serotonin's inhibitory action in the brain prevents excess nervous stimulation at night, so sleep can occur. Serotonin is thought to be an inducer and regulator of sleep. It also controls states of consciousness, mood, and may reduce sensitivity to pain and have tranquilizing effects.[10]

Serotonin is also a growth hormone releaser. Growth hormone is crucial for growth and repair as well as stimulation of the immune system. It normally reaches peak levels during sleep, but these peaks are frequently even smaller or absent in elderly and obese people.[11] Read more about the growth hormones in the *Men's* chapter (Chapter 13).

Natural Products to Help
with Depression and Anxiety

Anxiety can be the result of either physical or psychological factors. For example, extreme stress can definitely trigger anxiety and so can certain stimulants like caffeine. According to Melvyn Werbach, M.D., there are at least six nutritional factors that may be responsible for triggering anxiety. He said we need to avoid alcohol, caffeine, and sugar, which can go a long way in relieving symptoms. Anxiety may even be caused by food allergies. It may also be caused by a deficiency of the B vitamins, niacin (B3), pyridoxine (B6), thiamin (B1), calcium or magnesium.[12]

Be sure to check your diet and the vitamins and minerals you are taking. To help you with stress and anxiety, consider the following.

Tryptophan and anti-anxiety 5-HTP

Tryptophan is an essential amino acid, which means that we are unable to make it within our bodies and therefore must depend upon our food supply to obtain it. Directly linked with the neurotransmitter serotonin, it was a very popular sleep aid in the '80s. In 1989, the FDA pulled the supplement form from the market because one batch from Japan was tainted. Tryptophan is now available only by prescription.

Tryptophan is not an easy amino acid to get from your diet, but good sources are milk and turkey. It is also found in soy protein and small amounts in brown rice, peanuts, pumpkin, lentils, and sesame seeds. Tryptophan is regarded by some as nature's weapon against depression and insomnia. A warm glass of milk before bed to help you sleep may not be just an old wive's tale, but may be an effect of tryptophan!

5-HTP. A modified form of tryptophan now available is called 5-HTP (5-hydroxytryptophan). It is derived naturally from seed pods (*Griffonia simplicifolia*). 5-HTP is the direct precursor for making serotonin in your brain. It works by increasing the cell's production of serotonin, which boosts serotonin levels. 5-HTP also raises levels of the neurotransmitters noradrenaline and dopamine, providing a tonic-like effect and a refreshing, restorative feeling. Thus, 5-HTP delivers a multiplicity of neurotransmitter bonuses without the risk or side effects associated with drugs. Increasing our serotonin levels can be important for our emotional health.[13]

In one study, researchers administered from 50 to 300 milligrams of 5-HTP to 107 patients with depression and found that 78 patients *take 5 H·TP*

(69 percent) were either cured or showed marked improvement.[14]

Weight loss. An Italian study on weight loss showed taking 5-HTP can also help suppress appetite. Those taking the supplement reduced their carbohydrate intake and felt satisfied sooner than the placebo group.[15] What a bonus! As we begin to feel calmer, we can also keep our weight and appetite under control.

5-HTP is safe. Published data indicates that 5-HTP is safe and produces relatively few adverse side effects.[16] It may be taken between meals or best if taken an hour before bed for a good night's sleep. Follow label instructions. It is available in your nutrition store.

St. John's wort: Nature's own version of prozac

St. John's wort, known scientifically as *Hypericum perforatum*, is the rising star in herbal medicine. It is a common wildflower with bright yellow flowers edged with tiny black beads. When the black beads are rubbed, the plant releases a red pigment that contains the hypericin, which is the active chemical. The name comes from the red spots of the plant and is said to symbolize the blood spilled by St. John the Baptist when he was beheaded. The plant blooms on the traditional birthday of John the Baptist. The term *wort* is an Old English word for plant.

It is most appropriate for the treatment of mild to moderately severe depression. At this time, there are not enough studies for severely depressed patients.

German physicians write about three million prescriptions a year for St. John's wort, based on the government's approval of the results of stringent clinical tests. It is the drug of choice for common depression. It outsells all other antidepressants combined and outsells Prozac by more than seven to one. These German doctors are knowledgeable about both medicines but clearly favor St. John's wort extracts standardized for 0.3 percent hypericin content. It produces equal or better results in relieving depression but, unlike prescription drugs, is relatively free of unwanted side effects.[17]

Studies from Germany and Austria show that about 60 to 80 percent of depressed individuals improve on St. John's wort. In a recent German survey of 3,250 depressed patients and their physicians, 80 percent reported an improvement or absence of symptoms after taking St. John's wort for four weeks.[18]

Many studies prove that St. John's wort is effective. In one study of 105 patients with depression, the researchers at the University of

Salzburg found that St. John's wort was 250 percent better than a placebo. Sixty-seven percent of the subjects taking 900 milligrams of St. John's wort daily improved dramatically within four weeks compared with 28 percent on the placebo. Jean Carper reports on St. John's wort, "This botanical antidepressant improved mood, emotional fear, and psychosomatic symptoms, such as disturbed sleep, headache, cardiac troubles, and exhaustion."[19]

St. John's wort sounds like a great natural product for those who are depressed. I would also suggest you begin a daily vitamin and mineral supplement program in adequate amounts, that you read the symptoms of hypoglycemia in the *Let's Put it All Together* chapter, follow the directions of small feedings often, and, of course, start exercising. Remember there is no "magic bullet." We need to follow a complete nutritional program, and this herb can be a great addition to the entire program.

RECOMMENDED DOSAGE. The adult dose for mild to moderate depression is one 300 milligram capsule of St. John's wort extract, standardized to contain 0.3 percent of hypericin, taken two to three times a day (600 to 900 milligrams) with meals. Maximum benefits are typically seen after six to eight weeks of continued use. Make sure you take the suggested dose as lower amounts may not be effective.

SAFETY FACTOR. Do not take St. John's wort if you are pregnant or lactating, and do not give it to children except on a physician's advice. Do not take in combination with prescription antidepressants except under medical supervision. For a more in-depth study, read *Hypericum & Depression* by Harold H. Bloomfield, M.D., a psychiatrist in Del Mar, California.

SAMe: A new treatment for depression

There is a new, naturally occurring substance called SAMe (pronounced "Sammy") and known formally as S-adenosylmethionine, and it is not an herb or a hormone. It is a molecule produced in each of our cells from the amino acid methionine and ATP (an energy storing molecule). Through some biochemical reactions in the cell, SAMe helps to maintain healthy cell membranes and make neurotransmitters work better.

Since the '70s, researchers have published 40 clinical European trials involving thousands of patients and SAMe has performed as well as traditional treatments for major depression, and is very effective for arthritis. The best news is that SAMe does not seem to cause adverse effects, even at high doses. Many are also using SAMe for their arthritis symptoms, which has been very effective.

In this country our Food and Drug Administration has not approved or disapproved of SAMe as it is considered a naturally occurring substance and cannot be patented as a drug. This does not mean it is untested. Doctors have prescribed it successfully for two decades in the 14 countries where it has been approved as a drug.

The herb St. John's wort has been used for mild depression, but SAMe has been tested against disorders that are far more serious. In one of several U.S. studies, researchers at the University of California, Irvine, gave 1,600 mg of SAMe daily to 17 severely depressed patients. It was a four-week course of either SAMe or desipramine, a well-established antidepressant. The SAMe recipients enjoyed a slightly higher response rate (62 percent) than the folks on desipramine (50 percent).[20]

A *Newsweek* article in July 1999 reported: "No one has found SAMe significantly more effective than a prescription antidepressant, but it is clearly less toxic. The drugs that predate Prozac (tricyclics and MAO inhibitors) can be deadly in overdose, or in combination with other medications. Newer antidepressants such as Prozac, Zoloft and Paxil are less dangerous, but their known side effects range from headaches and diarrhea to agitation, sleeplessness and sexual dysfunction. And SAMe studies suggest that, like other antidepressants, it may trigger manic episodes in people with bipolar disorder. Aside from that, the most serious side effect is a mild upset stomach."

Columbia University psychiatrist Richard Brown warns that severely depressed patients should not drop other treatments to try SAMe, as they may end up suicidal. However, Brown himself has treated several hundred patients with SAMe in recent years, sometimes combining it with other drugs, and he has never had a bad experience. "It's the best anti-depressant I've ever prescribed," he says flatly. "I've seen only benefits."[21] SAMe is also available at your nutrition store.

The omega-3 fatty acids and fish oil

It is amazing to know that your brain is 60 percent fat. It is made up of lipids, which are various types of fat-like substances. The fat you eat throughout life is constantly molding your brain. It is an exciting but sobering thought, considering the low-quality fat most of us feed our brain cells.

Jean Carper, in her wonderful book *Your Miracle Brain,* discusses brain-boosting fats:

- DHA: The top-gun omega-3 type brain fat. You get it from eating seafood, or taking supplements.

- EPA: The other high-potency omega-3 brain fat comes from eating fish or taking fish oil.

- Linolenic acid: The short-chain omega-3s that your body must transform to long-chain omega-3s to be beneficial to your brain. You get it in green leafy vegetables, nuts and flaxseed.

- Monounsaturated fat, as in olive oil: Contains some antioxidants, does not increase vascular threats, and has been found to benefit memory.

Failure to eat enough omega-3 fat is scientifically linked to an array of modern mental disorders and problems: depression, poor memory, low intelligence, learning disabilities, dyslexia, attention deficit disorder, schizophrenia, "senility," Alzheimer's disease, degenerative neurological diseases, multiple sclerosis, alcoholism, poor vision, irritability, hostility, inattention, lack of concentration, aggression, violence, suicide, according to Jean Carper.[22]

Depressed patients tend to have less omega-3 type fish fat in their blood cells. The blood level of omega-3 predicts the severity of depression. The lower the omega-3 levels, the more severe the depression.

Organic, unrefined flaxseed oil is one of the valuable keys to restoring the proper level of essential fatty acids. Flaxseed oil is unique because it contains both essential fatty acids—linolenic (omega-3) in high amounts and linoleic (omega-6). Flaxseed oil is the richest source of the omega-3 fatty acids, a whopping 58 percent by weight, more than twice the amount of omega-3 fatty acids found in fish oils.[23]

Dr. Andrew Stoll, a psychopharmacologist and assistant professor of psychiatry at the Harvard Medical School, found that doses of fish oil did indeed relieve bipolar (manic) depression in a group of patients. Dr. Stoll gave about ten grams of fish oil a day (14 large capsules) a combination of EPA and DHA. The results were so startling that Dr. Stoll stopped the study prematurely after only four months instead of the planned nine months. He found that 65 percent of the bipolar patients got better on fish oil compared to only 18 percent with the placebo.

One patient mistakenly picked up flaxseed oil instead of fish oil at a nutrition store. She took it for several weeks and felt so much better that Dr. Stoll now gives flaxseed oil to some patients. He isn't sure why, but he says that flaxseed oil also appears to work as an antidepressant and mood stabilizer.[22]

I recommend that we take at least one tablespoon of flaxseed oil a day. One tablespoon of flaxseed oil equals about 10 large capsules. It is easy to add this oil to your morning protein shake that I discuss in the *Let's Put It All Together* chapter. Flaxseed oil can also be used as a salad dressing. Because of their high level of omega-3 fats, and their wonderful effect on the brain, I also suggest you increase your intake of fish, particularly beneficial are the cold water fish such as salmon, mackerel, herring, and halibut.

A valuable amino acid: Tyrosine

The amino acids tyrosine and DL-phenylalanine are precursors of the catecholamines, which are adrenaline-like neurotransmitters. Norepinephrine and epinephrine are the neurotransmitters that are released in the "fight or flight" response. When confronted with a stress, these chemicals increase your heart rate, blood pressure, and level of arousal.

Tyrosine is a precursor to another important neurotransmitter called dopamine, which is vital for normal muscle tone. Abnormalities in dopamine concentration in parts of the brain lead to Parkinson's disease. Tyrosine is also essential for normal thyroid hormone production.

Tyrosine has been determined to be a safe and lasting therapy for depression, mood, hypertension, Parkinson's disease, low sex drive, appetite suppression, and therapy for cocaine addicts. It is also felt to be useful for those of us living high-stress lives.[24] Very little tyrosine is found in cereals, vegetables, fruit, or oils. The best dietary sources are meat, wheat germ, soy, and other animal proteins. Tyrosine can be purchased as a separate amino acid as L-tyrosine, "L" meaning the natural form.

Essential Nutrients for Healthy Brain Function

Scientific evidence is currently stimulating a resurgence of interest in the link between nutrition and cognition. Interest is focused on what is called "subclinical" malnutrition—which is a nutritional deficiency that is relatively mild. These subclinical deficiencies manifest themselves with very subtle symptoms, generally ones related to brain functions such as intelligence and memory.

Numerous studies have confirmed that a selective vitamin deficiency can cause mental problems at any age. Dr. Carl Pfeiffer was just one of several who studied the aged and found that when people of the same age are compared, those with senility are more likely to be deficient nutritionally. Malnutrition is one cause of reversible senility, as long as the senility has not progressed too far.

The vital vitamin B-complex and our brain

We know the B-complex vitamins are essential for all aspects of the nervous system, including brain function. The B vitamins need to be taken together in adequate amounts throughout one's life.

In a study of 228 individuals between 73 and 102 years of age, 30 percent had low blood levels of one or more B vitamins. These deficiencies occurred even though food intake was adequate and all were taking a daily vitamin supplement. This study suggests that absorption of B vitamins is impaired in a large portion of the geriatric population.[25] All of the B Vitamins help with brain function:[26]

- **Thiamin (B₁)**—the brain and nerves are the first areas of the body to show signs of a deficiency. It helps convert glucose into energy. It also mimics acetylcholine (a neurotransmitter involved in memory) and plays a role in brain functions related to memory and cognition. Symptoms may include mental confusion, subjectively poor memory, difficulty in concentration, and even mental illness. One study shows that a high dose of B₁ supplementation (3,000 mg to 8,000 mg a day) may actually decrease the deleterious effects of senility.[27] This high dose may throw off your B vitamin balance, so be careful.

- **Riboflavin (B₂)**—helps with cognitive impairment and mental deficit. This is probably the most common vitamin deficiency. A deficiency may be accompanied by trembling, lack of stamina and vigor, retarded growth, digestive disturbances, hair and weight loss, and possibly even personality disturbances.

- **Niacin (B₃)**—enhances memory and is a method of treatment for senility. A deficiency may also result in mental illness. Perceptual changes in the five senses are usually a key in determining if the person is deficient in niacin. In some, the ground moves when they walk, they hear voices, or words move when they try to read, or their faces seem to change when they look in the mirror.

☙ **Pantothenic Acid (B5)**—is essential to support the adrenal glands when a person comes under stress. A deficiency may lead to adrenal exhaustion, physical and mental depression, overwhelming fatigue, reduced production of hydrochloric acid in the stomach, allergies, some forms of arthritis, nerve degeneration, spinal curvature, disturbed pulse rate, and gout. It is essential to the production of antibodies that help fight off infection.

☙ **Pyridoxine (B6)**—is necessary for the manufacturing of valuable amino acid-derived neurotransmitters. Symptoms may be low blood sugar, numbness and tingling in hands and feet, neuritis, arthritis, trembling in the hands of the aged, edema (water retention) and swelling during pregnancy, nausea, air or sea sickness, mental retardation, epilepsy, kidney stones, anemia, excessive fatigue, nervous breakdown, mental illness, and acne (especially during menstruation). May provoke epileptic seizures in people prone to them, and may cause convulsions in babies.

☙ **Cobalamin (B12)**—increases the rate at which new material can be learned. Plays an important role in the formation of the myelin sheath around nerve fibers. Can cause pernicious anemia, nerve dysfunction—meaning weakness, poor reflexes, and strange sensations in the arms and legs—and impaired mental activity. May cause depression, especially in the elderly.

☙ **Folic Acid**—may help mental illness, including schizophrenia, dementia and senility. Necessary for the synthesis of RNA and DNA, which are proteins required for cell reproduction and division. Symptoms are much the same as those of a B12 deficiency. Birth defects are one of the worst results of a deficiency during pregnancy.

I want to explain a few of these in more detail for you.

The Importance of Niacin
in Preventing Senility

As a person ages, the importance of the B vitamins increases, according to Abram Hoffer, M.D., Ph.D., author of *Orthomolecular Medicine for Physicians*.[28] Hoffer cites vitamin B3—niacin and niacinamide—as being especially important in preventing or treating senility. As a Canadian psychiatrist, Dr. Hoffer has found vitamin B3 very effective in restoring memory, improving energy levels, lessening the need for sleep, and increasing alertness.[29]

Dr. Humphry Osmond, M.D., at the New Jersey Psychiatric Institute reported that a form of niacin was effective in treating 1,000 patients with schizophrenia. In medical journals for almost 40 years, Drs. Hoffer and Osmond have been reporting their almost miraculous results with schizophrenic patients (which is the most serious mental disorder). They found that 75 percent of their patients were cured with niacin treatment. "'Cured' is quite a significant word, one not often used with regard to this terrible mental illness that afflicts most of the patients in our mental hospitals," Hoffer said.[30]

Dr. Hoffer reported as early as 1962 in the *Lancet*:

> Niacin has some, though not all, the qualities of an ideal treatment: it is safe, cheap and easy to administer and it uses a known pharmaceutical substance that can be taken for years on end if necessary...Why, then have these benefits passed almost unheeded? One reason may be the extraordinary proliferation of the phenothiazine derivatives since 1954. These are tranquilizers. Unlike these, niacin is a simple, well-known vitamin that can be bought cheaply in bulk and cannot be patented, and there has been no campaign to persuade doctors of its usefulness.[31]

There are several forms of niacin available—plain niacin that can cause a flush to the skin, or "no-flush" niacin that is combined with inositol *(inositol hexaniacinate)*. Niacinamide does not cause a flush but is less effective.

Folic Acid Therapy

Surveys have found repeatedly that older people are often deficient in two B vitamins—folic acid and B12. Several investigators have reported that patients with symptoms of senility or dementia (the terms are synonymous) and who had low folic acid blood levels, showed improvement after therapy with folic acid.[32] Scientists in England found that supplementing the diets of patients with folic acid resulted in shorter stays at their mental hospital. Fortunately for the patients but unfortunately for acceptance within the medical community, this study was not a controlled study (which meant that it had no control group compared to an experimental group).[33]

Residents of nursing homes and chronic wards of mental hospitals are at considerable risk for folic acid deficiency.[34] These institutions, if they serve folate-rich green vegetables at all, are likely to do so in fairly unpalatable fashion. To compound the problem, many older people have chewing and digestive difficulties. Research shows a folic acid deficiency is often unrecognized in some elderly patients. Therefore, supplementation with B-complex vitamins, including folic acid and sublingual B_{12}, may be helpful to those in nursing homes, suffering from senility or dementia.

Vitamin B_{12} Therapy

Deficiency of vitamin B_{12}, which results in pernicious anemia, is a common vitamin deficiency. In the vast majority of cases, a person may be getting adequate B_{12} in his or her diet, but lacks a stomach-produced substance called the "intrinsic factor," which is necessary for absorption of the vitamin. B_{12} is difficult to absorb, which is why people are often given B_{12} injections.

A deficiency of hydrochloric acid (HCl) production in the stomach is known to impair vitamin B_{12} and folic acid absorption. Up to 50 percent of people age 60 and older experience seriously diminished hydrochloric acid production. Adding hydrochloric acid to the diets of the elderly normalizes vitamin B_{12} and folic acid absorption, according to Jonathan Wright, M.D.[35]

A vitamin B_{12} deficiency is related to some cases of mood disorders. Most elderly have symptoms of intellectual impairment, manifested as poor memory for recent events, difficulty in concentrating, and difficulty at work. Some will have symptoms of a burning sensation, unsteadiness, fatigue, and sometimes urinary incontinence. A broad spectrum of psychiatric symptoms from irritability to apathy to psychosis with hallucinations may also occur.[36]

A WIDESPREAD B_{12} DEFICIENCY? A deficiency in this vitamin may be more widespread than is generally recognized by the medical profession, because the range considered "normal" for serum cobalamin (B_{12})

is probably lower than it should be. In many cases, senile dementia of the Alzheimer's type and "chronic fatigue syndrome," which may very well be linked to a B_{12} deficiency, could be reversed through B_{12} therapy if diagnosed early enough.[37]

It may be that a high serum maintenance level is preferable to a merely adequate one, especially since the B-vitamins are water-soluble and any excess is excreted by our bodies through the urine.

NURSING HOMES. Recent studies suggest that a small but significant percentage of patients who are presently institutionalized in nursing homes or state hospitals for psychosis or senility actually have B_{12} deficiencies, a treatable condition.[38]

For many years, the medical profession held to the opinion that mental symptoms did not occur in the absence of anemic changes in the red blood cells. Thus, many physicians discounted the possibility of B_{12} deficiency as the cause of memory problems if the complete blood count was normal. We now know that the mental symptoms can occur before any changes are evident in red cells.[39]

VITAMIN B_{12} INJECTIONS. Vitamin B_{12} is a completely safe and inexpensive treatment. Dr. Alan Gaby says, "We usually forego the test in favor of a therapeutic trial of vitamin B_{12} injections. If the patient improves after a series of four to eight injections, we recommend continuing them on an as-needed basis."[40]

The usual recommendation is that a person take oral doses of B_{12} in the range of 1,000 to 2,500 micrograms a day. It is also available sublingually (under the tongue) that can deliver more of the B_{12} to the blood stream. As Dr. Gaby suggests, ask your physician about regular B_{12} injections for a few months.

Good dietary sources for vitamin B_{12} are organ meats (especially kidney and liver), eggs, beef, pork, fish and dairy products. Vegetarians are often deficient in B_{12} and need to take it in supplement form since it is primarily found in animal products.

L-Glutamine Is a "Brain Fuel"

When I was in high school, we already knew that glutamic acid, a nonessential amino acid, improved memory. My brother and I always took it while we were studying for tests and had great hope it would work. Research showed it could improve intelligence, give a lift when a person was fatigued, and help control alcoholism, schizophrenia, and a craving for sweets.

Since then, we have learned that the brain has a protective barrier that lets in very few chemicals. Glutamic acid is one substance that is "poorly" carried across the protective blood barrier, which is why so much of it has to be consumed for an effect to be registered.

Dr. Roger Williams has shown that another amino acid, the amide form of glutamic acid called L-glutamine, can cross the blood-brain barrier more readily, and once it has crossed the barrier, it is quickly converted into glutamic acid. The "L" indicates a natural form of the amino acid glutamine, which is used in this discussion.

L-glutamine's major function is that it serves as "fuel" for the brain. It is the only compound besides glucose (blood sugar) that can be used by the brain for energy. It has also been shown to improve the I.Q.s of mentally deficient children.[41]

MAY BE A HELP FOR ALCOHOLICS. Dr. Williams observed that L-glutamine protected rats against the poisonous effects of alcohol, but more importantly, it stopped their craving for alcohol. He found that experimental rats fed L-glutamine consistently decreased alcohol consumption.[42]

Not only rats, but nine out of ten alcoholics reported that after taking L-glutamine supplements, they had less desire to drink, less anxiety, and slept better. Relatives and friends observing them agreed. They did not do well on a placebo.[43]

One anecdotal report in the medical literature tells about an alcoholic who stopped drinking when L-glutamine was administered to him daily without his knowledge. The substance is tasteless and can be mixed with food or water without a person knowing it, which is apparently what happened in this case. Two years after the L-glutamine treatment began, he was still free from his craving for alcohol.[44]

Dr. Roger Williams recommends 1,000 to 4,000 mg a day. L-glutamine is a natural and harmless food substance without side effects. It is available in capsules or a high potency, tasteless powder.

There are reports that doses as high as 4,000 mg have been given to bone marrow transplant patients. All of the patients who received L-glutamine were statistically more "vigorous" and showed improvement in other areas as well. They felt less angry and less fatigued.[45] When you consider the sense of depression that accompanies most illness, you might ask whether depression could be diminished through the use of L-glutamine.

INCREASING GROWTH HORMONE. Back in high school I was excited about taking glutamic acid. Recently I read about a study reported in the *American Journal of Clinical Nutrition* in 1995, where scientists gave as little as 2 grams of L-glutamine to healthy athletes. Their blood levels of growth hormone rose 430 percent above initial levels 90 minutes after supplementation. In turn, growth hormone may promote greater muscle growth and the preferential use of body fat stores for energy.[46] Of course I want to experience increased fat burning and improved strength. How about you? (Refer to index for more information on L-glutamine.)

RECOMMENDATIONS. The most convenient and economical way to consume L-glutamine is to eat protein foods and/or you can also purchase pure L-glutamine in powder or capsules. I stir one heaping teaspoon of glutamine powder into my protein shake, or use juice or water. It is a taste-less, odorless white powder.

Ginkgo Biloba:
The Chinese Herb for the Brain

Perhaps the most remarkable nutrient for potentially improving memory and warding off senility is the Chinese herb Ginkgo biloba, derived from one of the most ancient trees known to mankind. The single Ginkgo tree can live for 1,000 years. Research shows that the leaves of this tree, taken in supplement form, provide remarkable pharmacological action to the circulatory and nervous systems.

Ginkgo biloba may be the most effective remedy available for short-term memory loss, slow thinking and reasoning, dizziness, ringing in the ears (tinnitus), and problems with vertigo and equilibrium. It is also being used to treat all types of dementia, cognitive disorders related to depression, absent-mindedness, confusion, lack of energy, Alzheimer's disease and senility.[47]

Ginkgo is the most widely used prescription medicine in Europe. More than ten million prescriptions are written each year for a variety of conditions, especially those related to the circulatory system.

Ginkgo specifically enhances circulation to the small blood vessels that are the farthest from the heart, and to arteries, veins and capillaries. Ginkgo actually stimulates the release of a substance that relaxes the microcapillaries, thus increasing blood flow.[48] It also reduces leg pain from low blood flow to the limbs and is important for male impotence. Read more about ginkgo and impotence in the *Men's* chapter.

A small double-blind study showed that ginkgo produced a significant improvement in long-distance vision for patients with macular degeneration, which is a frequent cause of blindness in the aged. It inhibits deteriorating vision due to oxygen deprivation to the retina.

Ginkgo affects mental alertness by changing the frequency of brain waves. Research has shown that ginkgo increases brain alpha rhythms, which are the brain wave frequencies associated with mental alertness. Increased mental alertness among volunteer subjects was evident after only three weeks of ginkgo therapy, and alertness continued to increase during the remaining three months of the study.[49]

Deterioration of cognitive functions

Ginkgo seems to be particularly beneficial for those people who are just beginning to experience deterioration of cognitive function. A German researcher, Dr. E.W. Fungfeld and his colleagues have concluded that Ginkgo biloba extract has promise in the treatment of Alzheimer's, as it appears to delay mental deterioration during the early stages of the disease. In fact, they contend that ginkgo may be able to reverse some of the disabilities associated with the disease and help the patient to maintain a normal life without hospitalization.[50]

Many studies using ginkgo have found that the leaves of the plant produce unique substances called flavone glycosides, which are powerful antioxidants. Scientific research regarding the therapeutic uses of the ginkgo extract are in full swing. A great deal of research has already been done in Europe, especially in France and Germany, to find more applications for ginkgo biloba in treating diseases that occur more frequently as we age.

Combats symptoms of aging

There are very few substances that combat the symptoms and signs of aging as well as this herb. Ginkgo biloba extract appears to fulfill all conditions laid down by the World Health Organization concerning the development of drugs effective against cerebral aging.[51]

SEVERAL FORMS OF GINKGO AVAILABLE

- Powdered leaves in capsules or tablets
- Liquid extracts, also called *tinctures*
- Powdered extracts (usually 6:1 or 8:1, which are unstandardized)
- Standardized extracts, 24 percent flavone glycosides[52]

It is important to note that only the highly concentrated extract form of ginkgo has been used in research studies: one kilo of extract being produced from 50 kilos of leaves (50:1). If you desire to purchase ginkgo biloba, find an extract that is standardized with 24 percent flavonoid glyco-sides, which is the active ingredient. Other less concentrated extracts are also available, but these have a much weaker action than that which has been tested conclusively. Most authorities recommend a dosage of 180 mg a day, which is 60 mg three times a day, or follow product label instructions.

Acetylcholine: A Major Neurotransmitter
Lecithin Converts to Acetylcholine

Years ago, Carlton Fredericks Ph.D., recommended giving choline, the vitamin B cousin, to increase the amount of acetylcholine in the nervous system. Acetylcholine is a major neurotransmitter that mediates our emotions and behavior and provides an important chemical bridge between nerve cells. Lecithin is the richest source of choline, which the brain converts to acetylcholine.

Soy lecithin granules

Lecithin comes from the Greek word *lekithos*, meaning "egg yolk," which, with soybeans, is one of its richest sources. Lecithin is a special type of fat called a phospholipid; its chemical name is phosphatidyl choline. About 13 percent by weight of the lecithin molecule is choline. The foods that are rich sources of lecithin are eggs, organ meats and other meats, whereas grains, fruits and vegetables are poorer sources.

Eliminating eggs from the average daily diet reduces the body's total lecithin intake by one third. Richard Wurtman, M.D., a neuro-scientist at the Massachusetts Institute of Technology, and other experts say many people are not getting enough lecithin and choline in their diet.[53]

Throughout her career, my Mother, Gladys Lindberg, placed all of her clientele on soy lecithin granules. She did so because of her textbook knowledge of its importance. Convinced of the value of lecithin, she would say, "it is like a detergent that keeps cholesterol soluble in the blood." Subsequent studies and scientific research proved her right, as lecithin has a cholesterol-lowering ability.[54]

Lecithin and choline improve memory and learning. Phosphatidyl choline (lecithin), the precursor of acetylcholine, has been given to patients to correct an acetylcholine deficiency. Short-term memory was improved in some patients who took daily doses of phosphatidyl choline for four months. Supplemental choline also enhanced short-term memory.[55]

When choline was fed to pregnant rats, their offsprings showed significantly better memory in maze tests than rats whose mothers were not fed choline. The improved memory was maintained at a level comparable to that of much younger rats even after the rats grew old. The beneficial effect probably relates to lecithin's function in nerve membranes and to the need for choline to make the neurotransmitter acetylcholine, which enables signals to go from nerve to nerve.[56]

Human studies suggest lecithin and choline may also benefit memory. In one study researchers gave 61 healthy older adults, (aged 50 to 80 years) either two tablespoons of lecithin or a placebo for five weeks. By the end of the study, memory test scores of the lecithin group improved significantly, exceeding those of the placebo group. The lecithin group also reported a 48 percent decrease in memory lapses. The researchers concluded that "the cost of lecithin is so low, the negative side effects so minimal and the potential benefits so positive, that we would recommend...all persons experiencing memory problems take lecithin granules as food supplements."[57] I personally feel all of us should take lecithin, even if we don't have memory lapses. Let's prevent them.

Increasing the amount of acetylcholine in the brain may open the way to improving mental function, particularly memory. Researchers at Ohio State University found that mice fed a diet laced with choline-rich lecithin or phosphatidyl choline (PC) had much better memory retention than animals given regular diets. When their brains were examined under a microscope, the lecithin-fed mice showed fewer signs of aging.[58] Specifically, the lecithin-fed mice had brain cell membranes that were less rigid and with fewer fatty deposits in them. As the brain ages, its cell membranes become more rigid with fatty deposits and they lose their ability to take in and release brain chemicals and to relay messages. This can cause memory loss and confused thinking.

As we age, brain cells also tend to lose parts of the nerve cells (dendritic spines) that convey impulses to the nerve cells in the body. These chemical receptor areas are very important in transmitting information. This loss in nerve cells results in a condition that may be analogous to a bad telephone connection—messages tend to be distorted or lost. However, lecithin-fed mice in the study above had the same number of dendritic spines as younger mice.

Psychological disorders

Lecithin also has been useful in detoxifying some of the severe side effects of the neuroleptic drugs and major tranquilizers used in the management of psychological disorders such as psychosis, according to Dr. Sheldon Hendler. One of the worst side effects of these drugs is tardive dyskinesia, which is characterized by involuntary movement of the neck, head, and tongue. When used for six months or longer, these drugs deplete the brain of choline and acetylcholine, resulting in deficiencies that can last even after the neuroleptic drugs are no longer taken. Supplemental phosphatidyl choline can often arrest the involuntary movements of tardive dyskinesia. It has been used with some success in patients with other neurological diseases such as *Gilles de la Tourette's* syndrome, *Friedreich's ataxia*, and a form of dyskinesia caused by the anti-Parkinson's disease drug, *Levodopa*.[59]

When lithium has failed

Choline and phosphatidyl choline (from lecithin) have also been employed in managing some forms of mania. In fact, these nutrients have been successful in cases where the mineral lithium has failed. In one study, the combination of lecithin and lithium significantly reduced the severity of manic episodes. However, when lecithin was discontinued and the patients were getting only lithium, 75 percent had a worsening of their problem.[60]

Recommendations

Each tablespoon of our brand of lecithin granules contain 1,725 mg of phosphatidyl choline; 1,050 mg of phosphatidyl inositol; phosphatidyl ethanolamine 1,500 mg, essential fatty acids (linoleic acid) 2,195 mg, plus other nutrients. Check your brand and make sure it contains enough of these essential nutrients.

The easiest way to consume lecithin is to mix it into juice, our protein breakfast shake or use on dry or cooked cereal. It can even be added to salads or into salad dressings. Lecithin granules are much more economical and potent as it takes approximately ten large lecithin capsules to equal one tablespoon of granulated lecithin. All forms should be available at your nutrition store.

Phosphatidyl Serine (PS): A remarkable brain cell nutrient

Phosphatidyl serine (PS) is a naturally-occurring phospholipid and is similar to other phospholipids that include phosphatidyl choline (PC) and phosphatidyl inositol (PI). Until recently, commercial lecithin contained only trace amounts, but new products include enriched powdered compounds, softgel capsules, and even liquid blends. Recent breakthroughs in technology have made phosphatidyl serine (derived from soy) available commercially in a concentrated form. It is considered an important dietary supplement for the support of brain function.

Essential functioning of all cells of the body

The concentrated phosphatidyl serine (PS) derived from soy phospholipids and clinical studies have shown that when it is taken on a regular basis, it can help adults maintain and improve learning and memory. Phosphatidyl serine is essential to the functioning of all the cells of the body, but it is most concentrated in the brain. Human research studies dating back to the '70s indicate that phosphatidyl serine tends to decline with age and that supplementation can benefit many cognitive functions (the capacity to think and reason). Some 35 human studies span almost three decades, according to Parris M. Kidd, Ph.D.

Numerous other studies involved subjects with existing, measurable losses in memory, judgment, loss of abstract thought, and loss of other higher mental functions, and in some cases, changes in personality and behavior. The results of the studies showed conclusively that, in mature adults, PS helped maintain cognition, concentration, and related mental functions. The dosages of these studies ranged from 200 mg to 300 mg a day.[61]

Subjects showed significant improvement

In two of the studies conducted in 1991, Thomas Crook, Ph.D., of the Memory Assessment Clinics, Bethesda, Maryland, studied 149 subjects between the ages of 50 and 75. The patients received either a placebo or 300 mg of phosphatidyl serine (100 mg three times a day) in a double-blind study for 12 weeks. The subjects showed significant improvement with the following functions:

- Name-Face Recall: Learning and matching of names with faces.

❧ First-Last Names: First and last names presented, then last names given for pairing with the first names. Also assesses verbal memory.

❧ Face Recognition: A test of visual memory.

❧ Grocery List: To help assess verbal learning and memory.

❧ Telephone Dialing: Memorize and retain a telephone number, under different conditions of delay and distraction.

❧ Misplaced Objects: Placement and recall of keys, glasses, other common household objects—"verbal-visual associative memory."

❧ Divided Attention: Simulates driving a car, also recall of radio reports while driving. Reaction time and verbal vocabulary memory.[62]

Reduced cognitive age

The benefits were greatest in those with the most impaired memories. The benefits persisted at least four weeks after the supplementation was discontinued. The researchers noted that phosphatidyl serine (PS) reduced the "cognitive age" of 64 to the cognitive age of 52—roughly 12 years of improvement! This was a win in the case of name-face recognition.[63]

I met with Parris M. Kidd, Ph.D., in 1996 at the Natural Products Expo West convention in Anaheim, CA, and again at a convention in Nashville where he spoke. He said that when phosphatidyl serine is taken orally, it is rapidly absorbed and readily crosses the blood-brain barrier. Normal aging can bring about neurotransmitter disturbances, metabolic decline, and nerve connection dropout.

Dr. Kidd believes PS makes clinically measurable contributions to all of these brain functions, and furthermore, toxicological studies have shown it to be completely safe without side effects.[64]

Dr. Kidd pointed out a study in 1993 by an Italian doctor who carried out a major, randomized, double-blind, placebo-controlled study of 125 subjects aged 65 to 93. They came from 23 institutions in northern Italy and all suffered from moderate to severe cognitive decline.

Following six months of phosphatidyl serine supplementation, scores on memory and learning improved significantly. In addition, scores on standardized neuropsychological tests for withdrawal and apathy also improved. The investigator concluded, "These observations are remarkable, particularly since...the large number of subjects enrolled...represents the geriatric population commonly encountered in clinical practice."[65]

At the conclusion of an Italian study the author stated, "Phosphatidyl serine appears to exert an action in two distinct contexts: one relating to the cognitive effects of vigilance, attention and short-term memory, and the other relating to behavioral aspects such as apathy, withdrawal, and daily living."[66]

Supplements are necessary

Since phosphatidyl serine is not found readily in common foods, supplementation with the concentrated product may prove to be highly desirable, particularly to mature adults experiencing a decline in mental ability. Phosphatidyl serine may be taken in combination with a healthy diet, vitamins, minerals, antioxidants, and other appropriate nutrients, as part of an integrated total nutrition program that includes exercise.

According to Dr. Kidd, to prevent or even reverse the symptoms of brain aging, it is a good idea to take this product for a period of time to see if you can obtain results. There are new "brain formulas" in your nutrition store that contain this product, or it can be purchased as pure phosphatidyl serine (PS) in softgels

L-Carnitine and Acetyl-L-Carnitine
Age Associated Memory Impairment

L-carnitine (LC) and Acetyl-L-carnitine (ALC) occur naturally in the body, where they transport fats across a membrane into the energy burning mitochondria of each cell. Acetyl-L-carnitine and carnitine are close relatives; they are naturally occurring nonessential amino acids. They play a critical role in maintaining youthful cellular energy, metabolism and blood flow. Since brain aging is a result of diminished brain cell metabolism and reduced cerebral circulation, the potential role of carnitine in protecting neurologic function is clear.

A cognitive enhancer

Researchers noted that elderly heart patients treated with carnitine demonstrated improved mood. This led to many studies on the effects of acetyl-L-carnitine (ALC) on cognitive disorders. ALC appears promising as a cognition enhancer for normal, healthy people, as well as a form of treatment for age-associated memory impairment and even

Alzheimer's disease.

Recently, Italian researchers published a landmark study that confirmed that ALC improved performance in young, healthy people. The research was conducted on 17 subjects who were given either 1,500 mg of acetyl-L-carnitine a day or a placebo for 30 days. They were tested before and after treatment, using video game style devices designed to evaluate attention levels and hand-eye coordination and reflexes. The reflex speed was markedly increased among those who received ALC, and their error rate and task completion times were reduced three to four times, compared to the control subjects. Those receiving ALC showed no adverse effects.[67]

For the elderly

Two other Italian researchers evaluated 236 mentally-impaired elderly people being treated with ALC in a large multicenter study. The treatment lasted more than five months, with subjects given either a placebo or 1,500 mg of ALC a day. All were tested for cognitive function, emotional state, and social behavior. Those who took ALC improved significantly, especially in memory, constructional thinking, and emotional state.[68] In several other studies, especially one at the University of Modena in Italy, the effects of ALC supplementation persisted long after the treatment ended.

Depression

Researchers in Italy studied the effects of acetyl-L-carnitine on 60 depressed people between the ages of 60 and 80. They were given either 3,000 mg of acetyl-L-carnitine or a placebo for 60 days and were tested repeatedly for depression and general well-being. ALC reduced the severity of depression and improved the quality of life significantly.[69]

Sleep problems

Researchers also found that acetyl-L-carnitine helped with sleep disturbances, which can disrupt the circadian rhythm (our biological "clock" or natural sleep/wake cycle) that can result in clinical depression. Circadian disturbances also can have a profound adverse effect on memory. Acetyl-L-carnitine appears to reduce sleep requirements while improving the quality of sleep.[70]

Many other studies have shown similar results with people with senile depression who were given acetyl-L-carnitine in doses ranging from 500 to 3,000 mg a day.[71]

Senility

Studies have also shown significant improvement and effectiveness of acetyl-L-carnitine (ALC) on people with senility.[72]

ALC is an effective treatment for mental impairment resulting from senile dementia. A study with 60 elderly patients concluded that subjects given 2,000 mg of ALC a day showed statistically significant improvement in the behavioral scales, memory tests, the attention barrage test, and a verbal fluency test.[73]

A study in *Neuroscience Letters* reported that ALC prevented the neurologic impairment that normally occurs in oxygen-deprived neonatal rats. The ALC treated rats did not suffer the memory deficits seen in the control group. The researchers suggested that ALC should be given to children who suffer from oxygen deprivation in the womb.[74]

Alzheimer's disease

Acetyl-L-carnitine is regarded by scientists and pharmaceutical companies as one of the most promising substances for the treatment of Alzheimer's disease.

Several studies showed ALC may retard deterioration in some cognitive areas in patients with Alzheimer's disease, significantly reduce the progression of the disease, or have a beneficial effect on some clinical features of Alzheimer-type dementia, particularly those related to short-term memory.[75] The only side effect noted was nausea in a few patients, particularly when acetyl-L-carnitine was taken on an empty stomach. Several other studies have confirmed that it improves memory, attention span, and alertness in Alzheimer's patients.[76]

ALC dosage

I recently came across the book *Smart Drugs II* by Ward Dean, M.D., and then met him at a convention and attended his lecture. I was glad to learn more information on acetyl-L-carnitine, as he is an expert in the field. Dr. Dean recommends a dose of 1,000 to 2,000 mg a day in two divided doses. You can find this product at your nutrition store in a 500 mg potency. This product is not recommended for those who are pregnant, lactating, or who are hypersensitive to acetyl-L-carnitine.[77]

Pregnenolone: A "New" Hormone for Our Brain

Pregnenolone is a hormone that is found in higher concentrations in the brain than in any other organ of the body. Pregnenolone is a key to keeping your brain functioning at peak capacity. *Some scientists believe it is the most potent memory enhancer of all time.* It appears to make us not only smarter, but happier, along with a heightened sense of well-being.

Pregnenolone has long been ignored by the medical community because it appeared to have no independent function other than to break down into DHEA (then the other hormones). Like all the other steroid hormones—pregnenolone is synthesized (made) from cholesterol. Cholesterol is first made into pregnenolone and used in the body in that form. What the body does not use undergoes a chemical change that "repackages" into DHEA. DHEA is then broken down into estrogen and testosterone. Because pregnenolone gives birth to these other hormones, it is sometimes called the "grandmother hormone." Pregnenolone provides the raw material for these other hormones. As the level of pregnenolone declines, so will the levels of the other hormones that are made from it.[78] William Regelson, M.D., has shown that pregnenolone is produced both in the brain and in the adrenal cortex. Like the other hormones, pregnenolone production declines with age. By the time you are 65, you are making approximately 60 percent less pregnenolone than you did in your 30s.

Pregnenolone proven safe and effective

It was one of the first hormones studied and was proven safe and effective. Back in the mid-'40s it was tested on students and workers and markedly improved their ability to learn and remember difficult tasks. It has been rediscovered in both animal and human studies, which indicate that pregnenolone may be the ideal memory-enhancing hormone and substance known, according to Dr. Regelson. This exciting research on pregnenolone and memory is being conducted jointly at two distinguished institutions, the Beekman Research Institute at the City of Hope Hospital and at St. Louis University School of Medicine.

In a 1992 animal study, Eugene Roberts, Ph.D., at the City of Hope, showed that *pregnenolone was 100 times more potent than any other agent in improving memory.* John E. Morley, M.D., from the University of St. Louis, involved in this study said, "It is clearly by far the most potent of the neurosteroids for improving memory by light-years. It has a much broader memory response than any of the other neurosteroids. This makes it almost an ideal agent for looking at memory and the consequences of the age-related deterioration of memory."[79] *Pregnenolone not only prevents impaired memory from declining further, it actually appears to restore it.*

Today we know that apart from producing other hormones, pregnenolone also minimizes inflammation, repairs damaged brain and spinal cord cells, allows our bodies to deal with stress more effectively, and as we said it is a potent memory enhancer.

Due to recent legislation, pregnenolone, like DHEA, is now being sold over the counter and is available at nutrition stores. Pregnenolone is effective, well tolerated, and causes no known side effects. Human studies of this hormone have shown improvements in concentration, reduction of mental fatigue, and elevation in mood. Dr. Regelson feels the right approach is to take pregnenolone with DHEA because hormones work best when they work in tandem. Make sure you read about DHEA in chapter 12, *Anti-Aging Therapies*. Since these are hormones, I feel they should not be taken by teenagers.

Magnesium and Brain Function

Low magnesium levels have been implicated in some cases of brain disease. One report in the scientific literature describes three patients who were suffering from brain disease and low magnesium stores, and eventually lapsed into a coma. They responded immediately to magnesium therapy, which brought about "prompt reversal of encephalopathy (brain dysfunction) and coma."[80]

Essential Fatty Acids and the Brain

A number of seemingly unrelated mental and psychiatric disorders, ranging from depression and hyperactivity to schizophrenia and alcoholism, often respond to essential fatty acid therapy.

Essential fatty acids are found in abundance in the lipids in our nervous system. They provide a source of the production of prostaglandins and the toughening of nerve-cell membranes. A deficiency of essential fatty acids has been apparent in many of the brain disorders studied. It seems logical to assume, therefore, that supplementary GLA (gamma linolenic acid) and EPA (eicosapentaenoic acid) might be effective in treating these disorders.[81]

GLA (omega-6) is found mainly in evening primrose oil, black currant oil, and borage oil. EPA (omega-3) is found in cold-water fish as well as in salmon, herring, mackerel, sardines, and sea bass. flaxseed oil is another wonderful vegetable source of the essential fatty acids. Flaxseed oil contains the omega-3, omega-6, and omega-9. All can be found in either capsule or liquid form.

DMAE and Brain Stimulation

DMAE (Dimethylaminoethanol), also known as Deanol, has become popular among brain stimulants. It is found in "brain foods" such as anchovies and sardines. Small amounts of DMAE occur naturally in the brain. It apparently stimulates the production of choline, which in turn alters the levels of acetylcholine (an important neurotransmitter we discussed). Research has shown that DMAE elevates mood, improves memory and learning, increases intelligence, and extends life span.

In one clinical trial by Dr. Carl Pfeiffer, patients received DMAE for chronic fatigue and mild to moderate depression. DMAE produced an increase in physical energy, personality improvements, and better sleep for those with insomnia.[82]

Another study reported in *Clinical Pharmacology and Therapeutics* showed that DMAE subjects had an increase in mental concentration and muscle tone after six weeks of taking the substance. The subjects reported more daytime energy, greater attentiveness at lectures, sounder sleep, and better ability to concentrate on writing papers or studying.[83]

DMAE is available in liquid or capsule form. No serious side effects have been reported. Those who take initial high doses may experience dull headaches, insomnia, tenseness in the muscles, but these symptoms subside when the dose is lowered.[84]

DHA: The Building Block of the Brain

DHA (docosahexaenoic acid) is a fatty acid—in precise terms, an omega-3 (long-chain) fatty acid—which is the main structural fatty acid in the gray matter of the brain and retina of the eye. The brain is 60 percent lipids (fat), and DHA is the most abundant lipid in both the brain and the retina. It is essential for brain and eye function.[85]

Humans obtain DHA initially through the placenta, then from breast milk, and later on through dietary sources such as fish (tuna, salmon, sardines, etc.), or cod liver oil, red meats, animal organ meats and eggs. Now the purest and least compromised source of this fatty acid is extracted from ocean-dwelling microalgae.[86]

An important conference on DHA was held in New York Hospital-Cornell Medical Center, entitled "Keeping Your Brain in Shape: New Insights into DHA." The researchers explained how DHA:

- In low levels correlates with changes in disposition, memory loss, and other neurological conditions.

- Helps prevent Alzheimer's Disease and memory loss in the elderly.

- Helps reduce or eliminate symptoms/behaviors related to Attention Deficit Hyperactivity Disorder (ADHD) in children and to hostility/aggression in criminals. Boys with ADHD had significantly lower concentrations of DHA.

- Ensures proper prenatal and postnatal infant neurological development.

- Helps prevent coronary heart disease.

- Helps prevent depression, and more.[87]

- Studies show that pregnant women taking DHA benefit from supplementation. Infants rely on their mothers to supply DHA for the development of their brain and eyes, initially through the placenta, and then through breast milk. It appears to be passed on to the unborn child for use in brain, neural and retinal development.[88]

- DHA could be helpful for neurological conditions: multiple sclerosis, schizophrenia, tardive dyskinesia, Zellweger's disease and Batten's disease.

Most of us have heard about Ginkgo biloba and how it improves memory, but many of us are unaware of the incredible array of benefits being ascribed to DHA. One of the richest sources is cod liver oil. Each tablespoon contains 450 to 500 mg of DHA. Look for Twinlab Emulsified Cod Liver Oil (emulsified means water soluble) for easier assimilation. There are new products with DHA but compare their potency and cost to cod liver oil. It is available at your nutrition store.

Insights into Alzheimer's Disease

Alzheimer's disease affects an estimated four million American adults, about ten percent of all people over age 65.[89] It is a progressive, degenerative disease that attacks the brain and impairs memory, thinking, and behavior. Alzheimer's disease is the most common and feared form of dementing illness, resulting in more than 100,000 deaths a year in the United States. That makes it the fifth leading cause of death in adults following heart disease, cancer, strokes, and prescription drugs. The disease is named after Dr. Alois Alzheimer (1864–1915), a German neurologist who observed the disease in his patients and initially reported it to the medical community in 1907.

Those affected with Alzheimer's disease become forgetful and confused. Although the progression is gradual and varies from person to person, the life span of a patient can be as much as 20 years after initial symptoms are observed. In addition to memory loss, there are other typical signs of the disease:

- language problems, such as trouble thinking of words
- problems with abstract thinking
- poor or decreased judgment
- disorientation in place and time
- changes in mood and behavior
- changes in personality

There is no diagnostic test for Alzheimer's disease. Physicians generally use a detailed medical history, conduct a thorough physical and neurologic exam, do mental status tests and psychiatric assessments, and other routine laboratory and neuropsychological tests.

The reason doctors find it so difficult to diagnose Alzheimer's disease is because not all patients follow the same pattern. Some people have a very rapid progression of dementia, others a much slower rate of decline. For this reason, some researchers believe the disease is actually several diseases. Part of the difficulty in conducting research for a cure lies in the fact that this disorder seems to be unique to human beings. Laboratory animals do not develop Alzheimer's disease.

DRUG RELATED CONFUSION

Over 30 percent of the elderly with Alzheimer's use eight or more prescription drugs daily.[90] Drug interactions probably play a greater role in dementia and confusional states than is currently realized.[91]

The disease can occur at any age, but most commonly after the age of 50. Many cases of dementia are entirely reversible.[92]

Every effort should be made to rule out these reversible factors. Over 80 percent of the elderly are deficient in one or more vitamins or minerals, which, if levels get too low, may induce dementia as we saw with vitamin B_{12}, folic acid and niacin.

Various research studies have shown positive benefits to supplementation with vitamin E, choline and lecithin, although much more research needs to be done in this area. It seems to me we should try all the nutrients we have just discussed at the first signs of trouble.

Aluminum and the Alzheimer's connection

In studying the brains of Alzheimer's patients who had died, researchers found one common denominator: *All had high concentrations of aluminum!* Neurons of the brain cells had four to six times the levels of aluminum found in normal brain cells. Changes in the nerve cells of the cerebral cortex made these cells look like tangles of filaments—such degenerated nerve cells could not possibly transmit nerve signals properly. Some researchers believe aluminum accumulations in the body may lead to many of the health complications and debilities of old age, not only Alzheimer's disease.

A great deal of aluminum pollution can be avoided by making wise decisions about products we tend to use as a part of our normal daily living. When we wrap our food in aluminum foil, it actually sticks to acid foods such as spaghetti sauce. *Aluminum is found in cookware, baking powder, buffered aspirin, antacids, aluminum cans, and even underarm antiperspirants*. When we apply antiperspirants to our underarms, we are rubbing aluminum right into our lymph glands. Your nutrition store carries deodorants that do not contain aluminum. They stop odor although they do not stop all perspiration.

There is no "proof" that aluminum contributes to the cause of Alzheimer's, but it has been hotly debated in the scientific field. Aluminum leads to a decreased synthesis of other neurotransmitters (dopamine, serotonin, epinephrine, norepinephrine) as well.[93]

Neuroscientists have tried to reassure us that this accumulation is the result of the disease rather than a cause. Still, when aluminum has been injected into the brains of animals, it produces tangled brain cells that are similar to the changes seen in human brain cells.[94]

The best way to remove aluminum from the body appears to be by displacing it with calcium, magnesium and vitamin D in the diet and using a high potency vitamin and mineral supplement.

Vitamin E: Better than the Alzheimer's drug

The use of antioxidants to protect against free radicals as a therapy for Alzheimer's disease has been extensively evaluated over the past decade. Vitamin E is perhaps the most studied because of its powerful antioxidant activity and its high fat solubility. The brain is more than 60 percent fat, and fat is at highest risk for free radical damage.

A landmark study was published in the *New England Journal of Medicine* in 1997. In this study, a total of 341 patients with Alzheimer's disease of moderate severity were divided into four groups. The first group received 10 milligrams of selegiline, a monoamine oxidase inhibitor, daily; the second group was given 2,000 I.U. of vitamin E daily; the third group was given both selegiline and vitamin E daily and the fourth group was given a placebo. The purpose of the study was to determine whether any of these therapies could slow down the progress of the disease so that patients would not deteriorate as rapidly. After two years, the researchers reported that the risk of reaching the most severe stage of Alzheimer's disease was 53 percent lower in the group taking vitamin E alone, 43 percent lower in the drug group, and 31 percent lower in the combination group than in the group taking the placebo. Of all these treatments, vitamin E alone worked the best.

Based on the growing number of studies that show vitamin E and other antioxidants can protect against so-called brain aging, vitamin E may prove to be useful in delaying the onset of Alzheimer's disease, or in some cases, even preventing it from occurring in the first place by protecting brain tissue against oxidative damage.[95]

DHEA—Important for Alzheimer's

Dr. Owen M. Wolkowitz of the Department of Psychiatry at the University of California at San Francisco has reported some small studies on depression accompanied by memory problems. Because of their positive results, they are now studying Alzheimer's disease with other researchers. Dr. Wolkowitz believes that DHEA may play a role in helping to prevent the inception or even the progression of Alzheimer's, but that it cannot reverse the disease once it has taken hold. "I think that it has more of a permissive effect; that is, if there is a neurotoxic degenerative process going on for whatever other reasons, having low DHEA levels could impair the body's natural ability to repair the damage. In other words, if there is some damage going on in the brain, having youthful levels of DHEA could facilitate recovery from the damage or hold the damage in check."[96] More information on DHEA is located in the *Anti-Aging Therapies* chapter.

Chelation therapy may be beneficial

Chelation therapy helps remove heavy metals such as lead,

calcium, and aluminum from the body. If started early, chelation therapy has shown very encouraging results, almost without exception, in treating patients who are exhibiting mild forms of dementia. As Richard Casdorph, M.D., Ph.D., told me personally, "We must see the patient before there is permanent damage to the brain. If dementia or Alzheimer's disease reaches an advanced stage, then the amount of improvement is limited. What we do see in our patients with early stages of dementia is that deterioration stops once they are started on treatment, and most patients bounce back and show some improvement in their intellectual ability." You can read more on chelation in the *Anti-Aging Therapies* chapter.

Alpha Lipoic Acid for brain function

Alpha lipoic acid is the subject of intensive worldwide study in neurodegenerative diseases because of its powerful antioxidant activity as well as its ability to regenerate other important brain antioxidants. It has the unique ability of being rapidly absorbed from the gut, and readily crossing the blood-brain barrier and enters the central nervous system. It serves to protect delicate neuronal cellular membranes against free radical damage. This blood-brain barrier is a protective layer of cells that excludes many chemicals from reaching the brain.[97]

In addition to its own antioxidant activity, alpha lipoic acid also facilitates the regeneration of all the other major brain antioxidants including vitamin C, vitamin E, and glutathione. We discussed under vitamin E how our brain is 60 percent fat, so you can also see the value of both of these excellent antioxidants for protecting the brain against free-radical damage.

Physical and mental exercise

Finally, two of the most important things to consider in maintaining active brain function throughout our life is physical and mental exercise.

Exercise increases the endorphins and dopamine levels in the brain. It is now known that endorphins are the neurotransmitters that are stimulated by morphine; they create a sense of well-being and even relieve pain.

Several scientific and anecdotal research studies in recent months have reported that those who continue to "learn something new" or who "exercise" their brains daily by doing puzzles, engaging in problem-solving exercises, playing chess, and doing work that requires mental activity appear to function much better, for much longer in life.

Stay involved in life. Passive mental activities, such as watching television, are no substitute for active mental activities. Volunteer your time to a hospital, school, nursing home, or get involved in something that interests you.

Consider taking a course at a local junior college or adult continuing education center. Learn to use a computer. You may even find such a course at your computer store or at your city adult school. Attend seminars that put you in touch with new information. Read, not only for fun, but to "learn." Choose to keep your brain active mentally, even as you choose to stay healthy and physically active.

Protecting Your Heart and Keeping It Healthy

Understanding Cholesterol, Triglycerides and Heart-Smart Nutrients

Our ancestors have been eating eggs, meat, and other good foods for thousands of years and the first mention of heart attacks in scientific literature was in the early 1900s. To blame heart disease on something that had always been a part of our diet doesn't make sense to me. It has to be something of more recent origin, such as the refining of flour and the introduction into the diet of processed, devitalized foods, sugar, and hydrogenated fats.

—GLADYS LINDBERG

Heart disease has reached epidemic proportions in our nation, in spite of our medical sophistication. Every year, millions of people succumb to the ravages of heart attacks and strokes, and millions more are left disabled. According to the World Health Organization, more than 12 million people die every year from cardiovascular diseases. In most nations of the world, every other death is caused by cardiovascular disease, both in men and women. In the United States, 1.5 million people will suffer a heart attack this year, and 300,000 of them will die suddenly before they reach a hospital or receive medical attention.[1]

The old adage "an ounce of prevention is worth a pound of cure" has never been so true as it is in heart disease.

Key Lifestyle Factors

These lifestyle factors can impact heart health in a positive way:

- normal weight
- reduced stress
- proper diet
- vitamin and mineral intake
- adequate antioxidants
- regular exercise
- smoke-free environment
- elimination of hydrogenated or hardened fats
- low sugar consumption
- normal homocysteine level

If you smoke, are carrying more than 20 percent additional body weight (above the normal range for your height and age), or are under heavy stress, you will need to make changes in your lifestyle if you want to have a healthy heart. There is a great deal we can do nutritionally and naturally to enhance the health of the heart and to prevent instances of heart disease. These measures are all well documented in the medical and nutritional research literature. Only a summary of key conclusions will be included here.

Understanding Cholesterol

Cholesterol is a waxy, fat-like substance that is absolutely essential to our good health, but there are two sides to this story. On the beneficial side, cholesterol is used in the body as a building block of our hormones and many complex chemicals. It is produced in many types of cells and is necessary for our bodies to function normally.

SOME FACTS ABOUT CHOLESTEROL

- Humans synthesize about 3,000 to 4,000 milligrams (mg) of cholesterol per day and receive a somewhat smaller amount in their food, mainly from eggs and animal fat.[2]

- The adrenal glands contain the highest concentration of cholesterol of any tissue in the body. Cholesterol is the starting material for the synthesis of adrenal hormones.

- The body must have cholesterol in order to function properly, and to manufacture vital hormones, including pituitary hormones, adrenal hormones, DHEA, pregnenolone and our sex hormones that include estrogen (female hormone) and testosterone (male hormone). This is important to remember so you don't improperly "cholesterol-proof" your children. Will they have enough of these necessary hormones to develop properly?

- The brain and spinal cord account for only 2 percent of total body weight, and yet they contain almost one fourth of the total cholesterol in the body. The brain uses cholesterol to make neurotransmitters that conduct nerve impulses throughout the body. Cholesterol is also an important building block of the insulation around nerves, which ensures nerve impulses are conducted appropriately.

- Your skin excretes excessive cholesterol by the normal, daily sloughing off of cells. The ultraviolet rays of the sun on exposed skin converts this cholesterol to vitamin D-3. Cholesterol is also the protective, insoluble skin molecule that resists water and prevents maceration (the softening and wearing away of skin in water).

- The body makes 80 percent of its cholesterol from fats, protein, and certain carbohydrates within the liver and intestines. The remaining 20 percent comes from dietary sources. If blood cholesterol rises above a certain level, the excess is converted into bile and excreted in the stool.

- ❧ Cholesterol is also found in the marrow within the bones where blood cells are formed.[3]

The good and the bad

Since 1950, a number of researchers have reported that people with high blood levels of a certain kind of fat did not get heart attacks. In fact, this fat, a kind of cholesterol, is so good for you that it greatly diminishes your chances of having a heart attack. It is a fat-protein combination referred to as high-density lipoproteins (HDLs).

In contrast, research reveals that people with high levels of another fat-protein combination called low-density lipoproteins (LDLs) were almost certain to have heart attacks. It is postulated that HDLs help protect against heart attack in two ways. They appear to interfere with the cells' ability to take in unwanted LDLs, thus stopping the buildup of fatty deposits that can cause atherosclerosis and heart attacks. And the necessary HDLs aid the body in excreting excess cholesterol.[4]

Dr. H. Loomis, writing in *Science*, described the HDLs as a garbage collector that sweeps up arterial cholesterol and takes it to the liver where it can be cleared from the body in the form of bile, which is lost in the feces.[5]

Although cholesterol is essential for the normal functioning of our bodies, we need to make sure we have adequate levels of the valuable HDLs. The next time you have a blood test, ask the doctor to measure not just your cholesterol level, but the ratio of HDLs to LDLs. Women generally have higher levels of the beneficial HDLs than men, and this may account for the lower incidence of heart attacks among women. Information on how to naturally lower LDLs and raise HDLs is found later in this chapter.

Proper blood cholesterol levels

The current magic number regarding blood cholesterol levels seems to be 200 mg/dl or less, according to the National Cholesterol Education Program. This number may change, however, according to a person's age and according to the opinions of medical researchers and physicians. (These numbers measure milligrams of cholesterol per 100 deciliters of blood.) Individuals with total levels of 200–239 mg/dl are considered to have a borderline risk of heart disease, while levels of 240 mg/dl and higher are considered higher risk.

Stress causes variance

People under stress have shown normal variances in their cholesterol of 10 to 20 percent. Other factors that impact cholesterol may be the time of day the blood is taken, whether the person has been resting or rushing prior to coming to the doctor's office, whether the person was lying down, sitting, or standing. All of these factors can impact a reading. A British study showed blood cholesterol levels will rise almost instantaneously if an individual is frightened, under anxiety, in pain, or exposed to an uncomfortably loud noise.[6] If your blood was sent to six different labs, you may have four different readings, as these lab tests are not always accurate.

My advice is to have several readings over a period of several weeks before you draw major conclusions about what to do regarding your cholesterol levels.

Truth about cholesterol from food sources

On the basis of research related only to lipoproteins, blood cholesterol levels and atherosclerosis, many authorities have recommended that certain foods be removed from our diet because they "have cholesterol." How many foods do we see on the market today that claim they have no cholesterol!

I certainly am not advocating that you ignore the dietary warnings you hear in the media. Rather, you need to monitor closely the *types* of fat you consume. *You should eliminate margarine, lard and hardened, heated, processed, man-made fat from your diet.* What you don't necessarily need to eliminate from your diet are foods such as eggs, low-fat dairy products, and lean meat. Edward Ahrens, M.D., a longtime cholesterol researcher at Rockefeller University, has summed up the case very well in my opinion. He said, "To deny everyone red meat, eggs, and dairy products when only a minute fraction of the population has a problem with high cholesterol reduces the joy of life unnecessarily."[7]

After conducting dozens of major epidemiological studies with thousands of animals, the renowned biochemist and researcher Richard Passwater, Ph.D., stated that no clinical study has conclusively shown that dietary cholesterol causes heart disease. He wrote in his book, *The*

New Supernutrition, "Although people insist on examining all the diets of the world looking for one component, such as cholesterol, to blame as a cause of heart disease, they would be doing better to look for the absence of one component, such as vitamin E. It is total nutrition, in fact supernutrition, that should be our main concern."[8]

The Famous Framingham Study

One of the most important studies regarding heart disease was conducted by a team of Boston University Medical School physicians. It was called the "Framingham Study" because the physicians picked Framingham, Massachusetts, for the project. This was the first large-scale project to study human heart disease that involved an entire town. The project began in 1948 and continues today.

Thousands of adults have participated in the study, which primarily is aimed at gathering information about the relationship between diet and heart disease. One of the study's directors, William Kannel, M.D., reported that there was no discernible association between the amount of cholesterol in the diet and the level of cholesterol in the blood. Half of the people who died of heart attacks in the time frame of his particular research *did not* have high blood cholesterol levels.[9]

In fact, over a 50-year period, thousands of adults in Framingham died without having elevated dietary cholesterol levels. *No correlation was found between heart disease and eggs or meat.* This is an important point. Cholesterol in the diet simply does not translate automatically into cholesterol in the blood! Our bodies have a feedback mechanism that decreases the amount of cholesterol we manufacture if we don't need as much.[10]

The much-maligned egg

It seems almost incredible to me that eggs, the most perfect food that God put upon this earth, the food for the embryo, the food associated with new life, has taken the brunt of the cholesterol scare. Years ago my nutritionally oriented pediatrician suggested I give my babies eggs, and he was the one who said, "It is the food for the embryo."

Carlton Fredericks, Ph.D., wrote, "Despite all the hue and cry, the case against eggs, which is the case against cholesterol, is in no way proved."[11]

Dr. Fredericks also observed that eggs are rich in the very substance, lecithin, that prevents cholesterol from working much of the mischief it is supposed to create in the arteries. Eggs are also rich in the B-complex vitamins choline, inositol, pyridoxine (B6), and the amino acid cysteine. These nutrients have all been used successfully in experimental medical treatments for preventing and reversing hardening of the arteries.

THE JAMA FINALLY SAYS IT'S OKAY TO EAT EGGS. My doctor son Douglas knew I would enjoy seeing this article where the *Journal of the American Medical Association* reported on April 21, 1999, research conducted by Dr. F. B. Ho from Harvard Medical School that revealed that *one or more eggs a day did not show any increased risk of cardiovascular disease.* This study included almost 118,000 men and women. Wow! Now we can finally set the record straight that you can eat eggs and not feel guilty. An egg is one of the most perfect sources of protein.

Very Low Cholesterol May Be Dangerous

Low cholesterol is often associated with malignant and other "wasting" diseases. The British medical journal, the *Lancet*, reported in March 21, 1992, that low serum cholesterol may be linked to increased suicide risk. The abstract states that middle-aged *people who have low blood cholesterol concentration may be at risk for suicide and other types of violent death,* although they are less likely to have coronary heart disease.

The *Lancet* also reported a study in which low cholesterol levels were associated with depression in a group of 1,020 white men aged 50 to 89. Those with cholesterol levels below 160 mg/dl were three times more likely to be depressed than men whose cholesterol levels were 200 mg/dl or higher. The researchers speculated that depression, suicide, and violent deaths in people with low cholesterol could be the result of low levels of serotonin, a chemical found in the blood that enables the blood vessels to constrict and contract. Serotonin, a chemical occurring naturally in the brain, suppresses harmful impulses such as suicidal or aggressive behavior. Fewer serotonin receptors decrease the amount of serotonin in the brain and may increase the likelihood of violent behavior.[12]

Understanding Triglycerides

Whenever cholesterol is discussed, knowledgeable people also talk about triglycerides. Triglycerides are chemicals produced in the process of converting excess carbohydrates into stored body fat and are linked to heart disease.

Blood triglyceride levels increase when you eat refined carbohydrates, products made with white sugar, such as cookies, cake, candy, donuts, ice cream, anything made with white flour, white sugar, and even sweetened fruit juices. Serum triglyceride levels from 70 to 150 mg/dl blood are considered optimal by many health-oriented physicians.

Individuals who consumed 30 percent of their calories from sugar—which is a little more than the average in the American diet—developed significantly higher levels of cholesterol and triglycerides in their blood than the control subjects in an experiment.[13]

Sweet and dangerous

Many authorities, including the biochemist and researcher John Yudkin, M.D., Ph.D., author of five books including *Sweet and Dangerous,* states that triglyceride levels are an important factor in predicting the likelihood of an individual developing a heart attack. Both triglycerides and cholesterol contribute to heart disease potential.[14]

Dr. Yudkin blames sugar consumption for increased heart disease in the industrialized nations and has a great deal of research to back up his claim. He contends that sugar is not only a cause, but the main cause. An article in the *American Journal of Clinical Nutrition* reported that the most consistent data dealing with diet and high triglyceride levels concerns sugar. When sugar is withheld, triglyceride levels fall. Diets high in complex carbohydrates such as cereals, breads, vegetables, and seeds do not have the same effect.[15]

Obesity is probably the major cause of mild elevated triglycerides. However, other situations that can lead to high triglyceride levels include alcohol abuse and the use of certain drugs, some diuretics, oral contraceptives, products containing female hormones, Acutane (an acne drug), and some drugs used for treating heart conditions.[16]

We know that sugar raises our insulin level and is related to diabetes. It is estimated that half of those with coronary artery disease and three quarters of stroke victims develop their circulatory problems prematurely as a result of diabetes. All of these factors seem to be related, in my opinion.

Vitamin C decreases total cholesterol

We need to increase our vitamin C intake since it is so beneficial to the cardiovascular system. Two to three grams (2,000–3,000 mg) of vitamin C per day, given over several months lowered triglyceride levels an average of 50 to 75 percent. This was only observed in patients with initially high levels of triglycerides. This fact shows that vitamins have primarily a regulatory effect; they lower blood factors only when necessary. Vitamin C decreases total cholesterol, harmful LDL cholesterol, and triglycerides, and it increases good HDL cholesterol.[17]

Hardened fats increase the amount of oxidation in the body, resulting in greater amounts of free radicals roving around in your body. To fight these free radicals, consume antioxidants such as vitamins E, C, A, beta-carotene, selenium, alpha lipoic acid, and L-carnitine (read chapter 3). We need better overall nutrition and must eliminate white sugar, white flour, overly processed foods, chemical preservatives, white fat on meats; and hydrogenated, hardened fats found in bakery products, fried foods and margarine. These principles are much more important than eliminating all lean meat, eggs, and dairy products from our diet!

Heart-Smart Nutrients

Among the foremost nutrients that help strengthen and revitalize the heart muscle are the antioxidants. Several of the antioxidants also have great benefit in lowering cholesterol, lowering blood pressure, and protecting the heart from damage.

Vitamin E: The great protector

Vitamin E is the oldest recognized biologic antioxidant. It may have even a more basic function, however—the production of energy. In these two capacities, vitamin E is of the utmost importance in maintaining good health at the most basic of levels. Natural vitamin E also appears to help slow the aging process and prevent premature aging. In fact, it has been called the "anti-aging vitamin."[18]

Vitamin E also decreases the need for oxygen in the tissues and organs of the body. Mega vitamin levels of vitamin C and trace levels of selenium also share this function. Additionally, vitamin E improves the transportation of oxygen by the red blood cells.

Much of the early research relating natural vitamin E (d-alpha tocopherol) and the heart has been done by Drs. Wilfrid and Evan Shute. I talked about their work in the opening chapter. Together, they operated a clinic in Canada.

Wilfrid Shute, M.D., reported a study he conducted at his clinic where he found that natural vitamin E in 300 to 3,200 IU doses a day was quite successful in helping both individual cells and tissues in general to function normally.

A number of years ago at a National Nutritional Foods Association convention, Mother and I had the privilege of hearing Dr. Wilfrid Shute discuss his work with 38,000 cardiac patients. During his lecture he showed fantastic color slides that I will never forget. Among them were pictures of patients with ulcerated amputated stubs, diabetic gangrene, terrible ulceration, and severe burns, all of which refused to heal. But, after natural vitamin E, usually 600 IUs daily, had been given to the patients, and vitamin E ointment had been used, all the patients were restored. Ulcerated and naked wounds healed more rapidly with vitamin E therapy, and the scar tissue did not contract and was not tender. Vitamin E was even shown to prevent disfiguring scars and to help heal old scars. Remember this if you need a scar to heal after an operation.

Your Heart and Vitamin E is the classic book by Dr. Evan Shute. He and other researchers have found that *only natural vitamin E* (d-alpha tocopherol) provides the following direct benefits to the heart:[19]

- *Dissolves clots.* An antithrombin helps dissolve fresh clots and prevents their formation in arteries and veins. It is useful in treating and preventing phlebitis (inflammation of the walls of the vein). As a preventive measure against strokes, vitamin E helps prevent arterial and venous thrombosis or clots in the circulatory system of the brain.

- *Restores capillary permeability.* It helps dilate the capillaries and thus helps circulation of blood throughout the body. This effect is of great value in conditions where there is a spasm in a vessel wall or a significant degree of vessel damage, either acute or chronic.

- *Increases collateral circulation.* Vitamin E steps up collateral circulation (alternative blood pathways), a process in which smaller vessels dilate to carry a larger volume of blood around a blocked vessel.

- *Decreases amount of heart muscle death.* In cases of heart attack, vitamin E in high doses appears to decrease the amount of heart muscle death.[20]

- *Lowers heart disease instances.* Dr. Richard Passwater, one of my favorite authorities, describes a study involving 17,894 participants who had taken various amounts of vitamin E for different periods of time. The heart disease rate of these participants was compared to that of the general population having identical ages. In all instances, where persons consumed 400 IU or more of vitamin E daily for more than two years, their rate of heart disease was significantly lower than normal (3 per 100 compared to 32 per 100). The amount of heart disease in any age group decreased proportionally with the length of time vitamin E had been taken. In fact, Dr. Passwater noted the length of time was more important than the dosage beyond the minimum of 400 IU taken daily.[21]

2. *Reverses arteriosclerotic damage.* Dr. Morgan Raiforth, a pioneering ophthalmologist, has shown with a series of published photos, that arteriosclerotic damage in the retinal vessels of the eye can be reversed by using 1,200 IUs of vitamin E, and three to five grams (3,000 to 5,000 mg) of vitamin C on a daily basis.[22]

PROTECTIVE BENEFIT AFTER BYPASS SURGERY. The School of Medicine at USC recently reported a study in which all patients who had undergone bypass surgery were carefully monitored for new fatty deposits in their arteries by angiograms—a type of heart x-ray. The angiograms revealed that patients taking the most vitamin E had much smaller lesions on their arteries than did those taking less vitamin E or none at all. The benefits were particularly noteworthy because the men taking larger amounts of vitamin E began the study with higher blood levels of cholesterol. Many researchers believe that cholesterol becomes dangerous only when oxidized in the absence of vitamin E.[23]

Since Vitamin E has virtually no side effects, a number of physicians are apparently beginning to prescribe vitamin E to their patients. I applaud their decision! Mother began recommending vitamin E to all her clients in 1949 after she had read Dr. Shute's original work.

Dr. Shute also recommended 400 IUs of vitamin E as a preventive measure. He would increase this dosage to 800 to 1,200 IUs daily. If you have extremely high blood pressure, increase your vitamin E very slowly, due to its blood thinning effect at higher doses and be under the care of a doctor who understands nutrition.

PROTECTIVE FROM HEART ATTACKS. A study of middle-aged men from 16 European countries, by the World Health Organization (WHO) in Geneva, Switzerland, reported that *low blood levels of vitamin E were a more important risk factor than either high cholesterol or high blood pressure in deaths due to ischemic heart disease (heart attacks).* In fact they said it was the *main risk factor.* Many people assume that lowering cholesterol is the most important thing they can do to decrease their risk of heart attack. This WHO study provides documented evidence that increasing important vitamins seems to be more than twice as important in protecting a person from heart attack.[24] Our vitamin E levels need to be maintained or increased!

HEART ASSOCIATION STUDY. The American Heart Association's annual science writers' meeting showed that vitamin E blocked negative changes in the bloodstream of men given 800 IU daily for three months.

The Heart Association president, Dr. W. Virgil Brown of Emory University in Atlanta, admitted, "Most of us in medicine have pooh-poohed megadoses of vitamins, but Dr. Ishwarlal Jialal's work has a good ring to it."[25]

Dr. Jialal's work proposed in his study that "fats in the bloodstream become lodged in the blood vessel walls and begin to clog arteries only when they have chemically combined with oxygen to turn rancid, the way butter does after being left out too long."[26]

Dr. Jialal supports the theory that heart disease begins when the dangerous low-density lipoprotein (LDL), the major cholesterol carrier, is oxidized by particles in the bloodstream called free radicals. Oxidized LDLs appear to begin the formation of blood vessel clogging plaque that leads to atherosclerosis (plaque in the inner artery wall) or hardening of the arteries.

You must get at least 400 IUs of vitamin E per day (800 IU is better) to keep cholesterol from going bad and beginning to damage arteries, yet our diet only contains between 8 IUs to 11 IUs per day.[27] And vitamin E does not just prevent heart disease, it can also reverse its progression, according to animal studies.[28]

REDUCING THE RISK WITH ANTIOXIDANTS. Dr. Jialal further suggested that antioxidant nutrients may be instrumental in preventing LDL oxidation and reducing the risk of atherosclerosis. "We found that vitamin C, vitamin E, and beta-carotene all inhibited the unwanted LDL oxidation and the early stages of plaque formation in our laboratory studies," he said. "Vitamin C and beta-carotene almost completely prevented LDL oxidation (95 percent and 90 percent respectively), while vitamin E inhibited oxidation by 45 percent." He compared the benefits of vitamin C to probucol, a cholesterol-lowering drug. Dr. Jialal concluded that both have antioxidant properties, but probucol is a drug and not free from side effects.[29]

VITAMIN E PREVENTS STICKINESS. Along with its antioxidant proper-ties, vitamin E acts as a surfactant (makes things slippery) so it minimizes the tendency of blood platelets to stick together and form clots. A significant decrease in adhesiveness (stickiness) of platelets was noted after only two weeks of daily supplementation with 400 IU of vitamin E. This has important implications for coronary artery disease. If platelets can be kept from sticking together to form clots, and also kept from adhering to vessel walls, the blood flow remains much more unobstructed and even.[30]

The Cambridge Heart Antioxidant Study, which was published in the *Lancet,* March 23, 1996, evaluated approximately 2,002 patients with a history of heart disease in a randomized, controlled trial. Half received 400 or 800 IUs of vitamin E daily, the other 1,000 heart patients received a placebo. They were followed for a total of 510 days (18 months), and the researchers noted a 75 percent reduction in new heart attacks (myocardial infarcts) in the vitamin E group, compared to the placebo group. Results of this study demonstrated that vitamin E supplementation significantly decreased the risk of cardiovascular disease and nonfatal myocardial infarction. The researchers explained the benefits of vitamin E was from supplements, not food sources.[31] What an exciting study, that the reduction of heart attacks was reduced by 75 percent. I strongly recommend you take vitamin E supplements daily, especially for its protection.

Beta-carotene cuts heart disease

Beta-carotene (the precursor of vitamin A) benefits the heart for many of the same antioxidant reasons as vitamin E. We once may have laughed at nutritional enthusiasts who insisted, "Eat your dark green vegetables" or "drink your carrot juice," but no more! These dark green and yellow vegetables are the richest sources of beta-carotene.

A Harvard researcher, Charles H. Hennekens, M.D., examined the relationship between dietary beta-carotene and vitamin E, and risk factors for heart disease. He studied a group of 333 participants in the U.S. Physician's Health Study who had stable angina (chest pain) and who had not had a previous heart attack or stroke. Dr. Hennekens concluded, "Those physicians who took 50 mg (equals 80,000 IU) of beta-carotene as a supplement every other day had (not quite) half as many heart attacks, strokes and deaths related to heart disease as those who did not."[32]

A MUCH LOWER RISK. In Dr. Hennekens' presentation before the New York Academy of Sciences in 1992, he reported on a study that followed 87,245 female nurses over an eight-year period. "Those nurses who consumed higher amounts of beta-carotene and vitamin E were less likely to develop heart disease. When we compared women in the top 20 percent of vitamin intake to women in the bottom 20 percent, we found the high vitamin group had a much lower risk of developing heart disease."[33]

The *Lancet* reported on July 8, 1995, that dark-green leafy vegetables are a rich source of micronutrients, but some people have trouble converting beta-carotene into vitamin A (retinol). The researchers cited the need in the diet for other foods that help overcome a vitamin A deficiency, such as the foods naturally rich in retinol (eggs, cod liver oil, whole fish, and liver) and fortified foods.[34]

The value of vitamin C

Linus Pauling, Ph.D., and Matthias Rath, M.D., along with other researchers at the Linus Pauling Institute of Science and Medicine now at the University of Oregon, evaluated the prevention and treatment of heart disease for a number of years. In 1989, Dr. Rath made a significant discovery. At the time, researchers assumed that cholesterol deposited in the arteries in atherosclerotic plaques was the dangerous LDL cholesterol and that the amount of LDL in blood serum was the major risk factor for heart disease.

Dr. Rath found, however, that the real culprit was another lipoprotein called lipoprotein(a)—a substance usually ignored in blood analysis. He concluded that lipoprotein(a) is the substance that is present in abnormally large amounts in patients with heart disease and that it is the greatest risk factor, not the bad LDL or total cholesterol level.[35]

In later studies, Drs. Pauling and Rath discovered that lipoprotein(a) and vitamin C are connected. They concluded that a low intake of vitamin C allows lipoprotein(a) to lay down these plaques, and thus a low intake of vitamin C may be the primary cause of heart disease![36] They suggested that vitamin C and other orthomolecular substances might prevent or even reverse plaque formation and angina pectoris.[37]

VITAMIN C AND COLLAGEN. In making their argument, Drs. Pauling and Rath pointed out that stores of vitamin C in the body directly determine the stability of the body's structural tissues, especially collagen, which functions in the body somewhat like steel reinforcement in a skyscraper.

When there is an acute vitamin C deficiency, the collagen dissolves and the body literally breaks apart at the cellular level. Although acute and complete vitamin C deficiency is virtually unknown in America today, chronic dietary vitamin C deficiency is widespread. The consequences of insufficient vitamin C intakes over decades can have a disastrous effect on the body, and especially upon the walls of the blood vessels.[38]

These two researchers believe that the deposit of plaque on the arterial walls is something of a desperate defense reaction on the part of the body. The arterial wall, having become fragile because of vitamin C deficiency, needs to be repaired from the inside. In depositing plaque, cholesterol and other clotting factors, the body is attempting to strengthen or build up the walls that have been weakened. They theorize that heart disease is actually an early stage of scurvy, which is a chronic vitamin C deficiency.

"THEY ARE BETTING ON THE WRONG HORSE."

Hundreds of millions of dollars have been spent by the National Institutes of Health, the American Heart Association and other agencies in support of studies of cardiovascular disease in relation to LDL and HDL cholesterol, triglycerides, saturated fats and unsaturated fats. Very little attention has been paid to vitamin C and other vitamins.

I think that these agencies have been betting on the wrong horse. It is fortunate that vitamin C is not a drug—it is an orthomolecular substance, normally present in the human body and required for life, and it has extremely low toxicity. You do not need to have a physician's prescription or the approval of the medical establishment to use it in the best way to improve your health and to prevent heart disease. Your knowledge may even be greater and your judgment better than theirs.[39]

—DR. PAULING

Matthias Rath, M.D., states that the main risk factor of human atherosclerosis is the instability of the vessel wall as a consequence of vitamin C deficiency. High cholesterol levels or other risk factors in the blood are a risk for heart disease only if the wall of the arteries is weakened by vitamin C deficiency.[40]

BLOOD PLATELET ADHESIONS. Impressive research from around the world shows that vitamins C and E reduce blood platelet adhesion—a very important discovery since blood clotting is one of the causes of many heart attacks. British and Swedish scientists have reported that vitamin C does this by reducing the stickiness of the blood.[41] You also read earlier that vitamin E decreased blood platelets from sticking together.

Researchers in Berlin, Germany, found that one gram (1,000 mg) of vitamin C daily normalized blood platelet adhesion and reduced the interaction of platelets within the arterial walls.[42] Yet another study showed that a group of patients with coronary artery disease who took one gram of vitamin C every eight hours for ten days significantly decreased platelet adhesiveness and platelet aggregation.[43]

IS HEART DISEASE A VITAMIN DEFICIENCY? Just when we thought cholesterol was the main culprit in heart disease, we are seeing research that indicates that the true culprit may be a vitamin deficiency!

Coenzyme Q10 and the heart

Coenzyme Q10—also called CoQ10, ubiquinol 10 or vitamin Q—is now being called a "miracle nutrient" by many. It is an essential component of the metabolic process involved in energy (ATP) production.

Dr. Karl Folkers, who was professor and director of the Institute for Biomedical Research at the University of Texas in Austin, has been recognized for years as the world's leading researcher on CoQ10. I had the honor of hearing Dr. Folkers lecture at the American Academy of Anti-Aging Medicine conference in 1996. When I told him about this book and that I'd quoted him, with a twinkle in his eye he said, "Oh, don't believe a thing I've said." He was over 90 years old and charming! During his lecture Dr. Folkers said, *I don't use the word 'cure' lightly but CoQ10 is the 'cure' for heart disease."*

He has conducted biochemical, biomedical, and clinical research on CoQ10 for some 35 years and has succeeded in establishing its structure and in isolating CoQ10 in human hearts. The highest concentration of the enzyme is in the heart muscle. His research shows a definite link between CoQ10 deficiency and human heart disease.[44]

PROGRESS IN CARDIOLOGY. At the conclusion of the 1986 conference where Nobel Prize winners reported on their research with CoQ_{10}, Dr. Folkers made the following remarks as he accepted the Priestley Medal, the highest award given by the American Chemical Society:

> We have heard that patients in advanced cardiac failure, who had only a few months to live, under close medical care, have revealed almost miraculous improvement after treatment with CoQ_{10}, and such is a step of progress in cardiology. Proof of effectiveness of CoQ10 in cardiology is now known to medical science...Proof of the safety of CoQ_{10} is known.[45]

Dr. Folkers reported dramatic effects of CoQ_{10} therapy for advanced cardiac patients—"For those who frequently experience discomfort with any physical exertion, and often have pain even when they are at rest. Such patients invariably do not survive long on conventional therapy."[46]

The use of CoQ_{10} to treat heart disease has become well established in Japan, where researchers began testing CoQ_{10} for heart disease in the 1960s, completing 25 studies, including two large double-blind trials by 1976. The results showed about a 70 percent improvement of the patients. By l987, more than ten million Japanese were estimated to be taking CoQ_{10} as a prescription drug for cardiac problems.[47] Here in the United States, CoQ_{10} is not a prescription drug and is available at your nutrition store.

The newsletter of the Linus Pauling Institute of Science and Medicine reported some of the many clinical studies on the treatment of congestive heart disease with CoQ_{10}, which support the following conclusions:

> *   The high correlation between occurrence and severity of congestive heart disease and the level of CoQ_{10} in the heart indicates that a deficiency of CoQ_{10} may be a causative factor of congestive heart disease. Cardiomyopathy (disease of the muscle of the heart) can be substantially, but not solely, a consequence of a deficiency of CoQ_{10}.
>
> *   This deficiency can be corrected by taking oral supplements of CoQ_{10}. An oral intake of 60 to 120 mg per day of CoQ_{10} has been shown to improve cardiac function, extend life

span, and increase the well-being of about 75 percent of patients with congestive heart disease. Therapy with CoQ10 can result in profound increase both in cardiac function and in the quality of life of a failing cardiac patient.

❧ The response to CoQ10 may take weeks or months. CoQ10 acts as a vitamin, rather than a drug. Thus, the therapy must be continued for weeks, sometimes months, before the positive benefits are realized. However, if the deficiency is large, the effects of CoQ10 may be seen in a few days. In many instances, the therapy may need to be continued indefinitely. If the CoQ10 therapy is discontinued, the improvement may cease and the condition may revert to its prior status.

❧ CoQ10 therapy improves cardiac function only when the CoQ10 level of the heart is low. There is little benefit in taking supplemental CoQ10 unless the heart has low amounts of this enzyme. However, maintenance of normal CoQ10 levels appear to be less likely as a person ages. Morbidity (death) tends to occur if the CoQ10 level of the heart is less than 75 percent of normal and survival is rare at 25 percent of normal.[48]

A STRONGER PUMPING ACTION. Researchers have treated heart failure patients with CoQ10 with considerable success. CoQ10 is said by these researchers to enhance the pumping capacity of the heart and to eliminate the major side effects associated with conventional heart failure drugs. Patients with very severe forms of heart failure seem to benefit the most, showing an *increase in pumping action of more than 200 percent after taking CoQ10*. In general, the more severe the heart failure condition, the greater the benefit.[49]

Another study reported an increase in the production of energy in heart-muscle cells. In this study, some 91 percent of the patients showed improvement within 30 days after beginning CoQ10 supplementation.[50] What exciting news this is! We should all be taking CoQ10 to support the integrity of our hearts. CoQ10 should be taken continuously to maintain heart strengthening benefits.

I have had the privilege of hearing cardiologist Stephen Sinatra, M.D., executive director of the New England Heart Center, lecture on the value of CoQ10 at several conventions. As a general heart-protective dose, Dr. Sinatra himself takes 180 mg daily, but for high blood pressure, he usually builds toward a daily dose of 180–360 mg, and for serious congestive heart failure, 360–400 mg daily. For preventive maintenance for someone without a specific heart problem, Dr. Sinatra recommends a dosage of 30–90 mg daily.[51]

Dr Julian Whitaker reports in *Health & Healing*, "If you are taking a statin drug, by all means protect yourself by taking 100 to 200 mg of CoQ10 daily (consider getting a blood test to determine your CoQ10 level and increase that dose, if indicated). And if any of your friends or family members are taking a statin, please tell them about the need to take supplemental CoQ10."

EFFECTIVE IN MANY OTHER AREAS. CoQ10 is also effective in many other areas such as periodontal (gum) disease, hypertension or high blood pressure, muscular dystrophy, cancer, athletic performance, weight loss, anti-aging, thyroid and thymus gland function and Parkinson's disease. Dr. Folkers has shown that CoQ10 strengthens the immune system, so read more in chapter 3.[52]

ANTI-AGING BENEFITS. The new promise for CoQ10 is its anti-aging benefit. CoQ10 supplements have been shown to re-energize aging tissues and to alleviate the effects of many aging related processes and age associated diseases.[53]

This vitamin-like nutrient appears to have great benefit to all of us. Many people find 60 to 120 mg daily supplementation to be effective. Other authorities recommend 120 to 300 mg a day, if the heart disease is severe. I consider taking CoQ10 an investment in the future, like an "insurance policy of good health" that will pay off in later years.

The value of L-Carnitine

L-carnitine is an amino acid-like compound found in all animal and human tissues, with the highest concentrations found in the adrenal glands and heart muscle. It is synthesized in the liver, where it is rapidly converted from the amino acids lysine and methionine. The process of conversion requires adequate vitamin C to be present.[54]

L-carnitine is critical for a strong heart because it helps to expand the blood vessels, making the heart's job easier. No other organ in the body has more L-carnitine in it than the heart. In fact, L-carnitine levels in the heart are approximately 100 times that of the L-carnitine levels in the blood. Interesting that the richest food source of L-carnitine is red meat.

Studies have shown that L-carnitine is an effective nutritional agent in managing ischemic heart disease (heart attack), abnormal heartbeat rhythm (cardiac arrhythmias), and elevated triglyceride levels. This safe and effective nutrient also raises serum HDL levels (the beneficial cholesterol). This can be important to patients who are unable to exercise.[55]

A minimum daily dose of 1,000 mg of L-carnitine is required. For therapeutic benefits, many recommend 4,000 mg. *This nutrient works so rapidly that triglyceride levels dropped to within normal limits in 15 days for 73 percent of the patients of one study.*[56]

MAY REDUCE RISK OF DEATH BY 90 PERCENT. In another study, 160 patients who had recently suffered a heart attack were divided into two groups. One group received standard care, while the others received standard care plus four grams (4,000 mg) a day of L-carnitine. After 12 months, 12.5 percent of those in the standard care group had died, compared to only 1.2 percent in the L-carnitine group. *L-carnitine treatment following a heart attack may reduce the risk of death by as much as 90 percent!* No other treatment so far has produced such dramatic results.[57]

L-carnitine has also been shown to be helpful to those who experience angina, symptoms related to mitral valve prolapse, and those who have hardening of the arteries in their legs.[58]

L-CARNITINE WITH CoQ$_{10}$. According to Dr. Julian Whitaker, "No studies have looked at what happens when both L-carnitine and CoQ$_{10}$ are used together. Because of their overlapping mechanisms of action, I believe that combining them would produce much better results than using either separately. Both L-carnitine and CoQ$_{10}$ have been shown to produce as good a result as standard drug therapy for angina."[59] Dr. Whitaker recommends taking 500 mg of L-carnitine twice daily and 30 to 100 mg of CoQ$_{10}$ three times daily.[60]

FAT BURNING AND WEIGHT LOSS. I enjoyed reading *The Carnitine Miracle* by Robert Crayhon, M.S. He discusses the value of L-carnitine for the heart, but I was thrilled when he discussed its value for weight loss. He feels as I do, that for weight loss we need a diet that allows for a lower insulin level, and that means a diet lower in carbohydrates and higher in protein. We need to exercise, but this will not solve the nutrient related problems.

Dr. Crayhon says, "Tuning up your metabolism with the right nutrients is essential for weight loss. There is significant scientific evidence that increased levels of carnitine in tissues leads to increased fat burning. Carnitine is a forklift that takes fat to the fat incinerators in our cells called mitochondria. Unless fat makes it into the mitochondria, you can't burn it off no matter what you do and no matter how well you diet. Once fat is inside the mitochondria, *fat is magically transformed into energy.* It's like turning bricks into gold. This is why carnitine both encourages weight loss and increases energy levels."

L-CARNITINE DOSAGE. Taking 1,000 mg to 2,000 mg of L-carnitine per day, low carbohydrate diets become much easier to stay on, for energy levels increase and cravings lessen.

You will notice in my Super Energy Protein shake in the *Let's Put It All Together* chapter that I have added 1 TB (1,000 mg) liquid L-carnitine to this shake. Many times I will take 2 TB (2,000 mg) in my shake as it tastes great. So now, I am not only helping you to protect your heart, but to help you take control of your weight, if necessary. The usual dosage is 1,000 to 4,000 mg a day in divided doses.

Magnesium: Essential for life

Magnesium is a major mineral component in our bodies. It is absolutely essential for life, and is required for every major biological process, including the electrical stability of cells in the heart, the maintenance of membrane integrity, muscle contraction, nerve conduction, and the regulation of vascular tone—all of which have direct bearing on the health of the heart muscle.

Magnesium appears to regulate the "gate" through which calcium enters the cells to "switch on" vital functions such as the heartbeat.[61] It is vitally important that magnesium and calcium be in balance for the heart to beat regularly.

Magnesium has been shown to improve different forms of irregular heartbeats and arrhythmias, including:

- rapid beating of the heart chambers *(ventricular tachycardia)*

- fibrillation of the heart chamber *(ventricular fibrillation)*

- irregular heartbeat originated in the smaller chambers of the heart situated above the main chambers *(supraventricular arrhythmia)*[62]

One of the causes of ischemic heart disease (heart attack) is that the coronary arteries fail to provide all of the oxygen the heart demands. The result is a spasm in the smooth muscles of the artery walls.

Inadequate magnesium has been related to greater susceptibility to muscle spasm. Thus, an increase in magnesium can be beneficial in heart disease to counteract vessel spasm.

Calcium-Magnesium Imbalance. This same principle applies to the overall heart muscle. Calcium is crucial for the heart muscle to work properly. If too many calcium ions enter the heart cells because magnesium is in short supply, then the effect can be disruptive, introducing toxic, killing forms of oxygen. Some researchers suggest that this may be the very root of heart-tissue death, and thus, of myocardial infarction (heart attack).

Sheldon Hendler, M.D., Ph.D., holds to this position and also believes that the resulting magnesium-calcium imbalance may also be the main obstacle to overcome in helping the heart to heal after a heart attack. Once calcium has the upper hand, it is all the more difficult for magnesium to promote the nucleic acid and protein synthesis necessary for the mending process in the heart muscle. Dr. Hendler says, "We do know that magnesium deficiency predisposes humans to potentially fatal disruptions of normal cardiac rhythm (cardiac dysrhythmia). Investigators have successfully treated ventricular dysrhythmias with magnesium. These disorders had not been improved by conventional drug therapy."[63]

Diuretics and Digitalis. These are known to diminish magnesium levels. Many times blood tests do not reflect a total body magnesium deficit. Cellular levels have often been found to be low even when blood levels of magnesium were within normal range. The cellular measure is a far more accurate gauge and should be employed more often, especially if a person is taking diuretics and digitalis. The problem is that there is no easy way to measure cellular levels. So if you are on these medications, discuss with your doctor whether you should add the minerals potassium and magnesium to your program.

Heart Attacks and Intravenous Magnesium. Recent studies in the *Lancet* have shown that those who have acute heart attacks have a much higher survival rate, or fewer life threatening dysrhythmia incidents, if magnesium is given to them right after the attack. I recently saw a very interesting television program on the Public Broadcasting System (PBS) in which a patient was rushed to an emergency room after a heart attack, and a doctor immediately began to administer magnesium intravenously. This stopped the attack and prevented further damage to the heart, according to the experts on the program. This is important since 300,000 heart attack victims die before they reach the hospital.[64]

Stephen Gottlieb, M.D., is quoted in *Emergency Medicine* as saying, "It's so safe and inexpensive that I can't think of a reason not to give it."

SIDE EFFECT OF TOO MUCH MAGNESIUM. If you overdose on magnesium it will cause a loose stool, as it will act as a laxative. This is not necessarily negative because so many people are constipated. If this is your problem, increase your magnesium level, and you will soon find your dose so you can have regular bowel movements several times a day.

Vitamin B6 has preventive value

Many researchers have shown, through carefully controlled experiments, that the B-complex vitamins are critical in avoiding heart disease. Pyridoxine (B6) has been shown to:

- combat the development of atherosclerosis
- reduce the risk of blood clots in coronary arteries
- normalize blood lipids (fats)
- reduce elevated homocysteine levels
- reduce the risk factor for heart attacks and strokes [65]

Vitamin B6 is a vital part of the coenzyme that helps form lecithin in our bodies, and lecithin is a known fat metabolizer with great benefit in helping lower cholesterol.

In one experiment, rhesus monkeys were fed high cholesterol diets. The monkeys developed human-like arterial plaques when they were deficient in B6, but not when they were well-supplied with the vitamin. Even though the cholesterol level of some of the monkeys was elevated to four times that of others, they didn't develop cholesterol plaques if they had adequate B6 levels. In fact, they had fewer plaques than monkeys fed far lower cholesterol diets, but that were deficient in B6. These experiments with monkeys were later confirmed by other researchers, and also were replicated using dogs and chickens with similar results.[66]

ARE YOU DEFICIENT? Vitamin B6 is indispensable for the manufacturing of coenzyme Q_{10}, a vital nutrient for the heart. Since a widespread deficiency of vitamin B6 among Americans has been well documented, it follows logically that a widespread deficiency of CoQ10 is very probable in the American population, especially among the elderly. If you are concerned about your heart, consider taking a complete B-complex vitamin that contains at least 50 to 100 mg of vitamin B6.[67]

Folic acid, vitamin B6 and vitamin B12 help lower homocysteine.

As long ago as 1969, Kilmer McCully, M.D., suggested that many Americans might have high levels of homocysteine, an intermediate metabolic amino acid, in their blood, either from their diet or because they inherited a genetic defect that required they consume sufficient amounts of these B-vitamins to keep homocysteine levels down.[68]

The likelihood of high levels of homocysteme can be reduced if methionine can be properly converted into cysteine. Folic acid, vitamin B6 and vitamin B12 are all important in this conversion. They are necessary for the metabolism of homocysteine.

The medical establishment wrote about the dangers of homocysteine when the *New England Journal of Medicine* (April 9, 1998) and the *Journal of the American Medical Association* (Dec. 18, 1996) published articles suggesting that vitamin supplements should be used to lower homocysteine levels.

These three important B-vitamins—*folic acid, vitamin B6* and *vitamin B12*—perform several functions in the body to help reduce the amount of homocysteine in the blood.[69]

Recently, researchers have found that a high level of homocysteine is an independent risk factor for cardiovascular disease. Elevated homocysteine is related to injured blood vessels, causing hardening of the arteries and thus, contributing to heart attacks and strokes. Folic acid supplements apparently can reduce blood levels of this amino acid to a safe range.[70]

The good news is that just about everyone's homocysteine levels will fall when they consume sufficient amounts of folic acid and vitamin B12, as they work in tandem in the body. Vitamin B6 also has a homocysteine-lowering effect, so take the entire B complex in sufficient quantities.

Taking supplemental folic acid, vitamin B6 and vitamin B12, quickly and effectively restores homocysteme to safe levels, essentially eliminating this very important risk, often within a few days (although the damage done by long-term elevated homocysteine takes longer to resolve).[71] Use the B12 sublingual lozenge (under the tongue) for better assimilation.

Natural and safe ways to lower cholesterol

A number of natural substances have been found to help many people reduce their cholesterol to safe levels. In this part of the chapter I recommend some safe alternatives for you.

The best approach is through diet and lifestyle modifications, but many times additional support is needed. Cholesterol-lowering drugs have many negative side effects, but fortunately, a number of natural substances can produce similar effects on blood cholesterol and triglyceride levels. However, if you are taking cholesterol-lowering drugs, do not stop using them without medical supervision, this is important.

NIACIN IS A LIPID-LOWERING AGENT. Niacin or nicotinic acid—vitamin B3—has finally been regarded as one of the substances of choice for lowering blood levels of cholesterol. A special form of niacin is *inositol hexaniacinate*. This form of niacin will save you from the side effects associated with the flush caused by the standard form of niacin. Inositol hexaniacinate, is composed of six nicotinic acid molecules bound to, and surrounding one molecule of inositol (a B-vitamin). Inositol hexaniacinate exerts the benefits of niacin without flushing or other side effects. Michael Murray, N.D., says, "It has been used in Europe for over 30 years not only to lower cholesterol, but also to improve blood flow in the treatment of intermittent claudication (a painful cramp in the calf muscle) and Raynaud's phenomena (a constriction of blood vessels to the hands)."[72]

"Although inositol hexaniacinate yields slightly better results than standard niacin, the big advantage is that it is safer and much better tolerated" according to Dr. Murray. No adverse reactions were reported in one study from 153 patients who took doses that ranged between 600 and 1,800 milligrams per day.[73]

Julian Whitaker, M.D., feels, *"the best single 'magic bullet' for high cholesterol levels is this same special form of niacin, inositol hexaniacinate.* If niacin were a patentable drug, this message would have been blasted over the airwaves. However, niacin is not patentable. So, most working to control their cholesterol levels will probably never hear about it," he says.

Dr. Whitaker's Guide to Natural Healing reports, "It's a simple prescription. It's simple to take. You can find this form of niacin in a nutrition store. Individuals with cholesterol levels above 280 should start with 500 milligrams, three times a day with meals, for two weeks. Then increase it to 1,000 milligrams three times per day thereafter. For individuals with elevated cholesterol levels below 280, the lower dose is all that is needed. After two months, check your cholesterol levels.

They may already be in the target range. If so, reduce the inositol hexa-niacinate dose by half, or just take it every other day. Check your levels in a month. If the levels have stabilized or are improving, you may no longer need this supplement. If they are rising, increase the levels," Dr. Whitaker feels that the evidence that supports this approach is compelling.[74]

Standard niacin is known to have side effects in many people at these high therapeutic doses. The complaints range from flushing of the skin to fatigue and some stomach irritation. For this reason, many physicians have stayed away from niacin. However, this safer alterna-tive (inositol hexaniacinate) is now available at most nutrition stores.

There are some great studies where the standard form of niacin was used, I am sure in divided doses. You will find when taking this form of niacin you will experience a "niacin flush," which is caused by arteries opening and bringing blood rapidly to the head, neck, and upper part of the body, making it very warm and in some cases, hot. Ladies, it is similar to a "hot flash".

However, in a Harvard University Medical School study, cholesterol was lowered 18 percent in over 100 heart patients taking a gram (1,000) of niacin daily. Niacin also improved the beneficial HDL. A dosage of 1,500 mg (1.5 grams) daily can result in a lowering of the dangerous LDL by 30 percent. Dosages up to 7,500 mg daily have been used to lower blood cholesterol levels an average of 45 percent. This (7,500 mg) is two drastic a dose to be unsupervised and should only be done under the guidance of a physician.[75] Researchers showed that 800 mg was found to be ineffective. But in some, a dose as little as 1,200 mg per day was found to be effective.

Dr. James D. Alderman, senior fellow in cardiology at Beth Israel Hospital in Boston, has concluded that niacin in doses up to two grams (2,000 mg) a day can "offer more lipid (fat) lowering benefits than traditional medication or diet alone."[76] Make sure you use a form of "flush free" or "no-flush" niacin at these higher doses.

The value of granulated soy lecithin

For almost fifty years my Mother, Gladys Lindberg, recommended the daily addition of one or two tablespoons of granulated soy lecithin to her clients' health routine. She knew it worked. Early research showed that lecithin is a powerful emulsifying agent and for this very reason is particularly important in cardiovascular health.[77]

Lecithin is a natural phosphatide, an essential constituent of all living cells of the human body. It is continuously produced by the liver, passes into the intestine with bile, and is absorbed into the blood. Lecithin is admired for its "soap-like" characteristics and the fact that it acts as a powerful emulsifying agent in the blood to help dissolve cholesterol. It works to rid the body of cholesterol in two ways:

- First, lecithin stimulates the transportation of cholesterol to the liver, before the cholesterol has a chance to accumulate or settle as plaque.

- Second, lecithin promotes the production of an enzyme that dissolves cholesterol that has already accumulated, and eases its transport to the liver. This process helps to prevent many cholesterol related diseases, such as atherosclerosis. The vital organs and arteries are protected from fatty build-up when lecithin is added to the diet.[78]

Lecithin serves as structural material for every cell in the body, particularly those of the brain and nerves. In a healthy person, it forms 30 percent of the dry weight of the brain and 73 percent of the total liver fat, both of which are greatly decreased in persons dying of heart disease.[79]

Our dear family friend and famous nutritionist, Adelle Davis reported, "All atherosclerosis is characterized by an increase of the blood cholesterol and a decrease in lecithin.[80] As early as 1935 it was shown that experimental heart disease, produced by feeding choles-terol to animals, could be prevented merely by giving a small amount of lecithin. Atherosclerosis has since been repeatedly produced in various species either by decreasing the blood lecithin or increasing the cholesterol. If enough lecithin is given, the disease does not occur regardless of how much cholesterol is fed. Even when atherosclerosis is far advanced, health is restored after lecithin is supplied in the diet."[81] This is tremendous news that health can be restored, reported in scien-tific literature almost 70 years ago!

Adelle also reported, "Many physicians have successfully reduced blood cholesterol with lecithin. For example, 4 to 6 tablespoons have been given daily to patients who had suffered heart attacks and been consistently resistant to many cholesterol-lowering medications, some for as long as ten years. Although no other dietary change was made, within three months the level of blood cholesterol dropped markedly, in one case from 1,012 to 186 milligrams. These patients felt more energetic, had an increased capacity for work, and were relieved of pain and other symptoms. After the blood cholesterol has once decreased, 1 or 2 tablespoons of lecithin daily have keep the blood fats at normal levels, though larger amounts have been taken over long periods with good results."

"Supplements of lecithin have also caused the pain of angina to disappear and have been especially beneficial to elderly persons who have suffered strokes or have cerebral atherosclerosis," according to Adelle Davis research.[82]

Lecithin is available primarily in three forms—granules, liquid, and soft gelatin capsules. The granular form is the most effective and also least expensive. It takes ten large lecithin capsules to equal just one tablespoon of granulated lecithin, and the liquids are heavily diluted with other oils, and therefore would not be as clinically useful. Granules are practically tasteless. Mix them into your protein shake, with orange juice, milk, water, or sprinkled on breakfast cereal or yogurt. One customer told me that he loved it on his salad with vinegar and oil dressing.

Note: *The good HDL cholesterol is manufactured partly from the body's natural emulsifier, lecithin.*

Nutrients such as polyunsaturated fatty acids, the B-complex vitamins, and the minerals magnesium and phosphorus are used by our bodies in the manufacture of lecithin. If we are deficient in any of these nutrients, our bodies will not make the right amount of the essential HDL.

Lecithin is a source of linoleic acid, as well as choline and inositol, which play a number of important roles in the body. Since linoleic acid cannot be produced by the body, lecithin's role as a source of this essential fatty acid is critical. Lecithin's primary role in cardiovascular health is its ability to lower cholesterol levels, but it also helps age-related memory loss. For more information on the value of lecithin for our memory, see chapter 7.

A personal testimony

Mary Lou wrote to me about her husband's remarkable recovery:

> Last year he suffered two heart attacks, had six clogged arteries and had two angioplasty operations. After leaving the hospital, his condition deteriorated. He was so weak

that he couldn't walk to the kitchen. Although he was in great pain, I was told there was nothing I could do to help my husband.

I read in a nutrition book that six tablespoons of granular soy lecithin could dramatically lower blood cholesterol levels in three months. So I gave my husband eight table-spoons of lecithin a day along with a protein drink and a high potency combination of vitamins and minerals. Within two weeks, his energy returned and his face regained its color. We witnessed a miracle! The lecithin took care of his cholesterol problem and it saved his life. We have renamed him *Lazarus*.

Mary Lou has since called me several times. Her husband is doing great and he now takes six tablespoons of lecithin! This is an example of a precious couple who got involved in their health and found a wonderful answer.

The chromium connection

I have always known that the value of chromium was for stabilizing insulin levels and therefore was very important for diabetics. Now we know that disturbances of carbohydrate metabolism are characteristic of other disorders. An added bonus from chromium is its action in reducing high blood levels of cholesterol and triglycerides, fats that accumulate in the arteries and often lead to heart attack or stroke.

According to a study first presented to the American College of Cardiology by Finnish researchers, high levels of insulin in the blood should be considered a risk factor for heart disease. In a group of 1,040 men between 35 and 64 years of age, high levels of the hormone (insulin) were associated with a two-to-three fold increase in the incidence of heart attacks.[83]

Another study tested blood levels of chromium in people with heart disease and people without the disease. The people with heart disease had consistently lower chromium status, while none of the people with normal blood chromium concentration had the disease. In fact, low chromium levels were found to be more reliable in predicting atherosclerosis than high blood levels of cholesterol and triglycerides, and high blood pressure.[84] Most authorities agree that the optimum daily intake for chromium is 200 to 400 mcg for men and women. Chromium picolinate and chromium polynicotinate are the best forms.

Is your thyroid gland functioning properly?

There is a very important connection between the thyroid gland, cholesterol and heart disease. People with low thyroid function have higher rates of coronary artery disease. This was described in Dr. Broda Barnes first book, *Heart Attack Rareness in Thyroid-Treated Patients.* If you have stubborn cholesterol, you may have low thyroid. Studies show that even mildly reduced thyroid function can cause elevations in "bad" cholesterol and decrease the "good" cholesterol. Be sure to read chapter 10, *Importance of a Properly Functioning Thyroid,* and take the simple, at home temperature test. This is an easy way to rule out part of your problem.

Latest Supplements for Healthy Cholesterol

Policosanol and red yeast rice are very helpful supplements for healthy cholesterol.

Policosanol

Policosanol is a natural supplement made from sugar cane. The main constituent is octacosanol. Octacosanol is an alcohol found in the waxy film that plants have over their leaves and fruit. The leaves and rinds of citrus fruit also contain octacosanol, and so does wheat germ oil.

Policosanol is a supplement that can normalize cholesterol as well or better than drugs, without the side effects, according to *Life Extension*, June 2001.[85] They report, "Efficacy and safety have been proven in numerous clinical trials, and it has been used by millions of people in other countries. Policosanol can lower LDL cholesterol as much as 20 percent and raise protective HDL cholesterol by 10 percent. This compares favorably with cholesterol lowering drugs that have the drawback of side effects such as liver dysfunction and muscle atrophy. Policosanol is free of these side effects."

Dosage for policosanol is usually 5 to 20 mg a day. It can be taken with other drugs,[86] and seems to enhance the effects of statin drugs, especially in conjunction with aspirin. No serious side effects have ever been reported for this cholesterol modifying supplement, and it cost 90 percent less than the leading cholesterol-modifying drugs. Policosanol is available in your nutrition store.

Red Yeast Rice

Red yeast rice *(monascus purpureus)* is native to China. It is a fermentation by-product of cooked non-glutenous rice on which red yeast has been grown.[87] It has been used by the Chinese as both a food and a medicinal agent since 800 A.D. Even during the Ming Dynasty (1368–1644), its therapeutic benefits as both a promoter of blood circulation and a digestive stimulant were first noted.[88]

Now it has been clinically investigated as a therapy for reducing cholesterol in human trials. In one trial, both men and women taking 1.2 grams (approximately 13.5 mg total monacolins) of a concentrated red yeast rice extract per day for two months had significant decreases in serum cholesterol levels.[89] In addition they had a significant increase in HDL (good) cholesterol and a decrease in LDL (bad) cholesterol. Elevated triglycerides were also found to be lowered.

At UCLA School of Medicine, a double-blind trial determined that red yeast rice in the amount of 2.4 grams per day (equals about 10 mg total monacolins) taken orally in capsule form, significantly decreased total cholesterol and LDL cholesterol levels in a sample of people with elevated cholesterol after 12 weeks of therapy. Triglycerides were also reduced in those taking red yeast rice. However, the HDL values did not increase substantially.[90]

Red yeast rice is generally well tolerated with possible temporary mild side effects such as heartburn or gas.[91] Do not take if you are pregnant or nursing. Consult your physician before using this product if you are taking any medications. It is available at your nutrition store.

Herbs for the Heart

Hawthorn berry—The heart herb

Hawthorn (*Crataegus monogyna* and *oxyacantha*)—both the berry and flower-tops extract—is widely used in Europe for heart problems. The heart benefit properties of this herb have been reported for centuries. Regular use is said to strengthen the heart muscle. The extracts have a combination of effects that are of great value to those suffering from angina, as well as other heart problems.

A number of studies have also demonstrated that hawthorn extracts are effective in lowering blood pressure and serum cholesterol levels.[92]

According to the *Encyclopedia of Natural Medicine*, the beneficial effects of hawthorn extracts are the result of improvement in two basic heart functions: heart metabolism and the dilation of coronary vessels, which increases the blood flow and thus oxygen to the heart. The recommended dosage of hawthorn extract containing 10 percent procyanidins is 100 to 250 mg taken three times a day.[93]

Garlic's benefit to the heart

What are garlic's specific benefits to the heart? Garlic prevents platelets (blood cells responsible for clotting) from sticking to each other and to artery walls. By preventing excess clotting, it may protect against coronary thrombosis (blood clots), atherosclerosis, and strokes.[94]

In addition, there's strong evidence that garlic normalizes fats in the blood by lowering harmful fats and raising protective lipids. In numerous animal and human studies, components of garlic have lowered cholesterol, triglycerides, harmful LDL levels, and dangerous very-low-density lipoprotein cholesterol (VLDL), while raising the beneficial HDL level.[95]

Many medical authorities feel that garlic can reduce high blood pressure, perhaps by acting as a vasodilator.

Garlic preparations are available in liquid extract, capsules, softgels and tablet form. Look for a high-potency garlic at your nutrition store.

Cayenne is more than a hot spice

Like many herbs, cayenne pepper *(Capsicum frutescens)*, also known as *capsicum*, is used for medicinal as well as for culinary purposes. In recent years, more than 650 studies of capsaicin (the "hot" property in cayenne pepper) have been published, including more than 100 clinical studies in human beings. Capsicum is excellent for equalizing blood circulation, which helps to prevent strokes and heart attacks. It increases the heart action, effectively increasing circulation without increasing blood pressure.[96]

Heart healthy oils

These essential oils are the omega-3 fatty acids (EPA) and should be part of your healthy heart and cholesterol-lowering program. Many researchers have reported on the value of eating fish to maintain a healthy heart. This includes eating all types of cold-water fish such as salmon, herring, mackerel, sardines and sea bass, all rich sources of the omega-3 fatty acids. Fish eaters are more apt to escape aging diseases, such as heart disease, cancer, arthritis, diabetes, psoriasis and bronchitis, studies consistently show. Fish eaters around the world live longer, such as the Japanese, who eat three times more fish than Americans, and hold the world record for longevity.

The omega-3 fatty acids mainly protect arteries by "thinning the blood," somewhat as aspirin does, thus discouraging blood clotting that triggers heart attacks and strokes, according to Jean Carper.[97] She says, "Such marine fat also lowers blood pressure and triglycerides, a potentially dangerous blood fat, raised good-type HDL cholesterol, regulates heart beats, makes aged arteries more flexible and helps block inflammatory processes that promote arthritis, cancer, psoriasis, diabetes and general cell dysfunction."

A study of men with high cholesterol examined the effects of supplementing their diet with omega-3 oils or eating cold-water fish. After five weeks, the beneficial cholesterol (HDL) levels in all the men increased and their triglyceride level decreased.[98]

Remarkable new research suggests that fish oil may be a marvelous supplement to help regulate heart rhythms and prevent fatal cardiac arrhythmias. Researchers feel that the most profound benefits from fish oil come directly from protecting the heart against electrical malfunction, that may lead to sudden death.[99]

Two major studies conducted in England and France indirectly *confirm the therapeutic ability of omega-3 fatty acids to suppress fatal arrhythmias after a heart attack.*[100]

In studies of about 1,600 patients, those who ate omega-3s as fatty fish or fish oil capsules were much less apt to suffer subsequent fatal heart attacks (but not necessarily nonfatal heart attacks) than those not consuming high levels of omega-3s. In fact, in one study not a single patient eating high amounts of omega-3s died of cardiac arrest.[101]

BODYBUILDERS AND DIETERS USE *FLAXSEED OIL*. It contains alpha-linolenic acid (omega-3) fatty acids same as fish, and is also a good source of linoleic acid (omega-6), and oleic acid (omega 9). Omega-3s are direct precursors to important anabolic hormones, so most body-builders use flaxseed oil for maximum muscle development. Dieters have found it a powerful aid in weight management and appetite control as well.

I have my clients add organic flaxseed oil to their *Super Energy Protein Shake* (see the last chapter) in the morning as it helps keep their energy level elevated. This Protein Shake is low carbohydrate, high protein and no fat, so it needs this natural oil to help keep you full longer. Flaxseed oil is valuable not only for your heart, but for beautiful skin and hair.

The Omega-3 oils are difficult to get from your diet since they are available mostly from fish. I recommend flaxseed oil since it has five times more omega 3s than any other oil.[102] Make sure that it is organic, and be sure you do not cook or heat this oil. Keep it fresh, as it turns rancid easily. Flaxseed oil should be in dark-color bottles in the refrigerated section of your nutrition store. This oil is great with apple cider vinegar and your favorite seasoning for salads.

Omega-6 oils (GLA) are found in evening primrose oil, borage oil and black currant seed oil.[103] In addition to supporting normal joint function and flexibility, these oils also help maintain healthy, moisturized skin, normal blood pressure and cholesterol, plus a healthy emotional balance during hormonal changes.[104]

Exercise Your Heart

The birth of the "exercise movement" could not have come at a better time in our nation's history. While exercise is not the only answer to heart problems, it surely aids in the prevention of heart disease.

Doctors are now realizing that people can benefit from, and need, a varied fitness program. Dr. Kenneth Cooper says, "We used to think exercise had to be three times a week with your heart rate at 60 to 90 percent of capacity for 20 to 30 minutes to get any benefit. We used to see it as all or nothing. But now studies are showing we can get benefits from other exercise prescriptions. People seem to have a favorable impact on health even from moderate walking."[105]

IMPORTANCE OF STRENGTH TRAINING. In studies at Tufts University, researchers found that strength—not aerobic capacity—was a significant factor in fitness. Dr. Miriam Nelson, a research scientist at Tufts has said, "What we see is that if you look at 20 to 40 year olds, their walking and running speed is directly related to their aerobic capacity, to their heart's ability to work. But for people in their 80s and 90s, walking speed is directly related to their strength. What aerobics can do for people under 60, strength training can do for people in their 60s and older."[106]

Note: *Chelation therapy may be very important in support of the heart. This information is discussed in the* Anti-Aging Therapies *chapter. In the same chapter there is information on the hormone DHEA, which shows positive effects in lowering cholesterol, preventing blood clot formation and protection against both heart disease and stroke.*

Conclusion

There is a tremendous amount of valuable information in this chapter to help you learn how to take charge of your health, and to keep your heart strong and healthy. Read my basic nutritional program discussed in the *Let's Put it All Together* chapter.

I pray this information will help you on your path to abundant health and vitality.

If the Pressure Is Up, Let's Turn It Down!

Natural Ways
to Lower Blood Pressure

People who are healthy feel well in body and mind. Free from aches and pains, they have robust energy, a spring to their step, bright eyes, good color, and a pleasant outlook on life. That is not to say healthy people don't have their share of situations that try their patience and temper. But when circumstances are difficult, healthy people are much more likely to cope in a calm, capable manner. They are usually fit in body, soul, and spirit.

—GLADYS LINDBERG

How do hypertension and stroke fit into the anti-aging puzzle? Studies show that years of uncontrolled high blood pressure damage delicate capillaries throughout the body, and it also appears to accelerate the development of atherosclerotic plaques in the arteries. Approximately one in six Americans suffer from hypertension—at least 38 million people—and hundreds of thousands more suffer its ill effects, include stroke, kidney disease, congestive heart failure, and eye disease.

You will not have the opportunity to enjoy your "golden years" and accomplish all you want to do in life if you allow these diseases to impair or shorten it unnecessarily.

According to an article in the *Journal of the American Medical Association*, "Treatment of hypertension has become the leading reason for visits to physicians as well as for drug prescriptions.[1] Yearly sales of blood pressure medications are estimated to be greater than 10 billion dollars. It is estimated that approximately 80 percent of patients with high blood pressure are in the borderline to mild range."[2] If in a borderline range, many experts believe that much may be done to help these people naturally. Do not, however, discontinue any medication prescribed for you, without your doctor's recommendation.

The Silent Killer—High Blood Pressure

Hypertension has been called the *silent killer* because it normally has no visible symptoms.

To understand high blood pressure, you need to know a few interesting facts about the heart. The human heart beats on average 70 times per minute, 100,000 times a day, and 2.5 billion times in a lifetime. With each heartbeat, about 2.5 ounces of blood are pumped through the heart—that is 1,980 gallons every day.[3] What an amazing organ our heart is!

Our blood pressure is actually the force exerted by the blood against the walls of the blood vessels. It is our blood pressure that forces oxygen or plasma—that is carrying glucose, amino acids, fatty acids, vitamins, and minerals—into the tissues through porous microscopic capillary walls. Normal blood pressure is vital to the nutrition of the cells. When the blood in the capillary beds becomes concentrated from the loss of plasma, the blood protein (albumin) attracts tissue fluids that carry waste into the vessels. This causes the quantity of blood to remain remarkably constant. Thus, by virtue of the blood pressure, all tissues are constantly bathed in fresh, nutrient-laden fluid. Also, the breakdown products from worn-out cells are removed.

When larger amounts of oxygen and nutrients are needed, the contraction of tiny muscles in the arterial walls causes the pressure to increase and supplies to be pushed more quickly to the cells. On the other hand, if few nutrients are required, these muscles relax, the pressure decreases, and food is conserved.[4]

What are the causes?

The causes of hypertension are numerous, but any of the following may make you a candidate:

- Highest risk is heredity (family history of hypertension), particularly for those of African descent.

- Smoking—narrows the arteries, decreases the blood's ability to deliver oxygen, and nicotine stimulates the heartbeat, increasing the need for oxygen-rich blood.

- Excessive drinking of alcohol.

- Those who are 20 pounds or more overweight—extra pressure is put on the heart to pump blood through the two extra miles of capillaries for every extra pound of fat.

- Too little physical exercise. Exercise relieves physical tension, helps keep the arteries flexible, and circulates the blood more widely and evenly.

- Negative emotions like anger, fear and anxiety.

- Eating excessive sugar—creating abnormalities of lipid, glucose, and insulin metabolism (leading to diabetes).

Obviously, if you have mild or moderate hypertension, and if any of these factors relate to you, you should try to remedy the factors that put you at risk. A change in your lifestyle can be your most potent, positive ally in achieving better health and longer life.

Norman Kaplan, M.D., professor of internal medicine and chief of the hypertension unit at the University of Texas Health Sciences Center in Dallas, has said, "I believe a non-drug approach should be the first treatment of mild hypertension, where the diastolic blood pressure (bottom figure and the reading that records the pressure of blood flow between heartbeats) is between 90 and 100 millimeters."[5]

Hypertension's effect on the heart

As the blood pressure goes up, the heart must work harder to push blood throughout the body. Just as with other muscles in the body, the heart can compensate for the extra work by getting bigger and stronger, but over the years the heart basically gets worn out. Two things usually happen to the heart as a result.

First, hypertension accelerates atherosclerosis by stressing and damaging the inside lining of the arteries, promoting plaque formation. Since the heart is working harder, it requires a greater blood supply. Too much plaque can slow or stop the supply to the heart, resulting in a heart attack.

Second, hypertension damages the capillaries throughout the body, including the heart muscle. As a result, the muscle cells don't get the oxygen and nutrients they need as easily, and the heart doesn't beat as strongly. Slowly, the heart chambers begin to dilate in an attempt to maintain the blood pressure, but eventually this fails. The heart becomes enlarged, floppy and ineffective in pumping blood, and the result is congestive heart failure.

The pressure of the blood in the main arteries rises and falls as the heart and muscles of the body cope with varying demands—exercise, stress, and sleep.

TWO TYPES OF PRESSURE MEASURED

- Systolic pressure, the high number in a blood-pressure reading, is the pressure created by the contraction of the heart muscle and the elastic recoil of the aorta (great artery) as the blood surges through it.

- Diastolic pressure, the low number in a blood-pressure reading, is the pressure when the ventricles relax between beats. It reflects the resistance of all the small arteries throughout the body and the load against which the heart must work.[6]

BLOOD PRESSURE VALUES

Normal ....120/80 or less

Borderline 140/90–160/100
Hypertension 160/104

A young adult has a blood pressure reading of about 110/75, which normally rises with age to about 130/90 at age 60.

THE IDEAL PRESSURE. More and more doctors are stressing not only the importance of checking your blood pressure periodically, but also the importance of intercepting "slightly elevated" blood pressures and addressing them nutritionally. By addressing a blood pressure problem early, a person is often capable of avoiding a lifetime reliance on drugs.

Stroke—The Brain's Equivalent of a Heart Attack

A stroke results from an interruption of the brain's blood flow. It is thus a blood vessel disease, the cerebral (brain) equivalent of a heart attack.

Strokes are the third most frequent cause of death in the United States among adults and the most common cause of neurological disability. Strokes and other cerebrovascular disorders affect about 500,000 Americans annually, with more than two thirds of these patients being 65 or older. Because more aggressive therapies for high blood pressure and heart disease have been developed and used in the last 30 years, stroke deaths have dropped from 89 per 100,000 to 30 per 100,000. Still, the mortality rate for those afflicted is high. An estimated one in four stroke patients dies within a month of their brain injury. Death from stroke is 93 percent in black men and 82 percent in black women, higher than among their white counterparts.[7]

Types and causes of stroke

Stroke may be caused by any of three mechanisms. Thrombosis and embolism both lead to cessation of the blood supply to parts of the brain, and thus to infarction (tissue death). Rupture of a blood vessel in or near the brain may cause a hemorrhage. Any part of the brain may be affected by a stroke. Accordingly, the symptoms vary considerably. These are the most common types of stroke:

- Cerebral Thrombosis. Blockage by a clot (thrombus) that has built up on the wall of a brain artery accounts for 40 to 50 percent of strokes.

2. Cerebral Embolism. Blockage usually by a clot (embolus) swept into an artery in the brain accounts for 30 to 35 percent of cases.

2. Hemorrhage. Rupture of a blood vessel and bleeding within or over the surface of the brain accounts for 20 to 25 percent of the cases.[8]

Symptoms of stroke

The symptoms of a stroke usually develop over minutes or hours, but occasionally over several days. Depending on the site, cause, and extent of damage, any or all of the symptoms may be present, in any degree of severity.

There may be warning symptoms prior to strokes. These are called "transient ischemic attacks" (TIAs), because the culprit is ischemia, or lack of blood flow, and because the interruption of circulation is brief. Brain cells survive TIAs and recover full function within 24 hours in most cases.

More serious cases lead to rapid loss of consciousness, coma, severe physical or mental handicap, or death, but some strokes cause barely noticeable symptoms. Among the more common symptoms are these:

2. weakness or paralysis on one side of the body (one of the more common effects of a serious stroke)
2. headache, dizziness, confusion
2. visual disturbance
2. slurred speech or loss of speech, and difficulty swallowing.[9]

Nutrients That Impact Hypertension and Stroke

A number of nutrients have been correlated with hypertension and strokes. While there is no "magic bullet" to use for either hypertension or susceptibility to strokes, there are a number of steps to take nutritionally that may help build up your health. Many important nutrients have been discussed in other chapters. The research reported in this chapter is only that which pertains directly to factors leading to high blood pressure or strokes.

Vitamins, minerals, and herbs have all been shown to have positive effects on the heart and blood vessels, with few if any side effects. Although prevention should always be our goal, these nutrients may be of benefit to those who already have heart problems.

The Relationship of Potassium and Sodium

For years, table salt (sodium chloride) has been considered a major culprit in aggravating high blood pressure, strokes, and other cardiovascular diseases. Recent studies indicate, however, that a generally low potassium intake may be one of the greater factors. Diets high in potassium appear to be protective against hypertension and stroke-related deaths.[10]

High potassium intake appears to have no effect on people with normal blood pressure, but high potassium intake does appear to lower blood pressure in many but not all with hypertension.[11]

The importance of dietary potassium against stroke

A study by Kay-Tee Khaw, M.D., and Elizabeth Barrett-Connor, M.D., found that a high intake of dietary potassium protected people against stroke and stroke-related deaths. In fact, they found that as little as one extra serving of a potassium-rich food, such as a fruit or vegetable, may reduce the risk of stroke death by up to 40 percent.[12]

These researchers based their findings on a study of 850 men and women in an affluent community in southern California. During the 12 years covered by their study, 24 stroke-related deaths occurred. These individuals were all found to have significantly lower potassium intake than survivors and individuals who died from causes other than stroke. They also found *the relationship between dietary potassium and stroke mortality was independent of blood pressure, as it also was of obesity, cholesterol level, cigarette smoking, alcohol, and blood sugar.* This was an amazing finding, as we generally associate strokes with high blood pressure. Rather, they found that a lack of potassium intake was the independent risk factor in these stroke-related deaths.[13]

One does not need to take a very big leap in logic to conclude that an increased intake of potassium lowers the risk of stroke, and a decreased intake raises the risk.

POTASSIUM TO SODIUM RATIO. A one-year study headed by James C. Smith, Jr., Ph.D., a chemist at the USDA's Agriculture Research service, found that the 28 men and women in their study ate too much table salt (sodium chloride) and not enough potassium, exceeding the safe and adequate daily ratio recommended by the National Academy of Sciences in Washington, D.C. That ratio is 600 mg of sodium for 1,000 mg of potassium. The adults in this study were consuming 1,300 mg of sodium daily for every 1,000 mg of potassium.[14]

RECOMMENDED RANGE. As a matter of general information, a teaspoon of table salt contains about 2,500 mg of sodium. The recommended range of potassium is between 1,900 mg and 5,600 mg daily.[15]

Vitamin and mineral supplements, by FDA regulation, are only allowed to contain 99 mg of potassium. To take a higher amount you need a prescription. How silly this seems when a medium-sized banana contains approximately 630 mg of potassium.

When people consume a high level of potassium in their diets, they excrete more sodium in their urine. But when the opposite is true, and they consume more sodium than potassium, they may retain excess sodium in fluids surrounding cells in the body. Urinalysis can determine if your potassium and sodium intakes are out of balance, and if either is too high or low.

INCREASING YOUR POTASSIUM. One easy way to increase your potassium is to drink 12 ounces of low-sodium V8 juice per day. This will give you a whopping 1,240 mg of potassium. Make sure it says "low sodium" on the label.

A 2002 *Lancet* study showed that increasing consumption of fruits and vegetables to at least five servings a day lowered blood pressure. They are one of our best sources of potassium.

THE BEST NATURAL SOURCES OF POTASSIUM

One cup potato ....1,747 mg
One cup baked butternut squash ....1,200 mg
One cup almonds, cashews,
        Brazil nuts, or peanuts ....780 to 1,000 mg
Half a cantaloupe.... ....885 mg
3–4 ounces of raw spinach......................................780 mg
1 banana..... ....630 mg
1 tablespoon blackstrap molasses...........................585 mg
Half cup of toasted wheat germ ....535 mg
Half an avocado..385 mg
One cup low-fat milk..377 mg
Medium orange...365 mg[16]

These natural foods can provide valuable protection against a stroke. Best of all, these are readily available foods and are easy to prepare and eat.

MONITOR YOUR POTASSIUM LEVELS. If you are using diuretics (herbal or prescription), or are on blood pressure medication, you may need a physician's prescription for extra potassium. It would be wise to have your potassium blood levels monitored regularly. Remember, when potassium is lost by a diuretic, so is magnesium. You may need to supplement this mineral also.

Calcium is very necessary

Research has shown that individuals with high blood pressure consume far less calcium than those with normal pressures. The diets of more than 10,000 adults were analyzed. Of the 17 nutrients examined, *low calcium was most consistently associated with high blood pressure.* In the analysis of 23 studies of 38,950 people, a consistent association of high dietary calcium intake and normal blood pressure was observed.[17]

Intakes of potassium and vitamins A and C were also lower in people with higher blood pressures, while cholesterol intake was not consistently different. These researchers, who reported their study in Science, concluded that diets that restrict the intake of calories, sodium or cholesterol may also reduce the intake of calcium and other nutrients that may be protective against hypertension.[18]

In a well-designed study, women with high blood pressure were given either 1,500 mg of calcium or hypertensive medication for four years. *The calcium-supplemented group achieved a significant drop in their systolic blood pressure. The unsupplemented group experienced a rise in their blood pressure, even though they were taking hypertensive medication.*

Calcium supplementation is free of the dangerous side effects of antihypertensive drugs. As the studies indicate, calcium supplementation can be an effective non-drug means of preventing high blood pressure in high-risk individuals.[19]

Calcium should be balanced with approximately half as much magnesium. (**Note:** *Some researchers say the ratio should be equal. Watch for further studies related to this. But the side effect of too much magnesium is a loose stool.*)

Magnesium is critical and essential

The *Journal of the American College of Nutrition* reported that magnesium supplements are essential for helping control the blood pressure in people with hypertension. The exact mechanism is not yet completely understood, but it is thought that magnesium helps drop pressure by regulating the entry-exit process of calcium in the smooth muscle cells of the vascular network. In combination, magnesium and calcium appear to help the blood vessels contract and relax properly.

The interaction of magnesium and calcium gives calcium the ability to get where it has to in the cells. Then, magnesium facilitates calcium in getting to the right place where it has a relaxing effect.[20] Hypertensives were shown to have significantly less magnesium in their blood cells than did normal people.[21]

The British researchers reported their findings in the *Proceedings of the National Academy of Science*. They noted that previous studies had shown magnesium supplementation to be an effective hypotensive (lowering) agent in some types of blood pressure.[22]

Vitamins A and C and selenium lower mortality

The *International Journal for Vitamin and Nutrition Research* reported that high intakes of vitamin C, or fruit and green vegetables that are high in vitamin C, have been related to lowered mortality from stroke and heart disease. The researchers suggested that ascorbic acid has a preventive effect on hypertension.[23]

In another study of adult males, higher blood levels of vitamin C and selenium were associated with lower blood pressure. This supports the hypothesis that antioxidants play a role in hypertension.[24]

A number of studies are available showing that low dietary intake of vitamin C increases the risk for high blood pressure. Dr. D.A. McCarron and his colleagues at the University of Portland analyzed the blood pressure of 10,372 persons of all ages in relation to their dietary habits. They found that the single most important factor associated with high blood pressure was a low dietary intake of vitamin C and vice versa.

Vitamin A deficiency was also found to increase the risk for high blood pressure, while the amount of cholesterol in the diet had no effect.[25]

SMOKERS, TAKE NOTE! Blood pressure increases can be measured immediately following cigarette smoking. If you are so addicted to cigarettes and can't seem to quit at this time, research shows you have some protection with at least 400 mg of vitamin C,[26] but I would recommend a minimum of 1,000 milligrams.

Coenzyme Q10 (CoQ10)

CoQ10 is an essential component of the metabolic process involved in energy (ATP) production.[27] Clinical studies have indicated that

CoQ10 is of considerable benefit in the treatment of hypertension and other cardiovascular diseases.[28]

Stephen Sinatra, M.D., cardiologist and Executive Director of the New England Heart Center, in Manchester, Connecticut, reports that, "As the heart muscle continually uses oxygen and consumes huge amounts of energy, heart muscle cells can greatly benefit from the energy boost of Coenzyme Q10. In fact, levels of CoQ10 are usually ten times higher in the healthy heart than in any other organ. This is why a CoQ10 deficiency is most likely to primarily affect the heart and contribute to heart failure. It is estimated that 39 percent of patients with high blood pressure have a CoQ10 deficiency," says Dr. Sinatra.

Dr. P. Langsjoen, M.D., treated 109 patients with an average dose of 225 mg of CoQ10 daily. The results were a steady increase in the functioning of the cardiovascular system and a decreased need for standard high blood pressure medications within one to six months. In fact, 51 percent of patients were able to discontinue up to three different drugs only 4.4 months after starting CoQ10, even though the majority of patients had been dependent on them for at least nine years.[29]

Dr. Sinatra recommends a heart protective dose of 180 mg daily, but for high blood pressure he usually builds toward a daily dose of 180 to 360 mg a day. Clinical research indicates it usually takes four to 12 weeks for CoQ10 to have a noticeable effect on blood pressure.[30]

See more information about CoQ10 in chapter 3 and chapter 8.

EPA or fish oil

Fish oils may help retard thrombosis, the deadly blood clots that cause strokes. The result can be fewer lethal blood clots. In addition, researchers at Harvard University have documented that these same fish oils reduce blood pressure, which seems to be a risk factor for both heart attack and stroke.[31]

New studies have reported that populations with high intakes of seafood, especially mackerel, salmon and other cold water fish, have a very low incidence of cardiovascular disease and hypertension. It is believed that the omega-3 fatty acids, or EPA, can reduce not only blood pressure (systolic and diastolic), but also help drop serum triglycerides and cholesterol. In one study, the addition of only three tablespoons of cod liver oil (omega-3 oil) a day to the normal diet was enough to lower blood pressure.[32] Omega-3 fatty acids are also available in supplements without the added vitamins A and D (found in cod liver oil).

It's a great idea to start eating fish, especially salmon, several times a week, thereby getting more essential oils in your diet. More information on oils is in the *Arthritis* chapter.

Garlic—To the rescue again

Garlic has been known for years to stabilize blood pressure. This conclusion was even reported in the prestigious British medical journal, the *Lancet*.[33] One reason may be found in garlic's high amount of selenium, a trace mineral that boosts protection against platelet adhesion.

Many cultures have used garlic to help keep blood pressure in check. Years ago, Dr. G. Piotrowski of the University of Geneva showed that garlic may dilate or open up the blood vessels and promote a free-flowing circulation that is the answer to hypertension.

Many recommend the equivalency of three to four cloves of garlic every day to lower blood pressure. Also, the enteric-coated capsules that are odor-reduced or odor-free, are very effective, especially since few people desire to eat that much fresh garlic a day. There is also a liquid aged garlic extract available. Follow the dosage recommendations on the label of the product you choose.[34]

Green tea also valuable

Several studies in Japan and China have shown that green tea helps control blood pressure. A research project with 9,510 women revealed that green tea drinkers reduced their blood pressure and slashed the risk of a stroke by one half over non-green tea drinkers.[35]

Most of the research on green tea has been focused on its cancer-preventive effects. Green tea polyphenols are flavonoids that are potent antioxidant compounds.

Hawthorn berry

The very active flavonoid compounds found in the leaves, berries, and blossoms of the hawthorn plant have an ability to increase intra-cellular vitamin C levels and decrease capillary permeability and fragility. Hawthorn berry extracts are effective in reducing blood pressure and angina attacks as well as other functions. It is used in Europe for lowering blood pressure and cardiotonic activity. Hawthorn extract's effect on lowering high blood pressure appears to be a result of dilating the larger blood vessels.[36]

Some cardiologists recommend hawthorn berry extract beginning at 500 mg daily, then increasing to 1,000 mg or 1,500 mg.[37]

Clinical studies have shown that hawthorn can help reduce blood pressure by reducing or blocking the constriction of blood vessels directly serving the heart. This is crucial because when blood vessels constrict, blood pressure rises.

What about diuretics?

Diuretics—water pills—are no longer heavily favored for lowering blood pressure. They work by removing fluid from the bloodstream, which reduces the pressure on the arterial walls. However, diuretics have a mineral depleting side effect—they cause vitally needed magnesium, calcium, potassium, sodium chloride, zinc, and iodide to be flushed away from the body along with the water! Loss of these minerals can invite greater dangers than hypertension—spasms in coronary arteries, stroke, irregular heart rhythms, and heart attack. Dr. W. J. McLennan has stated that 20 percent of the people over age 65 now take diuretics, and he noted that in this age group, *diuretics bring on more adverse side effects than any other prescription drug.*[38]

Nutritional therapy for high blood pressure

David Edelberg, M.D., an internist and medical director of the American Holistic Center in Chicago, has suggested the following as a nutritional therapy to lower high blood pressure:

- cut back on sugar, salt, caffeine, and alcohol
- reduce or eliminate red meat in the diet
- 500 mg of calcium, twice a day
- 400 mg of magnesium, twice a day
- one tablespoon of flaxseed oil a day
- 400 IU of vitamin E a day
- 30 mg of Coenzyme Q$_{10}$, three times a day
- one hawthorn berry capsule, three times a day
- one ginseng capsule, twice a day[39]

My personal modifications to this list would be as follows. You need more than just calcium and magnesium. You should include a complete mineral formula that provides: selenium, zinc, copper, chromium, iodine, boron, manganese, and potassium. It would be important to include a complete "stress" vitamin B-complex, vitamins A and D, and at least a gram (1,000 mg) of vitamin C, two or three times a day. I would also suggest fish several times a week, or fish oil capsules and flaxseed oil. Also high potassium fruit, vegetables and garlic would be beneficial.

Go back and read the *Heart* chapter, especially on CoQ10. Many doctors now give 300 mg of CoQ10 to lower blood pressure. Also read the last chapter, *Let's Put It All Together,* and consider my suggestions for a complete nutritional program, then check the potencies of your vitamin and mineral formulas and see if they are adequate.

Low Blood Pressure

As we have shown, blood pressure means the push or force of blood against the walls of the blood vessels. Only when the tissues of the vessel walls are strong can the blood pressure be maintained at its normal level. If these tissues become flabby and weak, they exert less force against the arterial walls, and adequate supplies of all the nutrients fail to reach the cells, resulting in fatigue and lack of endurance.

Low blood pressure is also called *hypotension*. In adults the pressure is usually less than 90 mm systolic (when the heart beats). In some people, their blood pressure drops when they rise from a horizontal position, which may cause light-headedness or brief loss of consciousness due to temporarily insufficient flow of blood to the brain. Severe hypotension may lead to inadequate blood circulation and shock.[40]

Since relaxation is greatest during the night, the person with low blood pressure finds that he/she is especially exhausted in the early morning, and just getting out of bed is a chore. They are usually sensitive to cold and heat, require more sleep than healthy individuals and develop a rapid pulse on exertion.

The thyroid connection

Low blood pressure is not necessarily healthy just because it isn't high. One of the common symptoms of hypothyroidism (low thyroid) is also low blood pressure. Take the Broda Barnes Temperature Test found in chapter 10 and see if your temperature reading is below normal. This may be the root cause or a key to your energy level. Low thyroid patients usually have trouble getting started in the morning; they are often fatigued, which varies from relatively mild to severe. They are usually sensitive to cold (especially cold hands and feet), and the symptoms go on and on.

The one point you need to remember is mild cases of low thyroid are often not detected in routine blood tests, so subclinical hypothyroidism mostly "falls through the cracks," according to Dr. H. Jack

Baskin. "Your doctor might try to convince you that your symptoms are 'a normal part of aging' or 'nothing to worry about.' Don't buy it," said Dr. Baskin. "It's your quality of life that is being severely compromised, and it is your right to get to the bottom of these 'minor' ailments."[41]

Low adrenal function

Adelle Davis, in *Let's Get Well*, recommends that the adrenal glands need to be fully supported since low adrenals play a part in both low blood pressure and low thyroid. Many of the symptoms such as feeling tired, can't get going, lack of energy, are very similar.[42] The B vitamin pantothenic acid is essential for adrenal support.

Our adrenal glands produce a powerful steroid hormone, aldosterone, which is a major factor in regulating salt and water balance in our bodies, making sure that our bodies "retain" enough salt for normal function, including normal blood pressure.[43] If the adrenals are weak, less than optimum amounts of aldosterone is produced, and blood pressure falls. Iodized sea salt, a natural salt with all the trace minerals, may be added to the diet. You can find this at most grocery and nutrition stores.

Years of prolonged stress, which increases the need for a proper diet and supplementation of all the vitamins and minerals, may have brought on low blood pressure along with low adrenals. Especially important are both pantothenic acid and the adrenal glandulars, which are valuable for adrenal support and discussed in the *Arthritis* chapter under "exhausted adrenal glands."

Vitamin B12 and anemia

Interestingly, hypotension is also one of the symptoms of pernicious anemia, believed to be caused by nutritional deficiencies of vitamin B12. Be sure to use the sublingual (dissolved under your tongue) B12 lozenge to help in the assimilation.

In a 17-year study of B12-deficient patients, researchers at Columbia-Presbyterian Medical Center and Harlem Hospital determined that pernicious anemia was the most common symptom of the deficiency. Other associated symptoms included muscle weakness, poor reflexes, mood swings and low blood pressure.[44] If these are your symptoms, it would be important for you to go back and read how essential it is to have enough B12 in your system. See chapter 7 on the *Brain*, which discusses this information on vitamin B12 and how it effects us in detail.

Taking Charge of Your Own Health

Nutritional supplements may aid in reversing the conditions that lead to hypertension, heart disease, heart attack, and stroke. Much can be done to prevent cardiovascular problems, which should be our primary concern. As is true for virtually all health problems, no one magic nutrient may help to correct this most serious situation. Preventive nutrition requires a multifaceted approach—nutrients, exercise, changes in lifestyle, all working together to synergistically put this country's population back on the road to better health.

The Importance of a Properly Functioning Thyroid

Recognizing Conditions Related to the Thyroid

It seems amazing that most of the people I speak with show so many symptoms of low thyroid. This may be the important key to unlocking the door of abundant health.
—GLADYS LINDBERG

*W*hen my clients come to me with various nutritional questions, I love to shake their hand as I welcome them. Many times, much to my amazement, their hands are very cold. Then this dear person tells me how tired they are, how they have no energy, and can't get going in the morning. Not only are their hands cold, but so are their feet. This brings to mind the seminars I've attended and the lovely dinners I've shared with the charming Broda Barnes, M.D. Cold hands are one of Dr. Barnes' major symptoms of hypothyroidism, or low thyroid function.

The Need for an Optimal Thyroid Level

Thyroid problems are far more prevalent in our society than one might think. "Low thyroid" is a condition that very often masquerades as other ailments, and the symptoms vary widely. The good news is that it can generally be addressed very successfully—if first you know what you are dealing with!

It may help for you to know a little about the thyroid gland, the most important endocrine gland in the human body. It controls the cell's metabolic activity and is responsible for keeping every cell and tissue in the body healthy.

The thyroid is a butterfly-shaped gland. It only weighs about two thirds of an ounce and straddles the windpipe just below the Adam's apple. Every hour, about five quarts of blood circulate through your thyroid gland, bringing iodide (a compound of iodine with a more electropositive atom or group) to the gland, as well as hormones from the pituitary gland that stimulate the thyroid into production. Iodide is the material your thyroid gland uses to make its hormone. The thyroid gland makes, stores, and discharges thyroid hormone into the bloodstream for delivery to your cells where and when it is needed. This hormone production is normally less than 1/100,000 of an ounce.[1]

Hypothyroidism is a condition in which a person has too little output from the thyroid gland. According to Broda Barnes, M.D., Ph.D., perhaps the most famous thyroid researcher and author of

Hypothyroidism: The Unsuspected Illness, along with other authorities reports that the symptoms related to low thyroid vary widely:

SYMPTOMS OF LOW THYROID OR HYPOTHYROIDISM

- Sensitivity to cold—especially in hands and feet.
- A young housewife who feels rundown, tires easily, is sleepy much of the time, and strangely oversensitive to cold weather.
- A child or adult unusually prone to infections, particularly respiratory infections, but not limited to them.
- Frequent bouts of cold or influenza.
- A victim of severe recurrent headaches.
- Poor circulation—due to heart not pumping with sufficient force.
- Fatigue, varies from relatively mild to severe. May come to accept fatigability as a virtually normal state.
- Coarse hair or hair loss.
- Dry eyes/blurred vision.
- Weight gain, inability to lose weight despite constant dieting.
- Digestion problems—irritable bowel syndrome or acid indigestion, constipation.
- Menstrual disturbances, painful flow, irregular, or sometimes excessive flow that suggests possible need for hysterectomy.
- Memory disturbances, concentration difficulties, severe mental depression, paranoid symptoms. Behavioral and emotional disorders, anxiety/panic attacks.
- The barren couple, both male and female, unable to conceive.
- Low blood pressure.
- Weak or dormant sex urge.
- Many skin disorders, including psoriasis and acne sometimes respond to thyroid medication. Dry, coarse, leathery skin.
- Swelling or puffy eyelids; lower half of eyebrow missing.
- High cholesterol and atherosclerosis.
- Wounds that heal slowly.
- Enlarged thyroid—goiter.
- Rheumatic pain—moderate to severe.
- Asthma and allergies.[2]

Each of these symptoms has been reported by people with low thyroid, as well as the feeling, "I just can't seem to get going." The effect of low thyroid is felt in each of the trillions of cells, in every organ and tissue of the body.

As early as 1957, Dr. A.S. Jackson, a nationally recognized authority on the thyroid gland, published a paper in the *Journal of the American Medical Association*, declaring that low thyroid function was the most common disease entering the doctor's office and was the diagnosis most often missed.[3] The situation is much the same today.

Laboratory tests fail to uncover low thyroid

A book written in 1960, *The Thyroid-Vitamin Approach to Cholesterol, Atheromatosis and Chronic Disease*, details a ten-year study. The author, Murray Israel, M.D., was founder of the Vascular Research Foundation in New York. In almost 40 years of practice, during which time numerous studies and experiments were conducted, *Dr. Israel observed that laboratory testing failed to uncover even a minute fraction of the people with low thyroid function.* He found the standard tests indicated that 85 percent of his patients had normal thyroid function, yet all of them showed marked benefits from thyroid supplementation, which increased body temperature, energy, and vitality.[4]

H. Jack Baskin, M.D., vice-president of the American Association of Clinical Endocrinologists, reports eight million Americans (seven times more women than men) have some sort of thyroid problems, but only half of those have been diagnosed. A vast majority of these have an underactive thyroid. Baskin went on to discuss the diverse conditions like the ones I have listed:

> While extreme hypothyroidism is rare and is easily identi-fied, mild cases are often not detected in routine blood tests, so subclinical hypothyroidism mostly falls through the cracks. Your doctor might try to convince you that your symptoms are "a normal part of aging" or "nothing to worry about." Don't buy it," Dr. Baskin said. "It's your quality of life that is being severely compromised, and it is your right to get to the bottom of these "minor" ailments.[5]

So it appears that after all these years this information is still being ignored. But, addressing this issue may very well be the key that unlocks the door to better health for countless people.

"The Biochemical Approach to the Aging Process" was a lecture given by Murray Israel, M.D., in New York in 1959. He is the doctor who did the ten-year study with thyroid and vitamins for chronic diseases. He said the subject could be discussed for hours and hours and went on to say, "The one aspect that seems at this time to be the most vital and the least understood; the hormone-vitamin approach to the control of the rate of aging—a recent development that is making it possible to prolong the better years."[6]

Dr. Israel continued, "In the human being, when the thyroid gland becomes inadequate, all the metabolic processes become disturbed. The person becomes tired, nervous, irritable, depressed. The metabolic pathways become deranged—the rate of aging becomes accelerated. And this can occur at any age. There are many other factors affecting the rate of aging besides thyroid hormone inadequacy. These factors, however, are of secondary importance and can only be considered after the thyroid deficiency has first been taken care of."[7]

The conductor of the metabolic symphony

"It is my opinion," Israel said, "therefore, that the thyroid hormone should be considered the conductor of the metabolic symphony. This does not mean that the thyroid hormone can conduct this symphony of all individuals and bring forth 100 percent cures or perfectly harmonious chords. If part of the members of the orchestra (such as the other glands of internal secretion that produce hormones) are not functioning, or are functioning very poorly, the resulting music will be discordant."[8]

Dr. Israel also concluded with his studies that "vitamin research has implicated a whole series of substances—chiefly members of the vitamin B-complex, for example, nicotinic acid (B_3) and pyridoxine (B_6), ascorbic acid (vitamin C) and lipotropic factors (choline, methionine and inositol from soy lecithin). These need to be given in standard amounts along with thyroid extract. To put it another way, thyroid cannot be successfully or safely administered without them."[9]

A Simple Thyroid Test

The earliest studies in England show that the hypothyroid (low thyroid function) patient consistently runs temperatures below normal. The body thermostat of a thyroid deficient person generally cries for more heat, essential for the oxidation of fuel in the body. In the thyroid deficient body, the temperature falls below normal because of inadequate oxidation. In hyperthyroid (high thyroid) too much thyroid is

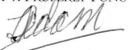

circulating, so much heat is produced that the body's thermostat cannot control the body temperature precisely and the result is a low-grade fever, or a high temperature.

Dr. Barnes studied 1,569 patients over a period of 20 years to determine the role of thyroid deficiency in heart disease. He also reviewed the medical literature, reading studies dating back to 1918 and 1925, which showed that thyroid therapy was an effective measure in preventing heart attacks.[10] How unfortunate that these early experi-ments, which clearly showed the relationship between thyroid deficiency and heart disease, were overlooked.

The basal temperature is not a perfect test for thyroid function. There are conditions other than hypothyroidism that may produce a low reading—for example, starvation, pituitary gland deficiency, or adrenal gland deficiency. Starvation is easy to rule out—and some thyroid is frequently indicated, anyhow, for the other conditions, reported Dr. Barnes.

Dr. Broda Barnes says, "Take your temperature."

He came to this conclusion as the result of studies involving more than a thousand college students, and later, thousands of soldiers during World War II. He concluded that a subnormal body temperature is a better indicator of hypothyroidism and the need of thyroid treatment than basal metabolic rate.

Although the basal temperature test is not 100 percent specific for thyroid function, the simple procedure is remarkably successful in uncovering hypothyroidism. Its results most often fit well with patient's symptoms.

The following chart shows the method that Dr. Barnes has suggested as an easy test for low thyroid function.

BARNES BASAL TEMPERATURE TEST FOR THYROID FUNCTION

Use a mercury thermometer (not digital). Shake it down well when you go to bed. When you awaken in the morning, slip the thermometer snugly under your armpit before you get out of bed and leave it there for ten minutes by the clock. Normal temperature for this method is between 97.8 and 98.2 degrees Fahrenheit. A temperature below 97.8—especially if recorded consistently over several days—strongly suggests low thyroid function. If your reading is above the normal range, you should be suspicious of an infection or overactive thyroid gland.[11]

Keep in mind that a woman's temperature varies in the different phases of her menstrual cycle. If you are menstruating, take your temperature on the second and third days of your period. Men, take your temperature for several consecutive mornings.

For small children who are likely to resist being quiet for ten minutes, more accurate readings often can be obtained by taking the temperature rectally for two minutes. The normal range in rectal temperature is about one degree higher than that of the armpit—98.2 to 99.2 degrees.

Thyroid blood tests may not be dependable

If your Barnes Basal Temperature Test reveals a consistently below-normal temperature, ask your physician for more than the usual thyroid panel of tests. Dr. Baskin stated, "For years, thyroid tests were a joke—you just about had to be dead before they showed anything. *Ask for the more sensitive TSH (thyroid-stimulating hormone) test, which is a much more accurate index of thyroid function.*"[12]

The standard test to measure thyroid activity attempts to determine the amount of hormone stored in the gland, or alternatively, the amount of thyroid hormone in the bloodstream. What these tests fail to do, however, is what really counts: indicate the amount of thyroid hormone available for use within the cells throughout the body.

If Your Blood Test Is Normal, What Next?

If your thyroid blood test comes back normal, but your temperature is low and you have a history of many of the low-thyroid symptoms, I suggest you read one of these books on the importance of maintaining adequate thyroid production:

- *Hypothyroidism: The Unsuspected Illness* by Dr. Broda Barnes and Lawrence Galton (Ty Crowell Co., 1976)

- *Solved: The Riddle of Illness* by Dr. Stephen Langer and James F. Scheer (McGraw-Hill/Contemporary Books, 2000)

After you have read either book, I suggest you take it to your physician and ask him for his advice in the matter. Many physicians are familiar with Dr. Barnes' method of treatment and his extensive list of publications in medical journals.

I am only able to give you a brief review of this important subject, but I have seen wonderful results when my family, friends and clients used natural thyroid. The turnaround in the way they feel has been amazing. If your thyroid function is low, a doctor must prescribe thyroid hormone tablets, as they are not available without a prescription.

The amount of thyroid hormone suggested

Dr. Barnes explains that, through a sensitive "feedback" mechanism, the amount of thyroid hormone in the bloodstream is maintained in an effective, narrow range. When thyroid function is deficient and the gland cannot respond adequately it is necessary to supply a small amount of thyroid hormone from the outside, just as insulin from the outside is supplied for a diabetic.

He also says, "The size of a proper starting dose of thyroid will vary with the age and size of the patient...A teenager or adult may safely be started on one grain daily. For a particularly large man or woman, two grains may be used—but no more than that at the beginning. The starting dosage should be maintained for about two months. After that, if necessary, the dosage may be increased."

If all symptoms have disappeared, the individual feels in good physical and mental health, and is adjusting well to work and other normal activities, the same dosage may be continued. However, Dr. Barnes says, "If symptoms have improved to some extent but have not disappeared entirely, an increase in dosage may be needed. If the blood cholesterol was high to begin with and has fallen to some extent but not to normal, the dosage may be increased if the basal temperature is still low.

"The proper dosage for an individual is the minimum needed to relieve symptoms. Most commonly in adults this is two grains; three grains sometimes are needed, rarely four grains may be required. The basal temperature may still be a little low, but one is treating symptoms, not temperature *per se*."[13]

The *Barnes Basal Temperature Test* can serve as an excellent guide not only to know when thyroid therapy is indicated for low thyroid, but also to monitor the therapy and to achieve the proper thyroid dosage.

Dr. Julian Whitaker says that in his practice, when a patient has symptoms consistent with low thyroid function, since both disease and age tend to reduce thyroid function, he starts them on a six-week therapeutic trial of desiccated porcine thyroid, regardless of what the blood tests show. He uses one half to one grain of Armour thyroid, and carefully monitors their well-being, and follows up with increasing the dosage by one-half grain, while measuring the blood level. He says if the symptoms get better, then continue the therapy. But if there is no improvement, the treatment should be stopped. "Even though this is an extremely safe therapy, you may have difficulty with your physician...the only solution to this is to shop around for a more open-minded physician," he explains.[14] Call the Broda Barnes, M.D., Research Foundation listed later for a physician in your area who understands this research.

Stimulating Thyroid Production

What can be done nutritionally to stimulate a thyroid gland into producing more thyroid hormone without a prescription?

Iodine and goiter

The thyroid needs iodine to function. A goiter may be caused by several factors. One is a lack of iodine, which causes the thyroid to swell. This can be seen on the front and side of the neck. Years ago, our government added iodine to salt (iodized salt) to prevent the tremendous number of goiters. Now that everyone is "off salt," I see so many tired, fatigued, and exhausted people. Could their lethargy be caused by low iodine, which caused low thyroid? Iodine is also found in seafood. We need such a small amount: women (100 mcg), and men (120 mcg).[15] Many fine, multi-mineral supplements include iodine as part of their formulas. Many people have been helped by taking kelp, a natural form of iodine that stimulates the thyroid.

In Japan, where residents consume about 4,000 times more iodine than Americans—mostly from large amounts of seafoods, kelp, dulse, and sea lettuce—incidences of hypothyroidism are rare.

Thyroid glandulars

Most nutrition stores carry a natural thyroid glandular. Glandulars do not contain the thyroid hormone, but Dr. Steven Langer stated at a recent National Nutritional Foods Association convention that many people with slightly low thyroid output have been helped by taking these glandular supplements. They apparently provide just enough support to the thyroid gland to stimulate adequate hormone production for some people.

L-Tyrosine

The amino acid L-tyrosine is a precursor of the thyroid hormones thyroxin and triodothyronine. Tyrosine supplementation, when health is good and iodide intake is adequate, may increase thyroid hormone levels. There may be a relationship between dietary tyrosine and thyroid hormone synthesis under the same circumstances. A slightly increased tyrosine plasma level is found in hyperthyroidism (high); a slightly reduced level is found in hypothyroidism (low).[16] There are many "thyroid" formulas that contain L-tyrosine, iodine, a few other minerals and B-vitamins to support thyroid function at your nutrition store.

Importance of vitamins

Vitamin deficiencies can result in low thyroid. Make sure you are taking a balanced "stress" B-complex with meals, which improves cellular oxygenation and energy. Vitamin B12 in particular should be taken in lozenge form (under the tongue) several times a day.

The lipotropic factors that Dr. Israel discussed—choline, methionine and inositol—would be helpful and are found in granulated soy lecithin. Dr. Israel said, "we found that these factors along with B6 enabled us to bring the patient to a higher maintenance dose of thyroid substance more rapidly than had been previously possible."[17]

Vitamin C can facilitate the production of the thyroid hormone. Vitamin E is also important for cellular oxygen. A person with low thyroid cannot convert beta-carotene into vitamin A, and when the body is low in vitamin A it cannot produce the thyroid stimulating hormone (TSH). A deficiency in vitamin A (from fish oil) also reduces the ability of the thyroid to take up iodine. Make sure your vitamin supplements include vitamin A or add several capsules of fish liver oil to your nutritional program. The bottom line is you need all the vitamins and minerals recommended in the last chapter. Also read about the antioxidants in chapter 3, which describes each of these vitamins in more detail.

Natural Form of Thyroid Hormone

Alan Gaby, M.D., has reported that nutritionally-oriented doctors now prefer a natural extract from an animal's thyroid gland. *Sold by prescription, this natural form of thyroid hormone is called desiccated thyroid or referred to as Armour thyroid (from Forest Pharmaceuticals).* This desiccated porcine thyroid (which more closely resembles our own thyroid hormones) contains not only T3 and T4, but other factors that we have yet to understand. This product was used long before the synthetic versions were available. This is the same Armour thyroid that Dr. Julian Whitaker prescribes.

Unfortunately, many physicians routinely prescribe the synthetic form of thyroid that is sold under the name of Synthroid. Synthroid contains only the thyroid hormone T4, only one kind of thyroid hormone. The second most prescribed thyroid hormone is a synthetic version of T3 sold under the name of Cytomel.

Dr. Broda Barnes reportedly used Armour thyroid in all of his studies. Both Dr. Whitaker and Dr. Gaby also use Armour thyroid. Ask your doctor to write your prescription for the Armour thyroid hormone, and then call the various pharmacies in your area until you find this form of thyroid, or ask the pharmacy to order it for you. If your doctor has any questions about the natural Armour thyroid, their web site is: *www.armourthyroid.com*. You may also contact *Patient/Physicians Questions: 1-800-678-1605. Women's International Pharmacy (1-800-279-5708) carries Armour thyroid and they can send it to you.*

Dr. Gaby has said, "I frequently see patients who are being treated for hypothyroidism with L-thyroxine (Synthroid), but who continue to experience typical hypothyroid symptoms, such as fatigue, depression, cold extremities, fluid retention, and dry skin. However, after switching to an equivalent (or sometimes even less equivalent) dose of Armour thyroid, their symptoms disappear rapidly."[18]

It is heartening to find an article appearing in the *Journal of the American Medical Association*, July 24, 1996, by researchers at John's Hopkins University who urge physicians to include testing for an underactive thyroid gland as part of routine physicals for patients after age thirty-five. The article discusses how low levels of the thyroid hormone can lead to high cholesterol levels, weight gain and depression, which often go undiagnosed. As you see, this information has been known for years and is just now beginning to be recognized and accepted.

As is true for most natural approaches, thyroid replacement therapy is never fast-acting. It might take several months for you to bring a low functioning thyroid up to normal.

Low thyroid and pregnancy

In our discussion on the importance of thyroid, I think an article published in the *New England Journal of Medicine* in August 1999 was fascinating. If a woman who has even a mild case of low thyroid (asymptomatic hypothyroidism) becomes pregnant, her child's cognitive development may be impaired as well. The study showed these children tested four to seven points lower on I.Q. tests than children of women with normal thyroid levels.[19] I think it is very important for all young women to have their thyroid tested. First, take the Temperature Test described by Dr. Broda Barnes a few pages back. If it is low, then have the TSH blood test taken. After reading this chapter, you will now know what to do. High on my list of things I wanted for my children was for them to be bright. Let's give this birth right to all the children.

Things to avoid

There are a few herbal stimulants that cause stress to the thyroid and adrenals, such as ma-huang, guarana, and excessive caffeine, all of which should be avoided.

It is really surprising to know that there are vegetables that are goitrogenic (causes a goiter) from the cabbage family that should be limited or completely avoided by people with hypothyroidism according to Ray Peat, Ph.D. These include broccoli, cauliflower, cabbage, turnips, mustard greens, kale, spinach, Brussels sprouts, kohlrabi, rutabagas, horseradish, radish and white mustard. These vegetables have been shown to *decrease thyroid hormone production as effectively as anti-thyroid drugs such as thiouracil.* Therefore, you need to include many other varieties of vegetables and supplement with kelp, iodine, all the antioxidants, cod liver oil or vitamin A, since beta-carotene is hard for hypothyroid individuals to assimilate.[20]

Cardiovascular Disease and the Thyroid Connection

Dr. Barnes believed what the early researchers found: They were able to prevent high levels of blood cholesterol and atherosclerosis by administering thyroid hormones. Dr. Barnes explains, "If their recommendations had been followed, cardiovascular diseases would have been conquered decades ago and much time and many lives would have been saved." Dr. Barnes noted, "By 1950, it was obvious that many cases of heart attacks were accompanied by high blood cholesterol levels. To most investigators, this suggested that the elevated cholesterol levels were causing the attacks, but to me they signaled possible thyroid deficiency."[21]

Dr. Murray Israel, in his ten-year-study, stated his severely atherosclerotic patients with a history of high cholesterol intake should be on a low cholesterol diet for the first few months. Also those with high cholesterol who had been on a low cholesterol diet needed to restrict cholesterol for the first few months until the thyroid was able to take effect. Israel said, "As the patient improves in his ability to utilize these lipoid elements, these restrictions become less important. The thyroxin improves his efficiency in processing lipoids and keeping them circulating, rather than deposited in tissues."[22]

For more information on hypothyroidism contact the Broda O. Barnes, M.D., Research Foundation, Inc., P.O. Box 98, Trumbull, CT 06611, phone 203-261-2101 or visit their web site at www.brodabarnes.com

High Thyroid Symptoms

The other side of the thyroid coin, of course, is "high thyroid," or hyperthyroidism. If your Barnes temperature test is above 98.2, it may indicate hyperthyroid. Certain diseases such as Grave's disease or thyroid inflammation, as well as stress or worry, may cause the thyroid to produce too much thyroid hormone. This results in high thyroid output—a condition that causes the body's motor to race, the heartbeat to increase (or beat irregularly), and blood pressure to rise. A person with this condition generally feels flushed and overheated, often to the level of a mild fever. A hyperthyroid person perspires profusely, feels nervous, is sleepless, and may suffer from weight loss or diarrhea. Although this condition is rare, a person may also suffer these symptoms if they take too much thyroid supplement.

Ruling Out Anemia

There may be reasons other than low thyroid for feeling cold. If your T3 and T4 tests return normal and you do not have a below normal temperature, you may want to have your doctor check you for anemia. Even a mild iron deficiency may result in anemia.

THE GENERAL SYMPTOMS OF ANEMIA

❧ pallor	❧ headache	
❧ weakness	❧ palpitation	
❧ easily fatigued	❧ labored breathing on exertion	
❧ persistent tiredness	❧ restless leg syndrome[23]	

ANEMIC PRESCHOOL CHILDREN'S SYMPTOMS:

- diminished coordination and balance
- lowered attention span
- reduction in intelligence quotient and memory

SYMPTOMS OF ANEMIA IN OLDER CHILDREN:

- difficulty reading
- poor learning and problem solving skills

A woman loses about 13.5 mg of iron through menstruation each month. For every milligram of iron lost, she needs to take at least ten mg to replace it. This is because the body usually can absorb only about 10 percent of the iron it ingests. The average American diet provides only 6 mg of iron per 1,000 calories. This means that a woman needs at least 8 mg daily (and more during pregnancy).[24]

The best dietary source of iron is red meat (especially organ meats such as liver). Other good sources are poultry, fish, ground soybean hulls, and blackstrap molasses.

Many foods considered high in iron are actually low in "iron availability"—foods such as spinach, and many green vegetables. Iron availability refers to the body's ability to absorb and use the form of iron that is in the food. Red meat is the most bioavailable form.

For those who will not eat liver, there are liquid liver softgels available by Enzymatic Therapy, where the animals are free of hormones and chemicals. Their "Liver Extract" softgels are rich not only in iron but folic acid, vitamin B12 and other natural blood building factors. Or, you may need to take supplemental iron. If so, chelated iron is the preferred form because the body more readily absorbs it. Avoid the ferrous sulfate form, although it is frequently recommended, since it destroys vitamin E and may cause constipation. The other forms often recommended are ferrous gluconate, ferrous fumarate, or ferrous citrate. I recommend the ferrous fumarate form of iron.

Anemia is not always a result of just an iron deficiency, but may be attributable to subtle, simultaneous deficiencies of all the vitamin B-complex, especially B12, vitamins C and E, and the minerals copper and magnesium.

May you regain your energy and a feeling of well-being as you now have a better understanding of the importance of your thyroid gland and all it accomplishes for you!

Nutritional Help for All Forms of Arthritis

Treating Arthritis, Carpal Tunnel
Syndrome, Joint Problems, Gout and
Related Conditions—Naturally

*Drugs work because they "whip" the adrenal glands to
produce cortisone, which pulls calcium out of the
bones, sugar out of the liver, and protein out of the
muscles. You feel better for a while…because you are
living on your own tissue. What you need to do is help your
body produce its own cortisone and other adrenal
hormones.*

—GLADYS LINDBERG

One of the greatest responses I have ever had from a television appearance was after we had discussed arthritis on the Trinity Broadcasting Network. According to the Centers for Disease Control and Prevention, this aging, crippling disease afflicts 50 million Americans—one in seven—the vast majority of whom are middle-aged or older. In fact almost everyone over the age of 50 has some signs of arthritis. One in three families is affected, at a cost of more than 8.6 billion dollars to the United States economy. Arthritis is one of the three major degenerative diseases among people in the western world as a whole. Its most common forms are rheumatoid, osteoarthritis, and gout.

Arthritis is not a single disorder, but the name given to a joint disease that has a number of causes. Arthritis may involve one joint or many in the body, and it can vary in severity from a mild ache and stiffness to severe pain and, ultimately, deformity.

The word *arthritis* comes from the Greek word *"arthron,"* which means "joint," and *"itis,"* which means "inflammation." The joint inflammation of arthritis generally manifests itself as swelling, a feeling of heat, redness of inflamed areas, and pain. Although not a direct killer such as cancer or heart disease, arthritis causes more years of pain and suffering than virtually any other disease. Its victims sometimes become virtual prisoners in their own bodies.

Up until now the general belief in the United States was that arthritis, particularly osteoarthritis, was incurable. That is why the commonly prescribed treatment was designed only to relieve the pain and make the patient more comfortable. But the root of the problem was never addressed. What was causing this crippling disease?

Of course we know that drugs doubtlessly save many more lives than are harmed. But these pharmaceutical toxicities are certainly one of the reasons why many are seeking natural alternatives. This is why the following information is so important for the arthritic sufferer, because the seemingly innocent, temporary pain relieving drugs, in many cases, have serious side effects.

Non-Steroidal Anti-Inflammatory Drugs (NSAIDs) and Arthritis

The Alternative Medical Alert: A Clinician's Guide to Alternative Therapies is a medical newsletter for physicians. In the November 1998 issue, discussing osteoarthritis (OA) it reported, "Nonetheless, the prospects of a nutritional remedy for the treatment or prevention of OA is compelling, particularly because no specific medications currently halt disease progression. The problem is enormous, because more than four out of five persons older than the age of 65 show some clinical or radiological evidence of the disease." "The current recommended treatment for OA is weight loss, physical therapy, and the use of pain relievers including acetaminophen and non-steroidal anti-inflammatory drugs (NSAIDs). NSAIDs have been reported to have positive and negative effects on cartilage metabolism...*NSAIDs and acetaminophen do not reverse OA.*"[1] This alternative medical article goes on to discuss the value of glucosamine sulfate that we discuss later in this chapter.

The negative side effects of NSAIDs

Dr. Julian Whitaker reported in his newsletter *Health & Healing* that about 25 percent of people who take NSAIDs develop ulcers. The Food and Drug Administration (FDA) statistics show that the number one category of adverse drug events is gastrointestinal complications from long-term NSAIDs use.[2] *Dr. Whitaker also reported that 20,000 people a year die from these complications.* He went on to report, "Believe it or not, the primary reason for blood transfusions in hospitals is not accidental injuries or replacement blood lost during surgery—it is for *gastrointestinal bleeding caused by drugs used to treat arthritis.* How could a therapy that causes so much harm possibly withstand the test of time?"[3] This statement was shocking to me, to think that we use these various drugs with such terrible side effects.

Dr. Whitaker went on to say, "Incredibly, NSAIDs block the body's mechanism for healing the joints and regenerating cartilage. Although they provide temporary pain relief, they tend to worsen arthritis in the long term by accelerating the rate at which cartilage is lost."[4]

The Natural Approach

There is no one answer, no "magic bullet," for the treatment of arthritis. The sound approach would be for a person to do that which is necessary to build up the body as a whole. The hope, of course, is that one or more of these natural approaches will greatly benefit the person with arthritis, gout, back and disc problems, osteoporosis, carpal tunnel syndrome, or autoimmune diseases. These natural therapies I will discuss are non-toxic, and many people have had fabulous results. They will also help a person build up their resistance to this disease, so over time they may minimize the severity of their problem and feel better.

Dr. Roger Williams, the researcher who discovered pantothenic acid and folic acid, also advocates this approach. He states, "Injuries, infections, allergic reactions, and psychological stresses may all play a part in the cause of arthritic disease. But the most probable underlying cause—poor nutritional environment for the cells and tissues involved—has, as usual, been neglected."[5]

Joint and Cartilage Involvement

Many difficulties associated with arthritic diseases arise from poor lubrication of the joints and all other movable structures in the body.

Joints are the areas where bones come together. Bone ends are shaped to fit together and are covered with *cartilage*, a rubbery protective cushion. The entire joint is enclosed in a capsule of dense fibers. The capsule is lined by the *synovial* membrane, which secretes a lubricating fluid in the spaces between the bone ends. When cartilage disintegrates, for whatever reason, bone ends rub against each other and put pressure on nerves, which causes pain.

Synovial fluid in the joints is thick, like mucous. It contains various mineral salts and *mucoprotein*. The mucoprotein, as other body proteins, must be produced in the body using raw materials from food and water. When any mineral, amino acid, or vitamin is deficient, or if the cells are poisoned by bacterial toxins or allergens, cells can become partially incapacitated. The result is poor mucoprotein manufacturing and, in turn, poor lubrication. It is vital, therefore, that we continually feed the body the nutrients it needs to manufacture mucoprotein.

Rheumatoid Arthritis—Inflammation

Rheumatoid arthritis and juvenile rheumatoid arthritis are types of inflammatory arthritis. Some two and a half million people in the United States have rheumatoid arthritis.[6] They are the most destructive, disabling, and unpredictable forms of arthritis. This persistent disorder begins with an inflammation of the lining that provides the lubrication of the joints. The disease then spreads to the cartilage, ligaments, muscles, and bones. The symptoms come and go, with stiff and swollen joints that are often more painful in cold weather. The disease can start at any age, even infancy, but usually manifests itself between the ages of 30 and 50.

Rheumatoid arthritis is an autoimmune disorder in which the body's immune system improperly identifies as foreign the synovial membranes that secrete the lubricating fluid in the joints. The immune system—which usually defends the body against bacteria, viruses, and cancer cells—loses its ability to distinguish between foreign invaders and the body's own tissue. It begins to attack the body, especially the joints. Inflammation results, and the cartilage and tissues in and around the joints are damaged. Often the bone surfaces are destroyed as well. The body replaces this damaged tissue with scar tissue, causing the normal spaces within the joints to become narrow and the bones to fuse together. Rheumatoid arthritis creates stiffness, swelling, fatigue, anemia, weight loss, fever, and often, crippling pain.[7]

No one knows with certainty what deceives the immune system into attacking its own body, but several theories have been advanced and are under investigation.

Exhausted Adrenal Glands

Studies have revealed that all forms of arthritis usually begin after years of stress, either physical or emotional. Dr. Hans Selye coined the word *stress* years ago and showed how stress exhausts the adrenal glands to the point where the adrenals no longer produce enough cortisone and other vital hormones. The adrenal hormones are essential for life. They are two glands perched atop the kidneys that manufacture the cortical hormones, which prepares us for "fight or flight."[8] The following chart lists some of the physical stress factors that exhaust the adrenal glands and run down our immune system:

FACTORS THAT IMPACT PHYSICAL AND EMOTIONAL STRESS

physical injuries	allergies
infections	chemical preservatives
cigarettes	antibiotics
caffeine	chemotherapy
alcohol	excess sugar

- drugs of all kinds
- crash dieting
- over-exercising
- emotional trauma
- prescription medicines
- lack of vitamins and minerals
- pregnancy
- x-rays
- intense noise
- extreme heat or cold
- insecticides

These stressors tend to overstimulate or "whip" the adrenal glands to produce cortisone. When this happens, vital calcium is pulled from the body's bones, sugar from the liver and protein from the muscles. Over time, the adrenals become exhausted to the point where no "whip" is big enough to get them going again in an adequate way.

Carl Pfeiffer, M.D., Ph.D., author of *Mental and Elemental Nutrients,* a world-renowned expert on nutritional medicine, has said, "Psychiatric theory claims rheumatoid arthritis is one of the stress-induced disorders. Poor nutrition, repeated bacterial infection, and a host of other causes are more apt to be the real cause of rheumatoid arthritis."[9]

Can a person have a healthy body and a disturbed mind? It is highly unlikely. When we are physically healthy, we have a greater ability to handle emotional trauma and will take better care of ourselves physically.

Let's rebuild the adrenal glands

The elements necessary for normal adrenal hormone production are protein, vitamins A, C, and E, and the entire range of B-vitamins, especially pantothenic acid. A diet deficient in these raw materials limits the ability of the adrenal glands to function under stress.

WHOLE, RAW ADRENAL GLANDULAR CAPSULES. These natural supplements help support the adrenal glands, allowing them to repair themselves so they can again secrete their own cortisone and other vital hormones. Raw adrenal glandulars have been very effective for many people and are available at your nutrition store.

PANTOTHENIC ACID FOR ADRENAL SUPPORT. It appears in the research that virtually every person suffering from an illness that is helped by cortisone—arthritis, lupus erythematosus, gout, and dozens of others—is likely to be deficient in the B-vitamin, pantothenic acid. Pantothenic acid protects the adrenal cortex from damage and stimulates the adrenal glands to increase production of cortisone and other adrenal hormones important for the body's reaction to stress.[10]

Pantothenic acid is made in several forms, among them pantothenol and calcium pantothenate. Actions are identical for all forms. Authorities recommend a range of 200 mg up to 1,000 mg in divided doses to build resistance to stress.

Dr. Agnes Faye Morgan was the first to demonstrate that a deficiency in pantothenic acid causes degeneration of adrenal gland tissue, with internal bleeding and, interestingly, premature gray hair in animals. Restoration of the vitamin to the diet caused repair of the gland and recoloration of the hair![11]

Dr. Roger Williams, who discovered pantothenic acid, has noted in his research that pantothenic acid consistently brought relief to sufferers of rheumatoid arthritis, although the improvement was not a complete cure. Mother, having read Dr. Williams' work back in 1949, added 200 mg of pantothenic acid to her B complex vitamin formulas. She was so very far ahead of her time.

VITAMIN C IS ALSO ESSENTIAL FOR THE ADRENALS. The adrenal glands have the richest concentrations of vitamin C in the body, and during great stress, the vitamin C content of these glands can be depleted within minutes.[12] The role of vitamin C in the chemistry of these glands is very complex, but what is vital for us to know is very simple:

- Vitamin C is essential for the manufacturing of the stress hormone adrenaline.

- Vitamin C not only increases the production and utilization of cortisone, but also appears to prolong its effectiveness.

- When vitamin C is rapidly depleted, restoration to an adequate level takes more time than the depletion took.[13]

Dr. Linus Pauling estimated that normal requirements for vitamin C should be between 250 and 2,500 mg per day. An arthritic is not "normal," however, and should definitely strive toward a higher amount, particularly since we know that adrenal dysfunction is part of their condition. I would suggest 3,000 to 5,000 mg of vitamin C in divided doses, to be taken with food in your stomach. At these higher doses I do not recommend the timed released tablets, as they stay in your stomach too long. Use capsules and include the bioflavonoids if possible.

VITAMIN C IS THE CEMENT THAT HOLDS US TOGETHER. Another reason to take vitamin C is that it helps in the synthesis and maintenance of collagen. Collagen is the intercellular "cement" that literally holds the cells in various organs and tissues together. Its various fibers form the connective tissue of the body. Collagen is found in skin, bones, teeth, blood vessels, eyes, heart—in fact, all parts of the body.[14]

Recent studies have also shown that when levels of vitamin C are high, the synovial (lubricating) fluid of the joints allows for greater mobility.

Smoking particularly destroys vitamin C, as do large doses of aspirin or the prescription drug, cortisone.

Nutritional Help for All Forms of Arthritis

Those with arthritis seem to have an imbalance of a number of minerals, further supporting the idea that this disease is linked to a poor nutritional environment.

Dr. Carl Pfeiffer cites a number of studies showing that copper levels are high in arthritis patients while zinc and manganese levels are low. The high copper level may be the result of a lack of elemental sulfur in the diet.

He says, "Rheumatoid arthritis patients should have zinc, manganese, niacin and vitamin C, with two eggs per day for their sulfur content." This was before the information came out on MSM (sulfur). Dr. Pfeiffer points out that arthritics should have a carefully balanced diet high in the B-vitamins, and he suggests taking ten tablets of brewer's yeast twice a day as part of his plan to help arthritics.[15]

Lead pollutants in the environment may contribute to arthritis in Dr. Pfeiffer's opinion, and he recommends vitamin C as a means of helping provide protection against this contamination.[16] Chelation also removes lead from our system and is discussed in chapter 12, *Anti-Aging Therapies*.

Crippling Arthritis in a Five-Year-Old

When I was president of the American Nutrition Society, I asked Robert Bingham, M.D., author of *Fight Back Against Arthritis*, to present to our audience the program he has used for decades to treat arthritics at his clinic in Desert Hot Springs, California. Dr. Bingham described a five-year-old patient with hips and knees so contracted "she could only lie on her side." She could not sit in a chair. For two years she had been a patient in a well-known hospital, but she had only grown progressively worse. Her parents were told to take her home with the prognosis, "There is no hope of any improvement or cure."

She was taken to Dr. Bingham's clinic, and this young girl was given fresh blended vegetable and fruit juices, eggs, and certified raw milk in five small meals a day. She received liquid vitamin supplements, including cod liver oil, vitamin C, and the B-vitamin complex "in therapeutic doses," which we would call megavitamin therapy. She was placed in a warm-water pool to relieve pain and improve circulation. The therapists exercised each of her joints under the mineral waters. Within four weeks, the pain and swelling of her joints had improved so that she could sit in a chair. Within six months she was discharged, able to walk and ride a tricycle.[17]

Dr. Bingham identified the following nutrients and doses as being essential for arthritis therapy:

- Vitamins A and D, the liquid form of cod liver oil.
- The B-vitamin complex, also natural sources of B vitamin, such as nuts, grains, brewers yeast and wheat germ.
- Vitamin C, with a starting dose of 2,000 mg daily.
- Vitamin E in an initial therapeutic dose of 1,600 IU and a maintenance dose of 800 IU daily.
- Calcium, magnesium, phosphorous, and other trace elements such as zinc, chromium, and copper.
- Digestive aids such as enzymes and hydrochloric acid.
- A high-protein diet.
- Plant extracts, especially yucca.

IMPORTANT COMMON DIETARY FACTORS. Dr. Bingham also stated that two common dietary factors are found in nearly every arthritis patient, regardless of diagnosis. This may be the main contributing factor in the cause of all arthritis:

- an abnormally low intake of protein
- an abnormally high intake of refined carbohydrates.

Niacinamide (B3)—Disappearance of joint pain

William Kaufman, M.D., Ph.D., who taught at the University of

Michigan Medical School and at Yale University, was a pioneer in the field of vitamin therapy for rheumatism and arthritis. He reported to the American Geriatric Society that most of his patients improved greatly on a regimen of 1 to 5 grams (1,000 to 5,000 mg) of niacinamide per day in divided doses (6 to 16 doses per day), continuing for as long as nine years. He observed no negative reactions in several thousand patients he treated during these years of continuous use. For those with restricted mobility of joints and manifestations of a deficiency of niacinamide, he recommended treatment with 4 to 5 grams (4,000 to 5,000 mg) of niacinamide per day.[18] It is important to give this amount in divided doses.

Many of Dr. Kaufman's patients showed a striking improvement in mental health on this niacinamide regimen. It is important to note that Dr. Kaufman used niacinamide, a form of the B3 vitamin, not niacin, which gives a flush to the skin.

Vitamin B6 brings relief

Another vitamin that brings relief for sufferers with rheumatism, menopausal arthritis and carpal tunnel syndrome is vitamin B6 (pyridoxine). This vitamin shrinks the synovial membranes that line the bearing surfaces of the joints. It thus helps to control pain and to restore mobility to the elbows, shoulders, knees, and other joints, according to Dr. John M. Ellis, a physician and researcher from Texas.[19]

The author of *Free of Pain*, Dr. Ellis reported that vitamin B6 is effective at an intake level of 50 to 100 mg per day, and more for some people.

Motion pictures taken before and after treatment with vitamin B6 give clear proof that it reduced swelling in hands and fingers, improved hand and finger dexterity, prevented transitory nocturnal arm paralysis, and halted nighttime leg cramps and muscle spasms. Shoulder pain was reduced or eliminated and shoulder and arm function was improved in his patients.[20]

All antioxidants are valuable

Successful antioxidant therapy for rheumatoid arthritis requires a synergistic combination of several antioxidants. In addition to the vitamins mentioned above, the minerals magnesium and calcium also supply the synovial (lubricating) fluid, as does vitamin A, C, E and beta-carotene. MSM, discussed later, is very valuable for rheumatoid arthritis.

SELENIUM—A CO-WORKER: Researchers have found a special benefit to selenium when combined with the other antioxidant vitamins A, C, and E.[21]

In a clinical trial using a formula containing selenium and these three vitamins, 64 percent of the patients reported considerable reduction in pain after only three months. Many of these patients were very severely afflicted. One of the patients told a newspaper reporter, "I thought that I would never get rid of the pain. Now I have full movement of my hip and no pain whatsoever."[22]

Other researchers have found that the greater the selenium deficiency in patients, the more severe their rheumatoid arthritis.[23]

In another study, patients reported increased mobility and significantly less pain when given 350 mcg of selenium with 400 IU of vitamin E for a two-week period.[24] But I feel it should be continued.

THE VALUE OF ZINC. Several reports in medical literature note that rheumatoid arthritics frequently have low levels of zinc in their hair (found in hair analysis) and blood, and there are confirming studies that cite improvement in arthritic conditions when zinc supplements are administered. Zinc is a powerful stimulant to the immune system, so much so that conventional literature in cancer research is now reporting its benefits.

Several researchers suggest that arthritis sufferers take a zinc supplement, perhaps 30 to 50 mg daily of zinc picolinate, gluconate or chelated zinc, to see if they have a positive response. Zinc should be balanced with the mineral copper at about a 10:1 or 15:1 zinc to copper ratio.

Osteoarthritis:
The Degenerative Joint Disease

Osteoarthritis (OA) is commonly called the "wear and tear" arthritis. It is the most widespread form of the disease, a slow progressive disorder characterized by a breakdown of cartilage and changes in bone. It is a degenerative joint disease sometimes caused by injury, excessive exercise or repeated strain. It may be caused by a defect in the protein that makes up cartilage. It very often afflicts the fingers and weight-bearing joints: knees, hips and spine.

The start of osteoarthritis can be very subtle; morning joint stiffness is usually the first symptom. As the disease progresses, there is pain in the involved joint with motion. Small bony growths, calcium spurs, and occasional soft cysts appear on bones and in the joints.

When osteoarthritis sets in, the cartilage (tissue that covers the ends of the bones) begins to break down and becomes thin and may even disappear. The normally smooth sliding surfaces of the bones become pitted and irregular. The tendons, ligaments, and muscles holding the joint together become weaker, and the joint itself becomes deformed, painful, and stiff. This change results in decreased fluid in and around the joints. When friction increases, pain results, but little or no swelling. Poor posture, fatigue, obesity, and stress seem to hasten its onset; however, improper nutrition or bacterial infection may also be involved.

According to the Arthritis Foundation, approximately 15.8 million Americans have osteoarthritis, with nearly three times as many women as men suffering from the disease. This is an enormous problem because more than four out of five persons over the age of 65 show some clinical or radiological evidence of the disease. Bone fractures become an increasing risk because osteoarthritis makes the bones brittle.

The good news is there are many natural products you can take to help the pain and stiffness of osteoarthritis. We just need to rebuild the naturally occurring substances found in high concentrations in the joint, which appears to be the best remedy for osteoarthritis. The following information will help you find a tremendous amount of nutritional help, not only for osteoarthritis, but all forms of arthritis.

The value of glucosamine sulfate

Glucosamine (glue-cose-a-mine) is made from glucose, the sugar that the body burns for fuel, and an amino acid called *glutamine*. It is a natural dietary substance that the body uses to help keep cartilage smooth, moist, and flexible. Sulfate is a salt of sulfuric acid. Most authors think that the glucosamine ion is the active principal, but at least some evidence suggests that a component of the glucosamine sulfate activity is related to sulfur residues, because sulfur is an essential nutrient for the stabilization of connective tissue matrix.[25] The tissues containing these glucosamine molecules include tendons and ligaments, cartilage, synovial fluid, mucous membranes, several structures in the eye, blood vessels, and heart valves.

Glucosamine sulfate is one of the biological chemicals that form all the major cushioning ingredients of the joint fluids and surrounding tissues. It helps to make the synovial fluid thick and elastic in joints and vertebrae. In other words, *glucosamine is responsible for stimulating the manufacture of substances necessary for joint repair.*

Glucosamine sulfate also helps increase the thickness of the gelatinous material found in the discs of the back. The discs cushion and support the vertebrae of the spine. Any injury or damage to these discs can cause the gelatinous cartilage to soften and may place pressure on nearby nerves, causing either pain or damage and loss of nerve function.

There have been numerous scientific studies showing the beneficial effects of glucosamine sulfate and its relationship with the symptoms of osteoarthritis, the most common form of arthritis.[26] Glucosamine sulfate has been shown to exert a protective effect against joint destruction and is selectively used by the joints tissue, exerting a powerful healing effect on arthritic symptoms.

Using glucosamine sulfate is a classic example of how a natural substance improves a condition by addressing the underlying cause and supporting the body's natural ability to heal itself.[27]

MORE EFFECTIVE THAN NSAIDS AND IBUPROFEN. Numerous double-blind studies have shown glucosamine sulfate produces much better results than NSAIDs (nonsteroidal anti-inflammatory drugs) in relieving the pain and inflammation of osteoarthritis and has better effects than the common arthritis drug *ibuprofen.*[28]

GLUCOSAMINE SULFATE IS NON-TOXIC. When given orally, it has been shown to relieve pain, joint tenderness and swelling, so that joint movement can increase.[29] Since it is *non-toxic* it can be used for prolonged treatment.

By getting to the root of the problem, glucosamine sulfate not only improves the symptoms, it also helps the body repair damaged joints. This effect is outstanding, especially when glucosamine's safety and lack of side effects is considered.[30]

It is interesting that most of the current data is derived from European and Asian literature. Six double-blind investigations in five countries all have documented statistically significant benefits without side effects.[31] There has been no medical information found in America.

GLUCOSAMINE DOSAGE. Take 500 mg of glucosamine sulfate 3 times per day (total 1,500 mg). Some may need slightly larger amounts if taking diuretics or if the body weight is over 200 pounds.[32] *Be sure you use glucosamine sulfate, the form with proven effectiveness in the world's scientific studies.* All of the medical studies for the treatment of osteoarthritis, in over 70 countries, used glucosamine sulfate. I always believe in using the form or products that the research was done with. Other forms are available, and some U.S. studies are now being carried out, but for two to three decades the sulfate form was used.[33]

TAKE NOTE, DOCTORS! The *Alternative Medicine Alert,* a magazine for doctors, recommends that "physicians should encourage weight loss, physical therapy, and regular exercise as the primary treatments for osteoarthritis. For patients seeking pain relief, an eight- to twelve-week trial of glucosamine sulfate, 500 mg three times a day, appears to be much safer and at least as effective as ibuprofen. Take 400 mg three times a day, for patients with mild-to-moderate osteoarthritis of the weight bearing joints. Patients should not discontinue their weight loss and exercise programs if they choose to add glucosamine; whether they continue taking an NSAID or acetaminophen while on glucosamine sulfate is an individual decision that the patient should make in consultation with his or her physician."[34]

OTHER ADVANTAGES. Glucosamine works not only in the strength and integrity of joints, but also in the formation of nails, tendons, skin, eyes, bones, ligaments, and heart valves. It plays a role in the mucous secretions of your digestive, respiratory, and urinary tracts.[35] Glucosamine sulfate has been shown to exert a protective effect against joint destruction and is selectively used by joint tissues, exerting a powerful healing effect on arthritic symptoms.

Chondroitin sulfate

Chondroitin (con-droy-tin) sulfate is a naturally occurring mucopolysaccharide found in the human body. Our diet contains chondroitin as it is found in most animal tissues, especially the "gristle" around joints. Chondroitin is the fibrous protein substance that binds water in the cartilage matrix, and is key to normal cartilage metabolism. Studies show that individuals with arthritis have abnormally low levels of chondroitin.

Chondroitin sulfate was also popularized by Dr. Theodosakis' book, *The Arthritis Cure,* and is right behind glucosamine in popularity. Dr. Theodosakis feels they work together synergistically.[36]

Chondroitin sulfate is completely non-toxic. A six-year study tracking people taking doses of 1,500 mg to 10,000 mg per day has shown no toxicity. So if the cartilage mechanism breaks down we can feel free to replace what the body fails to make.

SUGGESTED DOSAGE. Glucosamine sulfate, 500 mg three times a day (total 1500 mg per day), and chondroitin sulfate, 400 mg three times a day, (total 1200 mg). This is for a person weighing between 120–200 pounds. If your weight is higher, more should be used.

I find most of my clientele do better with the combined glucosamine and chondroitin, and others get relief from just the glucosamine sulfate. Remember, we are all biochemically different.

MSM—Organic sulfur

It has been reported lately on the news that "MSM" may be the new "miracle cure" for arthritis. MSM (methyl-sulfonyl-methane) is an organic source of sulfur—a nonmetallic element that occurs widely in nature. It is a white, odorless crystal, appearing similar to sugar. By weight, MSM is 34 percent elemental sulfur, making it one of nature's richest sources of natural organic sulfur. Sulfur is the fourth most plentiful mineral found in your body and is stored in every one of your cells. Sulfur is necessary for the manufacture of collagen, which helps to form bones, tendons, and connective tissue. It is also a constituent of keratin, the chief component of hair, skin, and nails.[37]

Because sulfur is necessary for the formation of connective tissue, MSM has been widely studied for its use in arthritis and other complications of joint inflammation. The results of several studies showed that when supplementing with MSM there was decreased damage to synovial tissue, decreased joint degeneration, and inflammation was significantly decreased.[38]

There was a tremendous testimony on several news shows from the actor James Coburn, who overcame crippling rheumatoid arthritis with the use of MSM. He said he had tried everything for 20 years while struggling with crippling pain. In an article in the 1999 *Journal of Longevity*, James Coburn said, "I took a teaspoon and a half of the crystals twice a day. Once in the morning, once in the evening. And three days later, no more pain. I could move!"[39] In the brand of MSM he was using, each teaspoon contained 4,000 mg, so his total for the day was 12,000 mg of MSM. It shows the importance of taking a large enough dose. It also contained a total of 720 mg of vitamin C. This is an encouraging testimony for someone who has suffered from rheumatoid arthritis. What a blessing!

BENEFITS OF MSM: AN ORGANIC FORM OF SULFUR

❧ MSM can be helpful for most types of musculoskeletal pain and inflammation including rheumatoid arthritis, osteoarthritis, tendonitis, and gout. It has shown helpful in lupus erythematosus and may be beneficial in other autoimmune disorders. It helps relieve pain.

❧ Sulfur is necessary for healthy nerves and proper brain function.

❧ Sulfur aids the liver in bile secretion and helps maintain overall body balance between acidity and alkalinity.

❧ Sulfur plays a role in carbohydrate metabolism, which is significant for hypoglycemia and diabetes. The lack of nutritional sulfur in the body can result in low insulin production. Sulfur is a component of insulin, the hormone secreted by the pancreas that is essential to the metabolism of carbohydrates.

❧ Sulfur plays an important part of tissue breathing, which is the process where oxygen and other substances are used to build cells and release energy.

❧ Nutritional sulfur helps keep hair, nails and skin healthy and is often referred to as nature's "beauty mineral." Vitamin C is also part of the essential structure of the skin and works with MSM.

❧ Sulfur protects the cells from airborne pollutants, such as car and airplane exhaust and factory smoke.

❧ Sulfur slows down the aging process in the cells and encourages the efficient production of protein.

❧ Sulfur helps to transport important elements such as selenium and zinc around the body, and in compound form has been found to protect the body against radiation.

❧ Sulfur is a crucial component of the tissues, hormones, vitamins, enzymes, antibodies and antioxidants in the body. We cannot maintain excellent health without it.[40]

❧ Sulfur is used as a treatment for bronchitis, slow wound healing, brittle nails, acne, constipation and many other health problems.[41]

2. MSM may also have some anti-cancer properties. Animal studies have found that it slows the growth of breast and colon cancer.[42]

DMSO AND MSM. MSM is a normal metabolite or by-product of DMSO (dimethyl sulfoxide). Many years ago DMSO was an alternative "wonder drug," a powerful pain reliever and anti-inflammatory widely used on animals. It rapidly transports other substances or nutrients through the skin and into the bloodstream. The only negative aspect of DMSO was its strong sulfurous smell, even when applied to the skin.

Stanley W. Jacobs, M.D., of Oregon Health Sciences University in Portland became intrigued with MSM, one of the active forms of DMSO in the body. Fifteen percent of DMSO is converted to MSM. The good news is that MSM provides the body with an important building block—sulfur—but does not retain the odor.

MSM IS NON-TOXIC. MSM has been widely studied for its toxicity level over several decades. It is one of the least toxic substances in biology and medicine, similar to the toxicity of water. Researchers have given rodents 8 grams (8,000 mg) per kilogram of body weight for six months and seen no toxic effects.

In human studies, researchers gave 1 gram (1,000 mg) per kilogram of body weight, orally and by skin, for 30 days with no serious toxicity, according to Dr. Stanley Jacobs. An unpublished Oregon Health Sciences University study of long-term toxicity of MSM over a period of 6 months, with more than 12,000 patients, showed no toxic effects at levels above 2 grams a day.[43]

If you take more MSM than you need, it simply passes through the body and is excreted in the urine. Dr. Stanley Jacobs, the pioneering researcher of MSM, reports he personally takes 30 grams per day and has done so for 20 years.[44]

TAKE NOTE, LADIES! It is reported that the only "side effect" of *too much sulfur (MSM) is fuller, thicker hair, stronger nails that grow quickly, and less wrinkles.* It is referred to as "nature's beauty mineral." I think we should all take it!

Note: *"Inorganic" sources of sulfur are sulfa drugs and sulfites, which are food preservatives to prevent bacterial growth. These are inorganic sources that many people are sensitive to and should avoid. MSM is an "organic" sulfur that is absolutely non-toxic.*

MSM DOSAGE. Dr. Jacobs reports that over the years thousands of patients have experienced healing benefits by taking daily doses of 2 to 3 grams (2,000 mg to 3,000 mg) of MSM per day. The amount was dependent on their gastrointestinal (GI) tolerance and their condition. Vitamin C added to this MSM regimen also greatly reduced symptoms of pain, swelling and inflammation.

Higher doses are typically necessary to experience therapeutic effects. You may need 3 to 8 grams (3,000 mg to 8,000 mg) of MSM a day to control allergic symptoms of sneezing, runny nose, and burning eyes during pollen season.

Dr. Jacobs reports, "We have recommended 40 to 60 grams and up in incremental daily doses for severe conditions, but in these instances patients were under our personal supervision."

He continues, "It is our opinion that the higher the dose you can take without developing an upset stomach, the quicker you will experience a healing response and the fewer symptomatic recurrences you will have. If you don't see a response, increase your dosage slowly." This information is reported in Dr. Jacobs' book *The Miracle of MSM: The Natural Solution for Pain.*[45]

It is best to take MSM with food. Do not take it before bedtime as it has a tendency to increase your energy, thus keeping you awake. I add these almost tasteless (slightly bitter) crystals to my protein shake each day. One teaspoon equals 4,000 mg, so I add almost 2 teaspoons to my shake. It is an easy way to add this essential mineral to my nutrition program.

I am receiving wonderful reports from my clients that MSM has solved their problems. These are classic stories from very happy customers, most taking 10 to 12 grams (10,000 to 12,000 mg) a day. If anyone tells me it doesn't work, I ask them how much they are taking which is usually just one capsule (1,000 mg). That is not enough! You may find MSM capsules, crystals, or powder at your nutrition store.

Best food sources of sulfur

Animal proteins have a high content of sulfur because of the essential amino acid methionine, found in fish, meats, dairy products and eggs. Methionine, cysteine, cystine, and taurine, known as the sulfur-bearing amino acids, are considered the building blocks of protein that are also found in grains and legumes. Egg yolk contains high amounts of the sulfur bearing amino acids, cysteine and methionine.

Garlic and onions are the richest plant source of sulfur and known by their odorous smell. Other vegetables, such as asparagus, red peppers, cabbage, Brussels sprouts, avocados, horseradish, mustard, sunflower seeds and broccoli have significant but not abundant quantities of sulfur. Unfortunately, most of the MSM present in these unprocessed foods is lost in the washing, cooking or steaming that are involved in preparing these foods for our consumption.

Natural anti-inflammatories

It would be important to take natural anti-inflammatories with the glucosamine sulfate and chondroitin sulfate. Then I would be sure to include MSM to your program.

A complete formula must deal with joint inflammation that causes swelling and pain. To combat inflammation naturally, precise amounts of enzymes and herbs are important. The National Institutes of Health just began a 5-year, multi-million dollar research project on the health benefits of these exact same herbs. Both tumeric and ginger have an impact on COX-2, an enzyme that triggers inflammation. COX-2 is what the latest anti-inflammatory drugs try to inhibit. The chart below lists some important anti-inflammatories.

NATURAL ANTI-INFLAMMATORIES

Bromelain—Bromelain, extracted from the pineapple, is an enzyme that interferes with a series of chemical reactions associated with inflammation. Less inflammation means improved joint flexibility and range of motion.

Pantothenic Acid—Pantothenic acid (vitamin B5) has long been recommended to combat the effects of stress on the body. It is critical to the production of adrenal hormones—your body's natural inflammation fighters. Pantothenic acid has also been shown to help many joint symptoms, starting with just 12.5 mg daily, but I suggest you take more.

Boswellia—The first important herb is boswellia. It is a tree sap (gum) extract historically used in Ayurvedic medicine for joint health. It affects inflammatory mediators (leukotrienes) without damaging normal joint tissues like many anti-inflammatory drugs.[46]

Tumeric—Tumeric has been used safely for centuries in cooking and as a traditional medicine. It contains curcuminoids, which are the active components. It impacts a key inflammatory mediator (cyclo-oxygenase 2, or COX-2) responsible for inflammation without causing harmful side effects.[47]

Ginger—Ginger is from the same family as tumeric and works much the same as tumeric. Recent studies have shown that it is a reasonable alternative to the popular anti-inflammatory drug, ibuprofen.[48]

Gout—Primarily a Male Disease

Perhaps the most painful form of inflammatory arthritis is gout. Fortunately, it is the form most readily controlled in most patients. Gout is primarily a male disease with about one million sufferers. For some reason, the big toe seems particularly susceptible, but smaller joints of the hands and feet may also be involved.

People once thought gout was the disease of kings—such as Henry VIII—because they associated it with foods that only kings could afford to purchase. Today, we know that gout can affect just about anybody, especially those under stress and who have an inadequate diet.

Victims of gout produce too much uric acid, or fail to excrete enough uric acid. Above certain levels uric acid forms microscopic crystals of sodium urate. These are shaped like needles and are just as sharp. When these needle-like crystals form in the joint fluid, they are "cleaned up" by special white blood cells. Unfortunately, when the white blood cells become full of crystals, they die, attracting even more white cells to clean up the debris. Deposits of crystallized uric acid salt in the joints causes swelling, redness, and a sensation of heat and extreme pain.

Consume plenty of quality water (not tap), as fluid intake promotes excretion of uric acid. Since gout is linked to stress, we must support the adrenal glands. We discussed aids for adrenal support earlier in this chapter. The following supplements and foods are helpful for gout problems.

Pantothenic acid

The body's supply of the B-vitamin pantothenic acid is responsible for converting uric acid into urea and ammonia, both of which are excreted in the urine. The nutritional approach is to help the adrenals produce cortisone by taking pantothenic acid, probably the most important vitamin for gout and stress. I would suggest 250 mg of pantothenic acid two to three times a day during a flareup. Include all of vitamin B complex. Alcohol should be entirely omitted from the diet because it increases uric acid production.[49]

Link to vitamin E

A deficiency in vitamin E causes the cell nucleus, where uric acid is made, to become damaged and uric acid is produced in excessive amounts. Rancid oils such as cooking oils, unrefrigerated mayonnaise, etc., all destroy vitamin E in our systems, causing an immediate imbalance of uric acid. Be sure to add at least 400 to 800 IU of natural vitamin E to your vitamin program.

Vitamin C

Ascorbic acid lowers serum uric acid levels. Read the information under the heading "Exhausted Adrenal Glands" in this chapter, which tells about the value of vitamin C.

I would suggest you take vitamin C with the bioflavonoids, (sometimes are combined with rutin and hesperidin), or add additional grapeseed extract or Pycnogenol. I recommend you take 3,000 to 5,000 mg of vitamin C daily in divided doses. Do not use time released capsules at these higher doses, as it stays in your stomach too long. You are "time releasing" it by using divided dosages throughout the day. You may also use buffered or Ester-C, but I would suggest capsules, not tablets.

Cherries, hawthorn berries and blueberries

These and other dark red-blue berries are rich sources of *antho-cyanidins* and *proanthocyanidins* (flavonoid molecules that give the berries their rich color). These compounds are remarkable in their ability to strengthen collagen.[50]

Studies have shown that consuming half a pound of fresh or frozen cherries a day decreases uric acid levels and prevents attacks of gout.[51] That sounds like a lot of cherries and not a very practical remedy, but the good news is that most nutrition stores carry a black cherry concentrate, which is deliciously sweet and contains no added sugar. It is very popular with my clientele. It can be added to plain yogurt or cottage cheese, or even mixed with water to make a delicious drink.

Systemic Lupus Erythematosus

Lupus is one of the more common autoimmune diseases that afflicts half a million Americans, and 90 percent of them are women. In this disease, antibodies attack the tissues of the body and organs. Some cases are mild, with minor problems, and some are extremely severe and crippling.

Many lupus patients have arthritic joint pain, swelling, and rashes, including the classic symptom, a rash on the cheeks. They also tend to have kidney problems and chest pain caused by inflammation in the lining of the heart and lungs and the other vital organs. The central nervous system is affected less frequently, but when it is, epileptic seizures, psychotic symptoms, and personality changes can result. Other symptoms may include unexplained fever, chills, hair loss, and progressive kidney disease.[52]

Autoimmune diseases are more common among older people, as the immune system begins to run down and becomes less efficient. It is not known what causes this autoimmune response to occur in these people. It may be triggered by an undetected viral infection; a genetic defect; a defect in the production or metabolism of sex hormones; or a combination of all these factors.

Numerous drugs have been thought to be responsible for causing lupus, among them tetracycline and other antibiotics, procainamide, birth control pills containing estrogen, sulfasalazine, and drugs used to lower blood pressure. If you are on these drugs, discuss this with your doctor.[53] If you have lupus our complete nutrition program should be used, plus the nutrients discussed for arthritis and osteoarthritis.

DHEA shows promise for lupus

Two successful studies from the Stanford University Medical Center have shown DHEA to be an effective treatment for lupus. DHEA in large doses was given to women patients with mild to moderate lupus. Eight out of ten patients reported that they were not only feeling and doing better, but showed improvement in their immune function. The encouraging part of the study was that patients were able to reduce their dose of prednisone, a corticosteroid used to control lupus symptoms. At this time the researcher from Stanford does not fully understand how it works, but he theorizes that it works by correcting certain abnormalities in the immune system.[54]

According to Michael Murray, N.D., the adrenal hormone DHEA, at a very high dose of 200 mg daily, can be of benefit in some cases of lupus. Do not try this large dose on your own. Lupus patients interested in taking DHEA should do so only under the care of a rheumatologist or trained physician, where the patient's blood levels can be closely monitored.[55] Currently, a large clinical trial testing DHEA's effectiveness on lupus is in progress, involving 25 universities and more than 200 patients. So far, the information looks promising for some of the people.

Back and Disc Problems:
Avoiding Surgery

Dr. James Greenwood, professor of neurosurgery at Baylor University School of Medicine in Texas, reported his observations on the effect of an increased intake of ascorbic acid (vitamin C) in preserving the integrity of intervertebral discs and preventing back trouble. He said that evidence from most patients indicated that muscular soreness experienced with exercise was greatly reduced by taking large doses of ascorbic acid. It increased again when the vitamins were discontinued.

Dr. Greenwood treated more than 500 patients and concluded: "It can be stated with reasonable assurance that a significant percentage of patients with early disc lesions were able to avoid surgery by the use of large doses of vitamin C. When the patients, after a few months or years stopped their vitamin C, their symptoms reoccurred. When placed back on the vitamin the symptoms disappeared. Some, of course, eventually came to surgery."[56]

Vitamin C, of course, is required for collagen production and collagen is the basic material in all connective tissue that supports muscles and bones. Glucosamine sulfate, vitamin D and all the minerals, especially calcium, magnesium, boron, and MSM (sulfur) should be taken.

Carpal Tunnel Syndrome:
Hand and Wrist Disease

Carpal tunnel syndrome is used to describe a number of symptoms that occur when the median nerve in the wrist is compressed or damaged. The median nerve controls the thumb muscles and is responsible for sensation felt in the thumb, the palm, and the first three fingers of the hand. The "tunnel" is the small opening below the surface of the wrist, where the median nerve in the hand passes through. This tunnel is lined with synovial membrane between the tendons and ligaments in the wrist, which is vulnerable to compression or injury.

Dr. John Ellis has shown that this disorder occurs about three times as frequently in women as in men, and it has a higher incidence during pregnancy and at menopause. Carpal tunnel syndrome is often associated with repetitive wrist motion, rheumatoid arthritis, obesity, diabetes associated with pregnancy, "tennis elbow," trigger fingers, and bursitis in the shoulder. Carpal tunnel is frequently diagnosed among those who work their wrists all day, such as computer operators, typists, postal clerks who sort mail, and so forth.

The symptoms can range from mild numbness and tingling to excruciating pain. Numbness is usually with the thumb and the first three fingers. The symptoms are usually worse at night or morning when the circulation is slowed down. It can affect one or both hands.

Vitamin B6—A controlled study

Vitamin B6 has been shown to shrink synovial membranes and has been used to bring relief to a number of people with carpal tunnel syndrome.

In a controlled, double-blind study of patients with carpal tunnel syndrome, those given 100 mg of B6 received great benefit, while those given a placebo had no benefit.[57]

Other research published in the *Proceedings of the National Academy of Sciences* stated that patients with carpal tunnel syndrome who were given 500 mg of B6 and 50 mg of B2 supplements experienced a complete disappearance of their symptoms.[58]

You should realize that 500 mg of B6 is considered a high dose, and should not be taken for a prolonged period of time.

All the vitamins and minerals I recommend for my clientele for all forms of arthritis should also be used. Remember, "healthy people don't have that, so let's make you healthy!"

Natural Oils for Arthritis

One of our friends was the late author Dale Alexander, who was dubbed the "Cod Father" because of his belief that cod liver oil could bring relief to sufferers of arthritis. He described these benefits in his book, *Arthritis and Common Sense.*

Fish oil contains EPA (eicosapentaenoic acid) and DHA (docosahexaenoic acid) that make body compounds that control inflammation and pain. Dale Alexander knew that cod liver oil helped thousands of arthritis sufferers. Today, a number of university laboratories are testing fish oils, rich in omega-3 fatty acids, as a means of helping arthritics. The resulting studies are encouraging, as the following chart shows.

FISH OILS HELP ARTHRITIS PATIENTS

☙ Animal studies at Harvard indicate that EPA helps protect the body against attack by its own immune system in autoimmune diseases such as rheumatoid arthritis and lupus erythematosus, as reported in the *New England Journal of Medicine.*[59]

    ✷   An article in *Clinical Research* reported that fish oil supple-
ments significantly improved symptoms in rheumatoid arthritis
patients. Forty patients were given 15 EPA fish oil capsules a
day for 14 weeks (approximately 1.8 grams of EPA a day). These
patients reported that they were in less pain, their joints were
less tender, and they made it through the day longer before
fatigue set in than those who were in a control group.[60] The
amount used in this study is equivalent to two tablespoons of
Max-EPA liquid.

    ✷   A study published in the *Lancet* showed that patients with
rheumatoid arthritis who received EPA for 12 weeks had less
morning stiffness and fewer tender joints. One to two months
after stopping EPA, their condition deteriorated to the prior
levels.[61]

    ✷   An Australian study in 1988 showed that 18 grams of fish oil a
day (18 capsules of 1,000 mg) for three months resulted in
fewer sore joints and measurable improvement in grip strength
in rheumatoid arthritis patients.[62]

    ✷   A number of studies have also shown a direct benefit from EPA
in lupus patients.

Omega 3 Oil

Usually one tablespoon of emulsified omega-3 oil provides over
1,000 mg of EPA and over 700 mg of DHA. It would take approximately
ten large softgels of EPA/DHA to equal just one tablespoon. Emulsified
means that the oil has been changed naturally to a water-soluble form.
The result is that it tastes better, with no aftertaste of oil, and it is easier
to digest. This form of omega-3 oil does not contain vitamins A and D.
DHA is very valuable for the brain, see chapter seven.

Cod Liver Oil

This valuable oil also contains the fatty acids, EPA and DHA, and it
also supplies vitamins A and D, as well as some natural cholesterol. The
emulsified form is the best tasting, easiest to digest, and most popular. The
recommendation is to take at least two tablespoons a day. Dale Alexander
insisted to me that the cod liver oil capsules were not effective for arthritis;
it must be used in the oil form or emulsified liquid form. Twinlab at one

time called their product *Dale Alexander Emulsified Cod Liver Oil*, which they named in his honor. It is available at most nutrition stores.

Flaxseed oil

Flaxseed oil is an excellent "vegetable" source of omega-3 fatty acids. Dr. Johanna Budwig, author of *Flax Oil As a True Aid Against Arthritis, Heart Infarction, Cancer and Other Diseases*, feels that mixing or blending flaxseed oil into good protein (like cultured, lowfat milk) will nourish the body better. She has repeatedly observed that the flaxseed oil and protein combination form special lipoprotein compounds that are easily digested, and the body will use them to build new tissues. She and other doctors in Europe use flaxseed oil mixed with non-fat yogurt or cottage cheese as an essential part of their successful dietary therapies for many modern maladies. It can be used in salad dressing, poured over vegetables or cottage cheese. Do not cook with this oil! One or two tablespoons a day would be an excellent addition to the daily diet. Be sure to use only the organic flax found in dark bottles, refrigerated at your nutrition store. Use the oil quickly to keep it fresh.

Omega 6 fatty acids (GLA) and evening primrose oil

Gamma-Linolenic Acid (GLA), part of the omega-6 family, is essential to good health. The body needs it to make a family of hormone-like compounds that control virtually every organ in the body. These compounds especially affect the heart and circulation, skin, immunity, and inflammation. The members of this vital family of compounds are called prostaglandins. Prostaglandins are so important to good health that the 1982 Nobel Prize in Physiology and Medicine was awarded to three researchers instrumental in the discovery of prostaglandins and their function in the body.[63]

Evening primrose oil, borage oil, and black currant oil are the richest sources of GLA. Since both EPA and GLA act as anti-inflammatory agents, and their mechanisms are slightly different, they work well together—each making the other more effective.

According to a study reported in the *Lancet*, GLA-rich evening primrose oil was found effective in controlling rheumatoid arthritis in a substantial number of patients. Some 90 percent of patients who took evening primrose oil felt better within two to four months, and more than 80 percent either stopped taking their anti-inflammatory drugs or were able to reduce the amount of drugs they were taking.[64]

In another study, rheumatoid arthritis patients were given

540 mg GLA and 240 mg EPA. After a year, those who received this dosage had reduced their amount of anti-inflammatory medicine significantly.[65]

Herbal Products May Help Arthritis

There are natural herbal products that may be helpful to arthritis patients.

Alfalfa helps stiffness

One of the herbals that Mother always recommended was alfalfa, taken in tablet form. A number of customers have said to me, "As long as I keep taking my alfalfa tablets every day, I have no more stiffness or pain in my hands."

ALFALFA: AN EXCELLENT SOURCE OF FIBER. Alfalfa *(Medicago sativa)* belongs to the legume family that includes beans, peas and clover. It is not a grass as some people believe. It is an excellent source of chlorophyll, potassium, magnesium and vitamins, especially beta-carotene. The reason alfalfa is so rich in vitamins and minerals is that, in its early stages of growth, the young roots have been known to penetrate as far down as 50 to 90 feet into the earth. The roots naturally "mine" precious mineral resources located deep in the soil.

Alfalfa tablets can be as beneficial to a person as eating a big green salad every day. They are an excellent way to prevent constipation, and it is essential that arthritics keep their bowels moving easily to prevent the buildup of toxins in their body.

Mother's recommendation was start with two or three tablets morning and night. Gradually increase that amount until you are taking as many as ten tablets twice a day. The tablets have a mild laxative effect with some people if too many are taken. You will soon be able to determine the proper amount for your body. If your elimination is sluggish, you should also consider adding acidophilus to your program.

Alfalfa has a superb calcium to phosphorous ratio, and it is the richest land source of the trace elements boron and silicon, both of which are valuable for bone integrity. One biochemist has observed that an essential alkaloid in the leaves of alfalfa works on the central nervous system to relieve minor pain. This may be part of the reason the plant has been helpful with arthritics.

Dr. Hans Fisher won a Nobel Prize for unraveling the chemical structure of hemoglobin from human blood. He was surprised to find that it was almost identical to chlorophyll, the plants' "blood." When Dr. Fisher separated the hemoglobin from the protein molecule to which it was attached, he found the main difference is that hemoglobin has an iron atom, and chlorophyll has a magnesium atom; otherwise they are identical.[66] *This has always amazed me—how God put this universe together. In other words, there is just a one-atom difference between the human blood supply and the plant "blood supply."*

Yucca as an arthritis aid

Dr. Robert Bingham started a revival of interest in yucca *(Yucca glauca)* after he reported the positive results of a one-year research program he conducted using yucca saponin (steroid compounds that are precursors to cortisone) in treating arthritis patients. Some believe that yucca saponins improve the body's ability to manufacture its own cortisone by supplying materials needed by the adrenal glands for cortisone production.[67]

The studies involved regular doses of yucca plant extract taken in tablet form. The patients reported there was less or even total elimination of pain, swelling, and stiffness. The patient should not expect sudden dramatic change. Yucca typically works over a period of time. It is not absorbed by the intestinal tract but acts indirectly on the intestinal flora, gradually eliminating or reducing harmful bacteria and encouraging the growth of favorable bacteria.[68] Diet and exercise were adjuncts to the yucca therapy.

Arthritis patients benefit from devil's claw

Devil's claw *(Harpagophytum procumbens)* is an herb that has been used to treat a variety of diseases, including gout and arthritis. Clinical research has shown it to have anti-inflammatory and analgesic effects, thus its benefit in relieving joint pain and decreasing uric acid levels.[69]

Devil's claw is a natural cleansing agent for removing toxic impurities from the body. It has been shown to be effective in helping hardened veins and arteries become elastic again, and it has helped patients with liver and gall bladder problems.

Using nature's aspirin—white willow bark

About 2,400 years ago, Hippocrates, the father of modern medicine, used white willow bark *(Salix alba)* as an effective pain killer. For centuries, before chemically synthesized aspirin was produced, people used white willow bark as a "natural aspirin."

The principal natural active agent in white willow is salicin. Salicin is an intermediate form of salicylic acid (or aspirin). Natural salicin seems to be converted into salicylic acid once it is in the body—with the same structure and function—except that salicin is mild on the stomach. In 1955 salicin was listed as an official botanical medicine in the *National Formulary*.

HISTORICAL USE OF WHITE WILLOW

Throughout history, white willow was used as:

- a fever lowering agent.
- a pain relieving (analgesic) agent, probably because it seems to depress the central nervous system.
- an anti-inflammatory agent for the treatment of rheumatism and arthritis.

Salicin, or white willow, is slower-acting than aspirin, but its action is stronger, longer-lasting, and safer than aspirin. As you may know, aspirin can cause adverse effects on the mucous membranes of the gastro-intestinal tract, including bleeding.[70] Although white willow is more expensive than aspirin, for many people it may be a safer product.

Eliminating the Nightshade Plants

Clinical evidence exists to lead some researchers to believe that an allergic reaction triggered by the "night-shade" family of plants appears to be the cause of arthritis. These foods contain solanine, a toxic substance that penetrates the immune barrier and creates a painful reaction, especially when consumed over a period of months or years.

Robert Bingham, M.D., who pioneered the research with yucca, believes that food allergies are a major problem in at least half of the people who suffer from arthritis, compared to only about 5 percent of healthy people having food allergies. He has stated, "Solanine may be the only cause of arthritis in some patients; in others, a secondary cause that interferes with their recovery."[71]

Our dear friend, the late Carlton Fredericks, Ph.D., lectured about this for years. In his book *Arthritis: Don't Learn to Live with It*, he details the need to omit nightshades from the diet.

Nightshades are various flowering plants, which include eggplant, tomatoes, peppers, potatoes, and tobacco. The substance that links these plants is *solanine*, a glycoalkaloid, which inhibits *cholinesterase*, an enzyme that provides agility in muscles. Studies have shown that elimination of this vegetable allergen for those who are allergic to it can control arthritis pain and relieve other symptoms of arthritis.

Norman F. Childers, Ph.D., the Blake Professor of Horticulture at Rutgers University, studied nightshades for years. He organized a group of thousands of individuals with arthritis who were willing experimentally to withdraw these foods from their diets. A large number of them became partially or totally relieved of their stiffness, aches, pains, and restricted joint mobility.[72]

In some instances, people were so badly crippled by arthritis they had to be confined to bed, or use walkers and wheelchairs. On a no-nightshades diet, they reported benefits ranging from relief to total recovery!

Eliminate these foods for a week or ten days and see if you are "allergic" to them. If you are allergic, it would be wise to eliminate them from your diet completely.

White potatoes

White potatoes were first introduced into Europe by 16th century Spanish explorers returning from the Americas, and were initially shunned because many people thought they were poisonous.

Glycoalkaloid and *solanine* are found throughout the potato, although the greatest concentration is in the peel. After eating white potato, some people experience a calming effect within an hour or so, but then aches tend to set in within the next day or two.

Potato products and potato starch are found in baby foods, inexpensive yogurts, gravies, and sauces. Potato chips are a special hazard for the solanine sensitive arthritic since the conversion of potatoes into chips increases the surface area of the potato exposed to light, which raises the solanine content. French fries drowned in ketchup is a particularly troublesome combination for the solanine sensitive since two offensive foods are included.

Sweet potatoes and yams are of a different family of potato entirely, and may be eaten.

Eggplant

This vegetable has only been used as a food in the present century. It was originally thought to cause emotional upset if it is eaten daily.

Tomato

The tomato was considered poisonous until the early 1800s. The solanine content was found to weaken the immune system and bring on arthritic disorders. Tomatoes are found in so many foods today— many prepared food items, as well as most Italian and many Mexican food dishes. We are a nation with a high intake of foods rich in tomatoes and peppers, from pizza to pasta to salads.

Tomato vines are poisonous to livestock. Just handling tomatoes or their vines causes some people to break out with sore, inflamed hands.

Peppers

The three main varieties of peppers that contain solanine: 1) sweet and bell pepper, 2) paprika and pimiento, and 3) chili and cayenne pepper.

Most of the Mexican foods on the market today include peppers of these types. Salsa with tomatoes and peppers is double trouble. Hidden sources of peppers include hot gravies and sauces, barbecue sauces, and certain medications that contain pepper oil. Chili peppers can often irritate the gastrointestinal tract or cause skin rashes. Black and white pepper are not of this pepper family and are acceptable.

Tobacco

Few people are aware that tobacco has toxic solanine content. Tobacco can affect the arthritic in two ways—with respiratory and cancer disorders, as well as injury to the immune system and antibody irritation, according to Dr. Fredericks.[73]

For more information on the nightshades be sure to read Dr. Carlton Fredericks' book, *Arthritis: Don't Learn to Live With It.* He covers all areas of arthritis and this would be a great addition to your library.

Natural Topical Preparations May Provide Relief

There are natural ointments and creams that, when applied topically, may provide relief. You may want to try the following:

Arnica *(Arnica montana)*

Rubbed on the skin, arnica is wonderful for the relief of pain due to muscle sprain, strain, injury or joint inflammation. Be sure to use arnica externally only, and never apply it to broken skin.

Capsaicin—Cayenne pepper

A cream containing small amounts of capsaicin, derived from hot peppers, seems to help symptoms of osteoarthritis. It can actually block the degeneration of synovial fluid in joints, according to studies reported in *Seminars in Arthritis and Rheumatism.* Chad Deal, M.D., of the Case Western Reserve University School of Medicine in Cleveland, said, "Topically applied capsaicin cream is an ideal analgesic therapy for patients with localized arthritis pain, offering proven efficacy with no systemic side effects...Relief occasionally occurs within a few days, but it may take a week or two to achieve full effect."

MSM

(Methyl Sulfonyl Methane) is an organic sulfur, a nonmetallic element that occurs widely in nature. MSM is important for your joints, hair, skin and nails.

MSM is also available in a cream used topically to aid skin disorders. MSM cream is helpful in treating arthritis pain, acne, psoriasis, eczema, dermatitis, dandruff, scabies, diaper rash and certain fungal infections.

Eucalyptus oil *(Eucalyptus globulus)*

When eucalyptus oil is rubbed on the skin it may provide relief against the pain of arthritis and rheumatism. This oil increases blood flow to the area, thus producing a feeling of warmth. It also may help soothe the stiffness and swelling associated with arthritis and rheumatism. Do not use this oil on broken or irritated skin and do not take it internally.

Commercially prepared liniments may also be used for muscle soreness or arthritis. Add eucalyptus oil to your bath, sauna and steam room treatments.

Other Considerations

HYDROCHLORIC ACID. Absorption of calcium in the gastrointestinal system depends partly on the presence of hydrochloric acid in the stomach. If an excessive amount of antacids or aspirin have been taken, or if there has been a shrinking of the gastrointestinal lining, a person may have a deficiency in the production of hydrochloric acid. Hydrochloric acid tablets may help not only with digestion, but also the assimilation of calcium and the other important minerals.

APPLE CIDER VINEGAR. The folk remedy of honey and apple cider vinegar for arthritis may be successful in part because it stimulates the formation of hydrochloric acid in the stomach. The acid in the vinegar also aids in calcium absorption. You can mix this remedy by combining one tablespoon of honey with one tablespoon of apple cider vinegar. You may want to use this as a salad dressing, or mix the honey and vinegar with vegetable juice. Some enjoy just drinking this combination in pure water every day.

CHRONIC CONSTIPATION. Many people with arthritis also complain of chronic constipation. They may have had trouble with their elimination for years. Consider taking alfalfa tablets and *Lactobacillus acidophilus*. It reimplants friendly bacteria into the intestinal tract that provides help with elimination. A friendly bacterium also helps remove toxins that can lead to infection. There are also many herbal colon cleansing products available in your nutrition store like *cascara sagrada* and *psyllium husks*.

DENTAL PROBLEMS. A number of arthritics report infections in their teeth that they have let slide for years. There are reports of arthritis clearing up after infected teeth have been pulled. Dr. Joseph Issels, a German cancer specialist, believes that root canals can be a major source of undetected infection in the body.[74] If you are experiencing arthritic symptoms, you may be wise to schedule an appointment with your dentist.

INFECTIONS. A large number and a wide variety of infections have been linked to arthritis.[75] They can be a contributing cause, or even the sole cause of arthritis symptoms or disease in many patients. Be sure to read chapters 3 and 4 on building your immune system with vitamins and herbal products. The program is outlined in detail in the last chapter, *Let's Put it All Together.*

OVERWEIGHT. It is accepted that excess weight puts more stress on the joints and can contribute to arthritis. Many insurance tables discuss what our weight should be but do not consider body composition. Because muscle is more dense than fat, a more muscular person is smaller in size than a "fatter" person, even though they are the same height and weight. Thus, your measurements, what size you wear, and how your clothes fit, are sometimes better guides for optimum weight. One doctor said he had several patients that avoided or postponed hip replacements "simply" by losing 20 to 30 pounds. So, weight loss may be the best place to start.

LACK OF MOTION. It is very important that you keep moving! A lack of motion seems to make arthritis symptoms worse. Although we tend to think of running as resulting in progressive wear and tear on the cartilage of the leg joints, studies have shown that many former long-distance runners have perfectly normal hip and knee joints, while their more sedentary friends are the ones plagued with degenerating joints.

I know of one woman who continued to type long letters to friends after she had retired from an office job because she found that the continued use of her fingers helped with arthritic pain. Swimming in warm water seems to help those who suffer from stiffness and pain in the hips and knees. Discuss with your physician the types of exercise that may be best for you to pursue...and then choose to stay active!

I pray that the above information will help you on the path to improved health, so that you may live free of stiffness and pain.

Anti-Aging Therapies

Slowing Down the Aging Process
with Various Hormones
Chelation Therapy and Cell Therapy

People have been searching for the "Fountain of Youth" for countless centuries. The more nutritional research that is being done, especially on hormone replacement, the closer we may actually be to finding such a "fountain."

—GLADYS LINDBERG

A number of new anti-aging therapies may prove very promising, especially when combined with methods that are more traditional. Conventional medicine is not generally accepting of these therapies, but remember that just a century ago, Louis Pasteur was ridiculed for suggesting that tiny organisms he called microbes could actually kill a man. And Ignaz Semmelweis in Vienna was persecuted and finally driven mad, because he said doctors should wash their hands before performing surgery.

This information is presented for your consideration. Realize that some are still in experimental stages. I am personally acquainted with a number of people, even my own family, who have benefited from many of these "anti-aging" therapies. Those who have used them are often highly appreciative and very positive about their effects.

The Importance of Our Hormones

The National Institute on Aging (NIA) conducts research with the goal of improving the quality of life and maintaining the independence and vitality of people well into their later years. In late 1992, the Institute launched a series of ambitious interventional studies to evaluate the safety and efficacy of certain hormones, especially human growth hormones and sex steroid hormones for older people.[1]

Hormone Replacement Therapy

These studies are taking place in several institutions across the United States, with additional research being conducted at the NIA Intramural Gerontology Research Center in Baltimore, Maryland. Scientists are conducting tests in order to explore the possibility that age-related disturbances can be slowed or partially reversed by the administration of these agents. Age-related decline includes changes in musculoskeletal function, body composition, and metabolic function, including weakening of muscles, bones, skin, nerves, and a number of organ and tissue cells. The researchers are investigating the value of combined hormone replacement therapy, with which they hope to return growth hormone and sex hormone levels to those typical of younger people.[2] They are hopeful that the additive or synergistic effects should improve both physical and psychological functions.

As we age, the production of the hormones DHEA, pregnenolone, melatonin, thyroid, estrogen, progesterone, testosterone and growth hormone declines. It is possible that hormone replacement may be an integral part of modern medicine in the not too distant future. Testosterone and growth hormones are discussed in the Men's chapter, pregnenolone in the Brain chapter, and thyroid in the Thyroid chapter.

DHEA—Anti-Aging Miracle?

DHEA exploded onto the market in March of 1996, and there were only one or two companies manufacturing it. However by our summer trade show convention, it seemed everyone had added DHEA to their brand of products. The list of research on DHEA is impressive. The New York Academy of Sciences; the Huffington Center on Aging at Baylor College; the National Institute on Drug Abuse (a study on DHEA and Brain Development, Aging and Memory); the University of California, San Diego; the Department of Microbiology and Immunology at Temple University; the University Hospital in Belgium and many other of the world's finest medical and research facilities have conducted extensive research into the biology, metabolism and effects of DHEA use and supplementation.

Most of the interest in DHEA was generated from articles in *Newsweek, Vanity Fair, Let's Live,* even the cover of *US News and World Report* which read, "Staying Younger Longer—How Scientists Are Pushing Back the Clock on Old Age." Even the *Wall Street Journal* and the *CBS Morning News* discussed DHEA. They have given it the title "The Mother of All Hormones." DHEA is here to stay and is an important anti-aging nutrient we should know about.

DHEA (dehydroepiandrosterone) is a naturally occurring steroid, a type of hormone distinguished from others by its unique chemical structure. A French chemist showed that DHEA is made from another hormone, pregnenolone, and that DHEA is, in turn, converted into estrogen and testosterone in both men and women.[3] DHEA is also produced by the adrenal glands (located on the kidneys) as well as by the brain and the skin. DHEA also converts to or stimulates the production of progesterone, cortisone, and the many other steroid hormones as the body needs them.[4]

We cannot ignore the rapidly expanding body of scientific research that indicates that DHEA may be helpful for preventing and treating a wide range of medical conditions. In fact, today nearly 5,000 in-depth scientific and medical studies on the use of DHEA have been conducted and completed in the laboratories of some of the top universities and medical research facilities in the world.

These studies have shown a direct relationship between low blood levels of DHEA and many diseases. Once DHEA has been released into the bloodstream, it is used in cellular metabolism and generates a wide variety of health and longevity benefits.[5]

I had the honor of meeting William Regelson, M.D., one of the nation's leading anti-aging doctors, at the American Academy of Anti-Aging Medicine convention. He is professor of medicine at the Medical College of Virginia and author of *The Superhormone Promise* and co-author of *The Melatonin Miracle* with Walter Pierpaoli, M.D., Ph.D.

DHEA APPEARS TO PROTECT THE BODY IN NUMEROUS WAYS.

Here are some of the reported benefits:

- Blood levels can indicate the present and future status of cancer and degenerative disease.
- Combats colon, breast, lung, and skin cancers in animals.
- Protects the immune system and thymus function to fight against infection.
- Fights obesity by rejuvenating a sluggish metabolism, reduces body fat and helps increase muscle mass.
- Helps chronic fatigue syndrome, Epstein-Barr, AIDS and shows promise with lupus.
- Lowers blood cholesterol and triglyceride levels thereby reducing the incidence of cardiovascular disease.
- Enhances memory, improves cognitive function, helps fight senility and early stages of Alzheimer's disease.
- Helps depression and learning problems.
- Stabilizes blood sugar levels and helps to prevent diabetes in adults.
- Appears capable of both inhibiting bone resorption and stimulating bone formation for osteoporosis prevention.
- Beneficial to those with Parkinson's disease and Grave's disease.[6]

Retard aging with DHEA

The secretion of this hormone markedly declines with age. DHEA appears in the bloodstream at about age seven, and then peaks at about age twenty-five. The secretion decreases progressively after that, and by age seventy it has diminished by 80–90 percent.[7]

Some age researchers agree that to retard aging, a person must maintain the peak serum level he or she had at about age twenty-five.[8]

It is currently being investigated as an anti-aging hormone. In essence, DHEA seems to rejuvenate the systems required for optimal functioning of the human body. The exciting part of the action of DHEA is that it may reverse many of the aspects of aging previously thought to be irreversible.[9]

Dr. Regelson says that his patients who are taking DHEA regularly to restore their youthful levels report they "feel more energetic, generally healthier, and also sexier than they had since youth. They feel this way on the outside because, inside their bodies, DHEA is actually correcting and reversing much of the deterioration to their organs and body systems—the "wear and tear"—that has been occurring since they reached middle age."[10]

Extending life-span

Some animal experiments have shown great promise in extending life-span.[11] So far there are no long-term studies on humans that show giving DHEA supplements can extend our life span. Nevertheless, I am sure these studies will take place.

Alan Gaby, M.D., reports that this age-related decline is not known to occur with any of the other adrenal steroids. It has therefore been suggested that some of the manifestations of aging may be caused by DHEA deficiency. In Dr. Gaby's experience, some elderly people who suffer from weakness, muscle wasting, trembling, and other signs of aging, experience noticeable improvements within several weeks of beginning small doses of DHEA (such as five to 15 mg a day).[12]

Feeling of wellness

Samuel Yen, M.D., a reproductive endocrinologist at the University of California in San Diego, reported that DHEA was "associated with a remarkable increase in perceived physical and psychological well-being." Among the volunteer subjects in his study, age 40 to 70, 67 percent of the men and 84 percent of the women reported feeling better. Dr. Yen found that they experienced increased energy, better sleep, and they felt more relaxed and able to handle stress. Those with arthritic symptoms also reported less joint pain. None of the study participants experienced any negative side effects. Dr. Yen says, "DHEA is a drug that may help people age more gracefully."[13]

Rejuvenates the human body

A fall in DHEA levels seems to be related to many forms of degenerative diseases including cancer, heart disease, diabetes, obesity, high blood pressure, and Parkinson's disease, to mention only a few. It has been proven to energize the body, restore sex drive, improve memory, lower blood cholesterol, fight obesity and heart disease, and strengthen the immune system. It relieves stress and may prove to be the most potent anti-cancer drug of all time.

People who take DHEA say they look and feel years younger. The theory, therefore, is that raising DHEA to more youthful levels through supplementation may help forestall the occurrence of these ailments, and we can battle all of these diseases and maintain health for a longer period of time.[14]

DHEA has also been shown to restore muscle mass, help with the beginning stages of Alzheimer's disease and other memory disturbances, rejuvenate immune system function including AIDS, battle chronic fatigue and create a sense of well-being in older people.[15] It may also be of value in preventing and treating osteoporosis.[16]

Memory enhancer

This powerful hormone also has a strong influence on the functioning of the brain. This is because there is more DHEA in the tissue of the brain than in any other tissue in the body. Optimal levels improve memory and mental acuity.

Forgetfulness is one of the first signs of aging. Dr. Regelson feels "several studies that have shown beyond any doubt whatsoever that DHEA has a direct and profound effect on the brain's ability to process and store information, and those results have now led some researchers to the belief that DHEA may play a major role in preventing the terrible mind and memory-robbing scourge we call Alzheimer's disease."[17]

Enhances immune response

DHEA may also enhance the body's immune response to viral and bacterial infections.[18] Our immune system is based upon the cooperation of several different types of cells, which learn to recognize and then attack infectious viruses and bacteria. Dr. Ronald Klatz, in *Stopping the Clock*, writes that one way DHEA may enhance immunity is by protecting the thymus gland, which regulates T-cells. These T-cells are the body's army for search and destroy missions of infectious agents. As we age our thymus gland shrinks, which scientists have linked with reduced immunity typical of the elderly. DHEA seems to wake up elderly immune systems to youthful levels of efficiency. DHEA may very well be responsible for decreasing age-related susceptibility to immune system "invaders" that can make us ill.

Animal research has shown that DHEA prevented thymic atrophy and improved the thymus' ability to control T-cells. Many researchers believe that DHEA supplements might also stave off the decline of the thymus in people. The immune-enhancing effects of DHEA still need further research as aging, infection and stress are all crucial factors that may affect its production.[19]

DHEA's immune enhancing power also affects diseases like AIDS. In an article in the *Journal of Infectious Diseases* (November 1991) researcher William Regelson, M.D., reported that only when DHEA levels drop do people with HIV develop full blown AIDS. In fact, low DHEA levels indicate twice the risk of HIV patients developing AIDS.

Anti-cancer effects

DHEA has protected against and slowed the progression of some cancers in animal work and in human studies. Some report it can actually block carcinogenic promotion.[20]

For example, the British medical journal the *Lancet* reported a study that followed 5,000 women and found that those who developed breast cancer had lower than average levels of DHEA in their urine as early as nine years before the development of cancer. The amazing part of the study was that all the women in the same age group died of breast cancer if their DHEA level was ten percent less than average, while those with higher than average levels remained cancer-free.[21]

In another experiment, Dr. Arthur Schwartz at the Fels Institute of Temple University gave rats a potent carcinogen that normally promoted tumor growth. He found, however, that when he gave the rats an injection of DHEA before introducing the carcinogen, they remained cancer-free. Surprisingly, it also increased the life span of these mice by an amazing 50 percent.[22] Dr. Schwartz is in the process of developing a DHEA-based drug that may prove to be the first anti-cancer pill.

Dr. Schwartz later reported on his DHEA animal studies, "Old mice regained youthful vigor and their coats resumed their former sleek and glossy texture; incipient cancers, whether naturally occurring or induced by artificial means, disappeared; obese animals returned to normal weight, and animals with diabetes improved dramatically."[23]

The good news, Dr. Regelson reports, is that DHEA and related steroids can block initiation or promotion of cancer depending on the model selected and can be thought of as chemopreventives. After a study of his advanced patients who had been diagnosed with terminal cancer, Regelson said, "The true leavening grace in this is that my patients were in stable condition and out of pain for most of their 'borrowed time.' Thus, although DHEA may not have 'cured' cancer, it improved the overall physical condition in patients and greatly enhanced the quality of life they had left."[24]

What exciting news as more research is continued!

Note: *Be sure to read about precautions on DHEA at the end of this chapter if you have cancer.*

DHEA may fight obesity

DHEA may prove to be the greatest weight loss boon to overweight Americans. Dr. Arthur Schwartz says, "DHEA is a very effective anti-obesity agent." DHEA induced weight loss in laboratory animals irrespective of how much food they consumed. DHEA appeared to stimulate the substance that signals us to feel full.[25]

Dr. M.P. Cleary found that even middle-aged rats lost weight when fed DHEA supplemented food. Diabetes, a typical complication of obesity, was also dramatically decreased. It appears from the most recent data that food deprivation, as dieting, is simply not necessary when using DHEA to lose weight.[26] This sounds almost too good to be true, but I sure hope it is!

This dramatic result has prompted researchers to study DHEA as a weight loss therapy for humans. In a human study the doctors at the Medical College of Virginia recently gave daily doses of DHEA for a full month to men with excess body fat. A control group of overweight men were given a placebo. Their diet and lifestyles remained exactly the same as before the study. The men in the DHEA group experienced an amazing 31 percent reduction in body fat and this lost body fat appeared to give way to new muscle. There was no change at all in the weight of men on the placebo.[27]

Another very common report from those who supplement with DHEA is that they lose weight and gain muscle. Some statistics have also shown that DHEA works as an appetite suppressant. But no matter the route, the evidence is clear that DHEA helps regulate body weight and body fat, to ensure that they are at healthy levels.

Osteoporosis prevention

Dr. Alan Gaby, author of *Preventing and Reversing Osteoporosis,* says that DHEA reads like the "who's who in osteoporosis prevention." His excellent book is suggested reading for those with or who want to prevent osteoporosis. DHEA functions as a precursor hormone, and can be converted by the body into other hormones including estrogen and testosterone, both of which play a role in the prevention of bone loss. In a study of postmenopausal women, administering DHEA increased serum levels of both testosterone and estrogens (estradiol and estrone).[28]

Bone-building effects

Also, DHEA may be capable of raising the levels of progesterone (a hormone manufactured by the ovaries). Dr. Gaby reports, "Although DHEA is not converted directly into progesterone, it may, through a feedback mechanism, indirectly increase the production of proges- terone. Both DHEA and progesterone are produced from the same precursor hormone, pregnenolone. If enough DHEA is present, then pregnenolone will be converted primarily to progesterone, rather than to DHEA."[29] DHEA might, therefore, augment the bone-building effect of progesterone. Preliminary results suggest that progesterone is at least as important as, and possibly even more important than, estrogen in preventing and treating postmenopausal osteoporosis. And as far as Dr. Gaby can tell, DHEA is the only hormone that appears capable of both inhibiting bone resorption and stimulating bone formation.[30]

Rheumatoid arthritis

In a study of 49 postmenopausal women with rheumatoid arthritis, DHEA levels (measured as DHEAs—the "s" stands for *sulfate*) were significantly lower than in healthy controls. DHEA levels correlated significantly with bone mineral density of the neck, of the femur (a bone in the hip), and the spine. The serum level of DHEA was able to predict bone mineral density, even after corticosteroid therapy was taken into account.[31]

Dr. Davis Lamson, a private practitioner in Kent, Washington, gave DHEA to several arthritic patients with low serum levels of DHEA. This treatment often relieved pain and morning stiffness, increased strength, and reduced the need for anti-inflammatory medication.[32]

In another study, Dr. Alan Gaby reported that 45 postmenopausal women being treated with corticosteroids were given 20 mg of DHEA a day, which resulted in an increased sense of well-being with no side effects.[33]

May prevent heart disease

A long-term study of 242 men between 50 and 79 years of age found that DHEA levels decreased with age as reported in the *New England Journal of Medicine.* Those with the highest levels of DHEA in their blood were only half as likely to die of heart disease as those with relatively little of the hormone, according to researcher Elizabeth Barrett-Conner at the University of California of San Diego.[34]

In a study at the Medical College of Virginia, patients who suffered from clotting problems were given DHEA. When researchers then examined the patients' blood, they found a significant decline in their propensity to form blood clots. By preventing excess blood clot formation, DHEA may protect against both heart disease and stroke, according to Dr. Regelson.

Those with histories of heart disease had particularly low levels of DHEA, and low levels, in general, were consistently associated with increased risk of death from any cause—even after adjusting for age, blood pressure, serum cholesterol level, obesity, fasting plasma glucose levels, smoking and history of heart disease. The connection between low DHEA levels and heart disease is a particularly strong one for men. According to Dr. Sheldon Saul Hendler this important study certainly suggests, but does not prove, that DHEA may confer some protection against several, and perhaps all, degenerative processes.[35]

Lowers cholesterol

After three months of taking DHEA, postmenopausal women showed an eight to ten percent decline in total cholesterol levels, which is quite significant given the fact that for every one percent drop in cholesterol, there is a two percent drop in the risk of developing heart disease. Other studies have since confirmed these findings.[36]

Improves sexual function

DHEA seems to turn back the aging clock when it comes to remaining sexually vital with advancing years. Men, particularly, report that it has revived their sexual interest, according to Dr. Regelson. Other doctors who prescribe DHEA report that many of their male patients experience an increase in libido and that many older men who did not have morning erections for years suddenly began to experience them after taking DHEA. We know that DHEA is converted into testosterone in both men and women, and that testosterone is known to enhance libido in both sexes. This would explain why those taking DHEA experience a heightened libido.

Although women also find that DHEA makes them feel better and more energetic, the heightened libido effect is not as apparent for them, possibly because women do not experience the same pronounced decline in libido that is common for men in their advancing years.[37]

Dr. Ray Sahelian, author of the book, *DHEA a Practical Guide*, has another opinion. He states that women in their 40s and 50s reported to him that DHEA gives them a powerful sex drive. He feels maybe it is even a minute increase in testosterone that may have this effect on women, whereas with men it would be hardly noticeable.[38]

DHEA for postmenopausal women

"It makes perfect sense that DHEA would be a useful treatment for menopause because DHEA is an estrogen precursor. This means that DHEA is converted to estrogen in the body. After menopause, when the ovaries stop making estrogen, small amounts of estrogen continue to be manufactured in the adrenal glands from hormones, including DHEA. Supplementing DHEA in postmenopausal women therefore appears to be a way of increasing estrogen levels naturally." Regelson also said that DHEA has some unique properties of its own that make it a boon for postmenopausal women.

Several clinical studies of DHEA's potential as a substitute for estrogen replacement therapy (ERT) are now under way, and several that have been completed have produced positive results. Preliminary findings indicate that DHEA offers many of the same benefits of estrogen without many of the potentially harmful side effects. Although DHEA may not do everything that estrogen does, it does do a lot in terms of relieving menopausal symptoms and protecting against disease, and it may even offer a few benefits that estrogen does not.[39]

A clinical study for menopausal women

In *The Superhormone Promise* by Dr. Regelson, he discusses some valuable information for menopausal women I want to share with you. Dr. Pierre Diamond reported on a study he conducted at Le Centre Hospitalier de l'Universit's Laval, Canada. He gave DHEA replacement therapy to 20 postmenopausal women, aged 60 to 70, for a year. None of these women were taking estrogen. DHEA was applied as a cream daily, and their blood levels were measured periodically to ensure that DHEA had been restored to 20-year-old levels. Nearly all reported an increase in energy and improvement in general well-being, but there were important physical changes:

- Dr. Diamond observed a reduction in both blood insulin and glucose (sugar) levels, reinforcing our belief that DHEA has a positive effect on insulin resistance. Since insulin resistance is a risk factor for heart disease, this suggests that DHEA shields postmenopausal women from heart disease, the number-one killer in postmenopausal women.

- Although the women's weight remained the same, they did show a change in "Body Mass Index," the ratio of fat to muscle. Their levels of fat decreased, and their levels of muscle increased.

- After menopause, women begin to lose roughly two to four percent of their bone mass each year. This causes many women to suffer from hip and spinal fractures. The good news is that while the women were taking DHEA, they showed a marked increase in bone density. In fact, after a year on DHEA, the average bone mass density of the women was increased at the hip and spine, two sites that are particularly vulnerable to osteoporosis.

- DHEA produced a modest drop in blood cholesterol of three to ten percent in the women. Even a modest drop can offer a significant reduction in heart disease.

- At least half the women in the study had suffered from vaginal atrophy, that is, a thinning of the vaginal wall (the endothelium), and a reduction in the production of vaginal secretions that lubricate the vagina, which occurs commonly after menopause. These changes not only

produce discomfort but they also promote vaginal infections and can make intercourse painful. DHEA may be a
good remedy, and appears to stimulate growth of the
vaginal endothelium and increase vaginal secretions, thus
restoring the vagina to its youthful condition.

Dr. Regelson said, "As an oncologist, what I find even more interesting was what DHEA did not do. Although DHEA did stimulate
growth of the vaginal lining, it did not stimulate the growth of the
uterine lining. In this regard, DHEA offers a distinct advantage over
estrogen replacement therapy."[40]

DHEA is no longer a prescription drug

It has now been confirmed with the Drug Enforcement
Administration that DHEA is not an anabolic steroid and is not a
controlled substance because it does not promote muscle growth.
DHEA is now classified as a dietary supplement according to an inter-
pretation of the 1994 Dietary Supplement, Health & Education Act. It
is sold in nutrition stores.

DHEA dosage

Opinions differ at the present time on the optimal dose of DHEA,
who should receive it, or when it should be started. Remember, we are
all biologically different. The following chart lists various approaches to
using DHEA.

OPINIONS AND RECOMMENDATIONS

 ❧ Dr. Alan Gaby considers a small dose, say 3 to 5 mg in the early
   postmenopausal period; and a larger dose, perhaps five to 15
   mg per day, in later years when adrenal output declines; and 3
   to 30 mg per day for the prevention of osteoporosis. He says
   much larger doses are being given to patients with cancer,
   AIDS, and other serious conditions.[41]

 ❧ Dr. Russe at University of California at San Francisco gave 50
   mg per day to individuals over 50 with declining memory, which
   had remarkable effects on well-being.[42]

 ❧ Dr. Julian Whitaker suggests the level of DHEA necessary to
   improve brain power appears to be 25 to 100 mg per day. All of

the human and animal studies on DHEA have found that it is exceptionally safe. The only side effect that has been mentioned with doses greater than 90 mg per day is infrequent and mild masculinization of women. This appears as facial hair or a drop in the voice timbre. These side effects go away with cessation or reduction of dosage of DHEA.[43]

Should I have my DHEA level measured before use?

Many feel it is important that one have his or her DHEA blood level tested before beginning a DHEA replacement program. This way the physician will know how much should be replaced. A second test should be drawn one month after beginning the treatment. There is no universal standard yet developed to determine an optimal dose. It is common practice, however, for a physician to use whatever dosage will bring the serum level of DHEA sulfate to 600 mcg/ml for men, and 400 mcg/ml for women.

There are saliva tests available so you can check your hormone levels. Many labs have these kits available, and you may be able to purchase these from your physician or nutrition store. These tests do not require the drawing of blood.

Most of the anti-aging researchers I have studied—Dr. William Regelson, Dr. Norman Orentreich, Dr. Samuel Yen, Dr. Edmund Chein, Dr. Ray Sahelian, and Dr. Ronald Klatz, to name a few—all agree that the DHEA levels should be monitored, to bring the levels up to "youthful age," and then checked periodically.

My friend and colleague, Marcia Zimmerman, M.Ed., C.N., who has reviewed the research on DHEA, feels that if we use the low doses, say 15 to 25 mg, it is probably not necessary to have our blood level tested. DHEA is generally well tolerated and quickly assimilated, but she does feel if we take higher doses, we should definitely have our blood levels checked.

Cautions

All of the research reports I have read suggest DHEA is safe in normal dosages. However, you need to know that adequate human studies have not yet been done on long-term usage of DHEA. Dr. Morton Walker warns that DHEA should not be taken by those lab tested with a suspicion of prostate cancer, due to the unproved but much *speculated* relationship between high testosterone levels (which DHEA may stimulate) and the onset of prostate cancer. This doesn't make much sense to me as every teenage boy would have prostate cancer. It seems to me that prostate problems develop in older men when testosterone levels are low. I am sure research will finally figure this out!

The *Life Extension Report* says, "patients with reproductive pre-cancerous conditions or reproductive cancer should not use DHEA, except under the strict monitoring of an experienced health care professional."[44]

This is not a product to be misused, and proper warning instructions should be followed. DHEA also should not be taken by any person who is under 40, pregnant, nursing, or taking any prescription medication. Persons suffering from any disease should consult a physician before using this product.

Melatonin May Reset the Aging Clock

Melatonin is a hormone produced in the pineal gland, which is situated deep behind the brain. Thirty years of laboratory research resulted in Dr. Walter Pierpaoli's landmark studies, which demonstrated that the pineal gland is our body's natural timekeeper and is regulated by the natural ebb and flow of the hormone melatonin. I had the honor of meeting and hearing Dr. Pierpaoli lecture on Melatonin at the 2nd International Anti-Aging Conference in Monte Carlo, Monaco. He feels that we may be able to slow the process of aging, turn back the hands of time, strengthen our immune system, and thereby heighten our resistance to disease and even prolong our sexual vitality by simply restoring the melatonin levels of youth. There are thousands of animal and human studies that suggest many roles for melatonin.

Melatonin was discovered in 1958, when Dr. Lerner at Yale University isolated the molecule. The other sex hormones I have discussed—estrogen, progesterone, testosterone, pregnenolone—are all made from cholesterol. Melatonin, however, is made from the amino acid tryptophan, an essential amino acid, meaning our bodies do not produce it. Instead, we must get tryptophan from the foods we eat. The best sources are found in the following: turkey, milk, whey, soy protein, cottage cheese, yogurt, fish, beef, liver, lamb, peanuts, pumpkin and sesame seeds, brown rice, and lentils.[45] The body converts these foods into the neurotransmitter serotonin, which is involved in controlling mood. Then at night serotonin is converted into melatonin.

The initial clinical studies on melatonin focused on problems related to the sleep-wake cycle or circadian rhythm of the body. But today melatonin ranks as one of the important hormones, stimulating the release of a wide variety of other hormones from the pituitary gland.[46] Many of the functions of melatonin sound similar to those of the human growth hormone (HGH). Melatonin can stimulate the release of human growth hormone. But recent studies indicate that in aging individuals optimal levels of melatonin cannot bring the human growth hormone levels high enough for you to experience maximum health.

Russell J. Reiter, Ph.D., author of *Melatonin: Your Body's Natural Wonder Drug* and Professor of Neuroendocrinology at the University of Texas, has been researching melatonin for more than 30 years. He has concluded that melatonin is the most powerful antioxidant molecule yet to be discovered. He considers it a hormone that possibly can "reset the body's aging clock, turning back the ravages of time."[47] Scientists may be on the verge of discovering the real "fountain of youth" that Ponce de Leon only dreamed about.

An interesting study on mice

Dr. Frank Varese of Laguna Hills, California, is the doctor that introduced me to the world of natural hormone replacement several years ago. To spur my interest in melatonin, he gave me a cassette tape on Dr. Pierpaoli's work. He is the premier researcher on the product. After hearing the fascinating tape, I then read the book. Here's what Dr. Pierpaoli, co-author of *Melatonin Miracle,* wrote about on a mice study he conducted:

> In fall of 1985, I began the first of what would be many experiments testing the effect of administering melatonin supplements to older mice. I selected healthy male mice that were 19 months old (human equivalent of about 65 years); they live to about 24 months. I divided the mice into two groups, one given melatonin in the evening drinking water, the other group regular tap water. Everything else, diet, living conditions, was exactly the same.
>
> At first, I could detect very little difference between the two groups of mice. Within five months, however, the

difference was astonishing. The untreated mice began to display the expected signs and symptoms of old age—of senescence. They lost muscle mass, they developed bald patches, their eyes grew cloudy with cataracts, their digestion slowed down, and so, generally, did they. In sum, they seemed worn out and tired—they were winding down and becoming old.

On the other hand, the melatonin-treated mice looked and behaved like their grandchildren. The mice on melatonin had actually grown more fur and continued to boast thick, shiny coats. Their eyes were clear and cataract-free, their digestion had improved and, instead of growing thin and wasted in the manner of the non-melatonin-treated mice, they maintained their strength and muscle tone. The vigor and energy with which they moved around their cage resembled the behavior of mice half their age.

Most importantly, they lived much longer! The untreated mice, having reached their expected life span of about 24 months (70 to 75 years in human terms), began to die. Yet the melatonin mice lived on and on—an astonishing six months longer, which in human terms would amount to gaining an extra 25 years of life, or living well past one hundred.[48]

Dr. Pierpaoli went on to determine the cause of death and found that most of the untreated mice had died of cancer, common for their breed and age. However, much to his surprise, the melatonin-treated mice had remained disease-free throughout their extended lives. He said their organs had shrunk, typical of old age, but they did not suffer or die from cancer.

Dr. Pierpaoli had succeeded in reversing the aging process in these animals, but what this experiment revealed about aging was even more remarkable:

> This experiment proved that disease is not an inevitable part of aging, and that it is possible for us not only to live longer lives, but to live them in strong, disease-free, healthy bodies. Senescence, the downward spiral that we have come to associate with aging, does not have to occur. Melatonin can stop the spiral.[49]

THE MICE GOT SEXY. Scientific protocol demands they repeat the experiment several times to make sure they can duplicate the results. Each time the results were the same. However, in one of Pierpaoli's experiments, they used male and female mice, and discovered something exciting.

Both the males and females displayed the sexual prowess of much younger mice. In fact, right up until their death, these mice were sexually active. He said this would be the equivalent of 100-year-old men and women showing the sexual interest and stamina of people a third their age![50] Amazing!

PREVENTS HEART DISEASE AND NORMALIZES BLOOD PRESSURE. Melatonin can lower cholesterol, thereby preventing the formation of plaque deposits that can clog arteries and block the flow of blood. Melatonin can normalize blood pressure and inhibit the action of free radicals, both of which are conditions that can destroy arteries and injure the heart. Melatonin can even blunt the destructive effects of corticosteroids—stress hormones that can inflict damage to the heart muscle and an otherwise healthy body, according to Dr. Pierpaoli.[51]

BOOSTS IMMUNE FUNCTION. One of melatonin's greatest powers is its ability to boost the immune system. The pineal gland, when secreting greater amounts of melatonin in a young individual, is able to restore the thymus to its healthy size. The thymus is the gland responsible for the production of T-cells, which fight off infectious organisms and cancerous cells. The thymus is also important in strengthening antibody response and increasing cellular activity. Our thymus undergoes a dramatic transformation as we age. It is largest during childhood, then begins to shrink and virtually disappears in old age. Melatonin appears to protect this gland by restoring it to its youthful size. This increases the number of T-cells available to fight off invading organisms as we grow older.[52]

Other studies have shown melatonin's immune-enhancing ability by knocking out viruses, moderating the effects of corticosteroid overproduction in response to stress, and rejuvenating thyroid function, which influences T-cell production. It also neutralizes some of the side effects of mammograms, x-rays, and surgery.[53]

Melatonin also protects against a variety of degenerative and age-related neurological conditions of the brain, such as Parkinson's disease, Alzheimer's disease, schizophrenia, and depression. It has also been shown to prevent cataracts.[54]

The cancer connection

Recent research has shown that melatonin combats cancer in many different ways. It not only strengthens the immune system's ability to spot and destroy abnormal cells that may turn cancerous, but it prevents the age-related decline in immunity that can leave a person more vulnerable to cancer.[55]

Studies have shown that women with low levels of melatonin are at greater risk for developing breast cancer. When the cancer does appear, the pineal gland starts pumping out greater amounts of melatonin to go to work fighting the invaders. In this way, melatonin not only influences the immune system, but acts as part of it.[56] Ironically and unfortunately, a traditional cancer treatment like chemotherapy suppresses the secretion of melatonin.[57] I hope the time will come when they combine melatonin with other promising anti-cancer treatments to see if a greater cure rate is possible.

Melatonin can dampen the effect of hormones that can trigger the growth of certain types of cancer, including breast, cervical, and prostate cancer.[58] In tissue cultures, melatonin has a direct, lethal action on melanoma cancer cells and estrogen-sensitive breast cancer cells.[59]

Melatonin as a sleep aid

This hormone controls our sleep-wake cycle, what scientists refer to as the *circadian rhythm*. Melatonin establishes the biological rhythm of each cell in the body. The presence of adequate amounts of melatonin induces sleep and may reduce anxiety, panic disorders, and migraines. A disruption of routine—shift work, travel across more than three time zones (jet lag), or even erratic daily schedules—can reduce melatonin levels and desynchronize (undo) the body's internal clock. The gland secretes the hormone melatonin during times of darkness and is suppressed by bright light.

Those who have trouble sleeping should try melatonin. Drugs such as NSAIDs (for pain of arthritis), sedatives, some tranquilizers, and anti-psychotic drugs can actually reduce melatonin levels. This may mean that a greater quantity of these drugs are needed over time to promote sleep. It also means that the REM phase of sleep may be interrupted. REM sleep is that which is required for a person truly to feel rested after sleeping. The use of melatonin, which is derived naturally from tryptophan and serotonin, may be the natural answer for giving you a sleep pattern that is healthy and doesn't leave you feeling drugged and unrested.[60]

Melatonin as a sex-enhancing hormone

Sexual arousal occurs when your brain and endocrine glands pump out sex hormones. The activity of these glands is controlled by the pineal gland and one of its chemical messengers, melatonin. The same messenger is also involved in signaling clues that tell us to touch and cuddle.

Libido is largely regulated by hormones. In men the male hormones, *testosterone* and *dihydrotestosterone*, among others, govern arousal and erection. In women, female hormones *estrogen* and *progesterone* and also male hormones or androgens are involved in the sex drive. In order to feel sexy, aroused and interested, you need to produce normal levels of these hormones, and it is the duty of melatonin to make certain we do.

Fluctuations in our melatonin levels stimulate the pituitary gland to release a number of hormones that regulate sexual activity. These hormones include *luteinizing hormone* (LH), which is involved in ovulation and the secretion of estrogen; *follicle-stimulating hormone* (FSH), which regulates the production of sperm in men and stimulates the maturation of the ovaries in women; and *prolactin* and *oxytocin*, which stimulate milk production and maternal bonding. The normal ebb and flow of hormones are essential to our ability to respond sexually.[61]

Heightens endorphins

Melatonin can also make sex a more pleasurable experience at any age. Melatonin heightens the effect of endorphins, the natural tranquilizers produced by our body that can relieve pain, stress, and create a sensation of pleasure and well-being. Melatonin's endorphin enhancing ability, which increases the pleasure of lovemaking, becomes even more important with each passing decade. As we age, we often lose our ability to experience pleasure. Through its effect on endorphins, melatonin can help relieve stress and thus create an environment that is more conducive to lovemaking.[62] Dr. Pierpaoli believes that taking melatonin supplements at bedtime later in life, starting at the time when natural levels begin to drop, may help restore these other hormones to more youthful levels and thus enable us to maintain our youthful levels of sexuality as well.

Melatonin dosage

The amount of melatonin a person should take is still being

debated. Some researchers believe it should be taken in small amounts, such as 0.5 mg a day, while others recommend larger amounts, 3 mg a day or more.

Drs. Pierpaoli and Regelson recommend the following dosages that are based on a person's age:

RECOMMENDED DOSE

Age	Dose of Melatonin
40–44	0.5–1 mg at bedtime
45–54	1–2 mg at bedtime
55–64	2.25 mg at bedtime
65–74	3.5–5 mg at bedtime
75 plus	3.5–5 mg at bedtime

If a recommended dose leaves you groggy in the morning, the dosage is too high for you. Reduce it until you find the right level for your body. Many authorities suggest that 1 mg a day should be adequate for a long period of time.

It is important that melatonin only be taken at night, about a half hour before bed. It is not known whether larger doses of melatonin are safe for long-term use. Hormones are extremely potent biological compounds that are usually effective in small doses. While melatonin shows great promise as an anti-aging hormone, we need to regard it with respect. Scientists will continue to explore its power. As of this writing, there are no known side effects.

Many doctors have said that melatonin has been shown to be completely harmless to the body. In other words, no matter how high the levels, melatonin apparently causes no side effects other than a natural drowsiness.[63] The aim is balance, and too much of any of these hormones throws off your body's functioning as much as having too little.[64]

CAUTIONS. Melatonin is not recommended for people under 40 years of age as you don't want to interfere with your own production of the hormone at an early age. It should not be taken by children, pregnant or lactating women unless under a doctor's supervision. You can find this "natural anti-aging nutrient" in several potencies at your nutrition store.

Chelation Therapy
for Blocked Arteries

Some on the forefront of nutrition research believe strongly in chelation therapy, and have solid evidence, research results, and statistics to back up their beliefs. Chelation therapy (key-lay-shun) is a procedure that costs about one tenth what bypass surgery costs, has minimal risk factors associated with it, and causes very little, if any, pain. It has a growing reputation as a "treatment of preference" for blocked arteries.

Chelation therapy is aimed at stripping lead, aluminum, mercury, cadmium, and unwanted calcium deposits from the arteries and other parts of the body in a way that allows these materials to be excreted through the kidneys. To accomplish this, physicians administer an amino acid solution called EDTA (ethylenediaminetetraacetic acid) through an intravenous drip into the bloodstream, for about three hours, two to three days a week. The number of treatments would be suggested by the physician, but usually 20 to 30 treatments are administered.

The therapy originated in Detroit, Michigan, in 1948 as a means of treating victims of lead poisoning. Physicians found that after the treatments, their patients showed marked improvement in their arteriosclerosis. Further experimentation resulted in the treatment we know today.

The word *chelate* comes from the Greek *chele*, which refers to the claw of a crab or lobster, implying a firm, pincer-like hold. EDTA floats past a hardened area in a blood vessel, and its strong attraction for calcium and lead causes it to literally "pick up" the offending mineral and pull it out of the area.

The treatment is given by member physicians of the American Academy of Medical Preventics (AAMP) in medical centers across the nation. Approximately six million infusions have been administered in the United States solely for the purpose of reversing degenerative diseases associated with hardening of the arteries. In the past 12 years of record keeping, not one death has occurred due specifically to chelation therapy when it has been administered by physicians who followed the standard protocol established by the ACAM.[65]

The medical literature contains some 10,000 articles about chelation, of which 1,800 were clinical studies. All but one of these many studies describe favorable results![66]

H. Richard Casdorph, M.D., Ph.D., Diplomat of the American Board of Internal Medicine, has been at the forefront of chelation therapy. I discussed chelation with him, and he told me that clinical studies on chelation have documented directly the effectiveness of this therapy in treating sclerotic heart valves, coronary heart disease, atherosclerosis, intermittent claudication (leg pains due to lack of circulation), gangrene, angina pectoris, heart attacks, stroke, senility, and even Alzheimer's disease. Studies have shown that the basis of most of these problems is poor circulation caused by hardening of the arteries.[67]

Chelation therapy: One of medicine's best kept secrets.

In this article by Gary Null it was reported that chelation has also been shown to help multiple sclerosis, arthritis, macular degeneration (a disease that causes blindness), hypertension, diabetes, and adverse reactions to environmental pollutants.[68]

Chelation has restored victims of severe angina to health, with complete freedom from pain and vastly improved tolerance for exercise. Many reported an improvement in intellectual function as chelation therapy improved the circulation to their brains.

The American Medical Association has not endorsed chelation therapy completely, ruling it is not useful because the effects are not lasting. The pharmaceutical and health insurance industries also stand in opposition to the therapy. Yet the Food and Drug Administration has approved EDTA for use in chelating lead and digitalis intoxication.

We should perhaps keep in mind that not all bypass surgery and angioplasty patients experience lasting effects unless they make significant lifestyle adjustments, including the addition of exercise and, very often, a change in dietary patterns.

Magnesium—A key mineral

Dr. Casdorph pointed out that magnesium is one of the key ingredients in the chelation formula, and it is added to every IV of EDTA solution. After the magnesium enters the bloodstream, it breaks away from the EDTA and serves to dilate arteries and relax smooth muscles so that the EDTA is more effective in its work of binding calcium, aluminum and other abnormal metals that should not be in the bloodstream, and then carrying them out of the body by way of the urine.

Mother was a great advocate of chelation therapy. She had a series of treatments several times as a preventive measure to keep her arteries clear. The benefit of chelation is that it provides an alternative means of treating blocked arteries in a preventive way, prior to emergency situations for which bypass surgery may be the only solution.

A cardiovascular surgeon's view

Ralph Lev, M.D., M.S., who is a clinical associate professor of surgery at New Jersey Medical School, has said, "As a practicing cardiovascular surgeon, I and many of my associates have patients who are not surgical candidates. These patients are then often relegated to a life of continued disability and pain. A member of my family fell into this group and was told to 'go to a nursing home and die.' He was instead treated with EDTA chelation therapy and is alive and comfortable three years later. I often observe similar benefits for patients in my own practice who have had chelation therapy. Those of us in academic medicine and surgery should put aside our blinders, open our minds, and delve further into any promise of improvement for those unfortunates who have no other hope."[69] Dr. Lev is also a vascular surgeon and chief of cardiothoracic surgery at John F. Kennedy Medical Center.

For lasting results

You can repair clogged plumbing, but for truly lasting results you need to correct the problems that created the clogged plumbing in the first place. Those who administer chelation therapy recommend to their patients certain lifestyle changes: cessation of smoking, intelligent choices of food, and proper use of vitamins and minerals. They frequently recommend an increased use of antioxidants, plus minerals, lecithin, garlic, rutin, and even kelp to help the thyroid.

More information is available in several good books: *The Chelation Way* by Dr. Morton Walker; *Toxic Metal Syndrome* by Dr. Morton Walker and Richard Casdorph, M.D.; *Bypassing Bypass: New Techniques of Chelation Therapy* by Elmer M. Cranton, M.D.

To find a physician who is competent in chelation therapy

Contact the American College of Advancement in Medicine (ACAM), 23121 Verdugo Drive, Suite 204, Laguna Hills, CA, or phone 1-949-583–7666 or 1-800-532–3688, or visit their web site at www.acam.org. ACAM lists more than 1,000 doctors across the nation who administer chelation therapy.

Cell Therapy

Cell therapy involves using "like cells" to treat "like cells." Cell therapy has been used with growing acceptance throughout the world in recent decades. It currently is not legal in the United States, but it is available in Switzerland, most other European nations and the Bahamas.

This type of therapy is actually quite old. Skin transplants from animals to humans were mentioned by Hippocrates, and physicians have long held the opinion that incorporating human or animal organs from a young and vital body may have a therapeutic benefits.

We had the pleasure of knowing Joachim Stein, M.D., from Heidelberg, Germany, and the privilege to visit his laboratory where the cells were freeze dried. The precautions and extent they went through to prevent contamination were really amazing. I was so impressed.

Dr. Stein points out that both Aristotle and one of the oldest known medical documents, the *Papyrus of Ebers*, mention a number of preparations made from animal or human organs. In the 16th century, Paraclesus offered this prescription: "Heart heals heart, kidney heals kidney."[70]

The Swiss surgeon, *Dr. Paul Niehans*, is credited with having developed cell therapy. The first cell injection in 1931 was a completely new method and a convincing success. A woman suffering from severe convulsions was transferred to Dr. Niehans' care following an unsuccessful operation on her parathyroid glands. He saved her life with an injection of a suspension of animal parathyroid glands.

As his research progressed he discovered that the cells from embryonic sheep tissues, injected into the muscles of an older or exhausted person, had a rejuvenating effect. He also observed that injections of animal cells from specific embryonic organs could improve the same organ in a human being. Thus, heart diseases were treated with heart cells, liver problems with liver cells, and so forth, just as Paraclesus had suggested.[71]

Dr. Niehans further found that the adult human body did not reject these embryonic animal cells. Cell therapy promotes physical regeneration and is used to stimulate healing, counteract the effects of aging, and treat a variety of degenerative diseases. The cell is a small, independent organism that has a life and metabolism of its own. As the smallest unit of life, the cell is the bearer of life. All human and animal organ cells are formed according to the same basic plan, have the same structures and physiologically the same basic functions. Even in specific organs there is no difference between the cells of humans and those of animals. In over 40 years of practical experience it has become apparent that the sheep is the best donor. Sheep are resistant to diseases, and sheep protein agrees well with humans.

Live cell therapy was originally used by Dr. Niehans, but he found it was impossible to control sterility and there was too much chance of contamination. Dr. Niehans developed and improved the method of freeze-drying for conserving cell preparations. These cell preparations are storable in ampules and will keep for at least ten years.

Distribution patterns of injected cells

Animal tests conducted by Prof. F. Schmid at Heidelberg University have established that, immediately following injection, the cells and tissue of the donor animal are transported by white blood cells (phagocytes) in the patient's blood to organs and tissues of similar type. There the specific organ cell elements are built into, and help to repair, the patient's damaged organs and tissues. The patient's organism is equipped with the capacity to recognize and accurately evaluate the implanted organ-specific cell elements from the donor material. Prof. H. Lettre of Heidelberg University proved this with tests utilizing marked cell material. For these tests the injected organ specific cells, previously marked with radioactive substances (isotopes), were traced along their path through the body of the recipient with a Geiger counter, to the designated organ.[72] Amazing!

Today there are over 900 scientific publications and more than 50,000 medical reports that record the effectiveness and successes of cell therapy in degenerative diseases and premature aging. Increasingly, cell therapy appears to provide a means of medically restoring lost vitality and making possible a complete, fulfilled life well into old age. I am sold on this process and wanted you to know about it. The only slight problem is, as of this writing some of the European clinics are now closed.

Men's Unique Challenges

Anti-Aging Therapies for Men
Testosterone, Human Growth Hormone,
Help for Impotence and Prostate Health

*There seems to be many therapies to keep aging men
with a spring in their step and a twinkle in their eye.
An excellent nutritional program with all the
vitamins, minerals and hormones seems to be the
bottom line.*

—GLADYS LINDBERG

*T*his entire book contains valuable information to help build your health. However, there are certain nutritional situations exclusive to men that may need extra attention that are included in this chapter for your consideration.

A darling couple in their mid–70s were discussing their nutritional needs with me. She was very enthusiastic and had been taking her supplements for years, but her husband was not very interested. I finally said to him, "Now you need to be able to keep up with your wife, so you can chase her around the house!" We all laughed. Later, he came up to me and whispered, "Do you have something to take in case I catch her?"

For Sex to Work, Things Have to Be Right Biochemically

Optimal nutrition clearly plays a role in determining interest in sex. Do you lack energy or sexual stamina? Do you have emotional problems, are you irritable, critical, nagging or depressed? Do you lack the energy to take a bath? This scarcely sets the stage for an evening of ecstasy. All of these seemingly insignificant things can prevent a fulfilling sexual relationship.

For sex to work, things have to be right biochemically. We need to go back to the basics; first of all, are you eating properly? What did you have for breakfast? It is important you have adequate protein in your daily dietary routine. Remember your muscles are made of protein. And, you need all the vitamins and minerals in adequate potencies.

My dear friend Adelle Davis reported in her classic book, *Let's Get Well*, that research is meager concerning nutrition and sexual performance. But she reports that it is known that protein, essential fatty acids, vitamin E, and several of the B vitamins are essential before the sex hormones can be produced. "A lack of protein causes a loss of sexual interest and a decrease in sperm count. Unless vitamin E is adequate, the testicles of all varieties of laboratory and farm animals degenerate; and there is a decrease in both the sex hormones and the pituitary hormone gonadotropin, which stimulate the sex glands. Vitamin E also protects the sex hormones from destruction by oxygen."

Adelle also reported, "Men deficient in vitamin B_6 have become impotent; and during stress, the sex urge and sperm production diminish. The motility and fertility of sperm are in proportion to the amount of vitamin E in a man's sperm."

Poorly nourished men and women of a sexually active age, upon autopsy, showed shriveled ovaries and testicles, a decrease in the cells that produce sperm or ova, vast areas of dead tissue, and much scarring; and the ovaries and testicles alike have been loaded with brown pigment characteristic of a vitamin E deficiency. The changes were similar to those seen in advanced senility and in animals deficient in any one of several nutrients, particularly vitamin E.[1]

The importance of zinc and sexual development

Zinc has numerous relationships with male sexual development and function all through a man's life. Zinc deficiency in childhood leads to impaired development of the male sex organs; the boy's penis may not develop to full size, and his beard and auxiliary hair may be less full than normal.[2]

In adulthood, zinc is vital to the testicles and for testosterone production. Even a marginal zinc deficiency can lower a man's libido. Adults may become infertile, and their sexual function impaired. Other symptoms of deficiency include poor wound healing, loss of hair, increased susceptibility to infection, reduced salivation, skin lesions, stretch marks, and reduced absorption of nutrients.[3] Check your mineral supplement to confirm you are taking at least 15 to 50 milligrams of zinc. Most authorities agree you should not take over 100 mg.

No magic bullet

There is no "magic bullet," but the following suggestions may be considered as an addition to your complete nutritional program. As we age, the production of DHEA, testosterone, melatonin and growth hormones decline. Men especially should be interested in these hormones since they help keep energy levels high and affect muscular strength and sexual stamina. We have discussed DHEA and melatonin previously. Be sure to consider those supplements in this regard.

Testosterone: The Male Sex Hormone

Scientists of ancient days knew that the removal of the testicles would take away the vitality and aggression of men and beasts. Historically, castration (removal of the testes) was performed on male slaves who guarded Muslim harems. It was also used on some male singers during boyhood to preserve a high-pitched voice.[4]

The testicles are male gonads, or sex glands, that produce sperm and secrete *androgens*. The production of androgens by the testes is controlled by certain pituitary hormones, called *gonadotropins*. The most important and active of the androgen hormones is *testosterone*, the male sex hormone. Testosterone is produced chiefly in the testes, but also in small amounts in the adrenal glands and in the ovaries of women. It stimulates bone and muscle growth and is responsible for the development of male secondary sex characteristics at puberty, including enlargement of the penis and the growth of facial and body hair.[5]

The effects of testosterone are most pronounced during puberty. It brings on the enlarged larynx, thicker vocal cords, new body hair, increased muscle mass, and increased oil-gland secretion by the skin commonly associated with puberty. After puberty, levels of testosterone drop gradually in men, with profound effects occurring later in life on physical health and well-being and particularly on mood and libido.

Testosterone is the hormone that makes men feel in their prime. If testosterone is restored to youthful levels, you will feel as you did when you were at your peak of physical and mental strength. You'll feel sexier, stronger, and healthier. In a real sense, testosterone is the ultimate aphrodisiac. Testosterone is responsible for the sex drive in both men and women, and it is the hormone that stimulates our desire for sexual activity and orgasm.

A low testosterone level is one of the most neglected hormonal difficulties in all of medicine, according to Herbert L. Newbold, M.D., in *Mega-Nutrients for Your Nerves*. Dr. Newbold taught neurology and psychiatry at Northwestern University Medical School and authored a textbook on psychology (which is used in medical schools around the world). He now considers himself a nutritional psychiatrist, someone who recognizes that the results of vitamin, mineral, hormonal, and other deficiencies are generally not taught in medical schools.[6]

Dr. Newbold routinely tests serum testosterone levels of all his male patients, and he finds that a large number (20 to 30 percent) suffer from a deficiency. The lack of testosterone could be the result of emotional illnesses, testicle damage, male menopause (where they experience a gradual decline of hormonal output), or excessive alcohol or marijuana consumption. He recognized early on in his research that his patients with low testosterone levels had grossly deficient diets. Dr. Newbold said, "Recently it has also been discovered that male homosexuals, as a group, have significantly lower serum testosterone levels than heterosexual males..."[7]

"Male menopause" or andropause and the importance of testosterone

Men who are experiencing "male menopause," known as *andropause*, are now interested in testosterone and what it can do for them. Andropause does not happen as quickly in men as menopause does in women. While andropause and menopause share similarities, the rate of the fall of total plasma testosterone is much slower than the rather rapid drop in estrogen levels associated with menopause.

Dr. Ronald Klatz is President of the American Academy of Anti-Aging Medicine. I have attended almost all of their conventions in Las Vegas and have heard Dr. Klatz lecture many times on hormones. In his excellent book, *Stopping The Clock*, he reported a large scale epidemiological study of male sexual behavior called, The Massachusetts Male Aging Study. It looked at a cross-sectional random sample of 1,709 men, between the ages of 40 and 70 years. They found that the mean testosterone levels decline by about one percent per year. Fifty-one percent of the normal, healthy males in this age group reported experiencing some degree of impotence. Several organic factors contributed to this impotence in up to 80 percent of the men affected. Diabetes, hypertension (medications used), smoking, chronic alcohol use and high cholesterol were cited as major factors in male potency loss.

While the total testosterone of a male does not drop drastically, the free testosterone, which is the biological active part of testosterone, does drop precipitously with aging. In fact, a significant drop in free testosterone can occur as early as the forties causing impotency or libido problems.[8]

William Regelson, M.D., in *Super Hormone Promise* said, "Testosterone can stop and reverse the physical decline that otherwise robs men of their energy, their strength, and their libido. Testosterone can restore muscle tone and improve stamina. For men who have lost interest in sex—and perhaps in life itself—testosterone can restore healthy sexual excitement and desire."[9]

Low testosterone can also predict susceptibility to abdominal weight gain (increased waist-to-hip ratio), the men you see with a large stomach. This is a pattern of obesity that is also associated with heart disease and diabetes. Testosterone, like estrogen, is a hedge against osteoporosis. It also seems to be associated with better sleep quality, and a deficiency in senior men may account for the familiar sleepless-ness of older age.

Dr. Gerald Phillips of Columbia University Medical School states, "A low testosterone level may lead to atherosclerosis, and that testos-terone may protect against atherosclerosis in men through an effect in lipoprotein—HDL. Administration of testosterone to men has been reported to decrease risk factors for heart attack".[10]

Testosterone occurs naturally in adult women at a level around one tenth of that found in men. Women's adrenals pump out other andro-genic hormones like DHEA and androstenedrone, also considered longevity hormones.

Health advantages of high testosterone

Studies show that men with high testosterone levels live longer, healthier lives and maintain sexual potency. Testosterone goes far beyond just promoting aggression, body and facial hair, and male pattern baldness. It has also been shown that testosterone has a protec-tive effect against autoimmune disease. Testosterone is anabolic, meaning that it promotes muscle growth. Loss of lean body mass is a major feature of aging in both men and women. Testosterone offsets this loss.

The most significant study about the correlation between high levels of testosterone and reduced risks of cardiovascular disease was reported in May 1994, when the Department of Medicine at Columbia University found that low levels of free testosterone are a risk factor and correlate directly with the degree of coronary artery disease in men.

Increased/inhibited by lifestyle

There are certain factors that can promote or inhibit testosterone levels. A low fat diet limits testosterone production, since the choles-terol molecule is the building block for male sex hormones. Additionally, vigorous exercise promotes testosterone, but over-training may diminish it.[11] Sexual activity also boosts testosterone, but severe stress or depression may lower it. Many older men can still sire children but sperm production may be reduced.

The history of testosterone

The following chart gives a brief history of the research studies that show the variety of benefits of testosterone:

HISTORY OF TESTOSTERONE

- In 1934 scientists isolated the testosterone molecule and illustrated the structure. They received the Nobel Prize in 1935.

- In 1938 the beneficial effect of testosterone on impaired glucose tolerance was discovered.

- In 1939 scientists found it can improve intermittent claudication and reduce angina pectoris and confirmed that it can cure gangrene.

- In 1945 another scientist showed it was able to stop angina pectoris.

- In 1951 it was shown that testosterone can improve nitrogen balance and increase lean muscle mass.

- In 1960 another scientist discovered it can lower cholesterol.

- In 1962 scientists normalized the abnormal electrocardiograms of 2,000 cardiac patients with synthetic testosterone.

- In 1963 a study showed it can improve diabetic retinopathy.

- In 1964 scientists showed testosterone can lower the insulin requirements of diabetic patients and decrease the percentage of body fat.

- In May 1994 the Department of Medicine at Columbia University reported that low levels of free testosterone are a risk factor and correlate directly with the degree of coronary artery disease in men.[12]

Administration of testosterone

There are several forms of natural testosterone and growth-hormone that can be administered by a physician, preferably an expert in hormone replacement therapy. I suggest that your physician test your blood for levels of testosterone and growth hormone. The test should determine the level of "free" or "unbound" testosterone because this is the form of testosterone actually available for use in the body. Testosterone is available only by prescription.

Synthetic testosterone taken orally or by injection, for the most part, causes liver toxicity (hepatotoxicity) and its use is not recommended.[13]

In the past, doctors were hesitant to supplement testosterone levels in healthy men for fear of increased risk of prostate cancer. Recent data suggests that testosterone is not a causal factor in development of prostate cancer. The research showed no significant differences were found in age-adjusted total testosterone or free testosterone before diagnosis. This data suggests that there are no measurable differences in testosterone levels between men who were destined to develop prostate cancer and those who did not develop the disease.[14]

Dr. Ronald Klatz reports, "Most physicians today prefer to use natural testosterone rather than synthetic testosterone. Natural testosterone can be delivered by intramuscular injections, suppositories, a patch attached to the scrotum, a cream applied to the scrotum, oral micronized capsules or sublingual lozenges. Administration of testorone in the form of a precutaneous gel (absorbed by skin into the bloodstream) is currently used in Europe and has been shown to be very effective in mimicking the natural mode. The least effective method seems to be via the oral route, since studies have shown the testosterone to inactivate."

DHEA is converted into testosterone

Dr. Regelson believes that for many midlife men whose testosterone levels are normal for their age, testosterone is not necessary if they are already taking DHEA. This is because DHEA is converted into a small amount of testosterone in the body and this, Regelson believes, will provide enough of a testosterone boost to counteract the decline. He also believes that because DHEA is what we call a testosterone precursor, it may at least postpone the need for testosterone. Thus a man in his 40s or 50s may do well on DHEA alone until he reaches his 60s or 70s, at which point he may require testosterone.[15]

Stimulate Your Own Anabolic Mechanisms With ZMA

What do Olympic level athletes and Navy SEALS have in common? They suffer from exercise-induced mineral loss that robs them of strength, endurance and growth. ZMA is the only non-steroidal, natural dietary supplement clinically proven to increase free testosterone levels and strength in training athletes. ZMA replaces minerals lost during strenuous exercise. And it has been shown to improve strength, endurance and muscle recovery. In a recent study Insulin-Like Growth Factor (IGF-1) levels increased by 4 percent whereas the placebo group decreased by 10 percent!

ZMA is a patent-pending formula containing highly absorbable zinc, magnesium and B_6 to maximize your body's own anabolic functions. A study of strength-training collegiate football players showed ZMA increased free testosterone more than 40 percent!

After 8 weeks of strength training, nightly ZMA supplementation was shown to increase quadricep strength 250 percent greater than a placebo![16]

The best time to take ZMA is on an empty stomach before bed to ensure peak absorption and maximize anabolic hormone production at night. ZMA should not be taken with any calcium-containing supplements or foods, which will impair its absorption. ZMA can be purchased at your nutrition store under different brand names.

Human Growth Hormone Therapy

Human growth hormone (HGH, GH or somatotropin) is the most abundant hormone made by the pituitary gland. It hits its peak in the body during adolescence and is responsible for the rapid growth spurt experienced at this time. It promotes lean muscle tissue and decreases body fat. Studies suggest that low levels of HGH are responsible for shrinkage of vital organs and may be linked to increased risk of cancer and heart disease. Also the latest studies from Johns Hopkins show that by maintaining youthful levels of human growth hormone the immune system strengthens, muscle and bone regain strength and size, the skin thickens and becomes firm again.[17] This research on the value of hormone replacement is anti-aging medicine at its finest.

Amazing results!

The conservative *New England Journal of Medicine* published in 1990 a landmark article, "Effects of Human Growth Hormone in Men over 60 Years Old," headed by Daniel Rudman, M.D., and his colleagues at the Medical College of Wisconsin. In their study they selected 21 healthy men aged 61 to 81 and injected 12 of them with human growth hormone three times a week for six months. The rest of the men were untreated and served as a control.

The HGH receiving group experienced an 8.8 percent increase in lean body mass, a nearly 15 percent decrease in fat tissue, a 7 percent increase in skin thickness, and a 1.6 percent increase in lower spine bone density.

Based on his study Dr. Rudman wrote: "The effects of six months of human growth hormone on lean body mass and adipose tissue mass were equivalent in magnitude to the changes incurred during 10 to 20 years of aging." In the study, the men's sense of well-being and ability to care for themselves was markedly enhanced, along with a return of sexual interest and performance.[18]

Thanks to Dr. Rudman, many serious scientists and physicians all over the world began to think about aging in a different way, to look at the possibility of growth hormone replacement in the treatment of aging and age associated diseases. Since his report, more than 28,000 studies have appeared in other journals in England, Denmark, Sweden, the U.S. and other parts of the world describing the benefits of growth hormone.

Dr. Ronald Klatz, in his book *Grow Young with HGH*, gives glowing reports on the benefits of growth hormone. In fact, he says it is the only age-reversing drug that has passed placebo-controlled, double-blind clinical trials with flying colors, not once, but many times over.[19]

The National Institute on Aging has funded a multi-million dollar effort in nine medical centers to determine if growth hormone and other factors can be useful in helping the elderly remain strong and vigorous. The studies are still in progress.

Dr. Regelson says, "I have studied growth hormone extensively through the years and believe there is a place for growth hormone in the superhormone pantheon of age-reversing agents." He also said, "Growth hormone has a very special role to play, and its benefits will be most acutely felt by those who are in greatest need and who are suffering from more severe problems. For these people I think the risk of side effects is minimal compared to what they stand to gain."[20] This doctor believes it is possible to gain the same beneficial effects using the other superhormones, particularly DHEA, melatonin, and testosterone, which are inexpensive, easily available, and have no unwanted side effects.

"Growing weak, growing frail, and getting sick is not an inevitable part of the aging process, and by restoring our superhormones to their youthful levels, we should be able to prevent the diseases of aging," according to Regelson. He also reported, "There are special circumstances when we need to restore a failing organ or stave off a serious illness. Growth hormone can revive a dying heart, stave off kidney failure, and reverse severe osteoporosis. It is strong medicine indeed and not, in my opinion, something for standard use."[21]

As you can see, there are many opinions on the value and long-term use and safety of growth hormone replacement therapy. Supporters say growth hormone therapy can be safe with proper doses and proper methods of administration. They say we do not have 20 years to wait for all the research to be completed. Its effects on health and well-being are so remarkable, and its age-reversing properties are so great, many say it is well worth the $9,000 to $12,000 a year it costs for daily injections.[22] I am sure this price will drop as use becomes more widespread.

In a 1994 review paper on the use of human growth hormone in hormone deficient adults, Drs. Rowen, Hohannson, and Bengtson of the University Hospital of Goteborg, Sweden, had this to say: "When one does not abuse or overdose human growth hormone, there is simply NO evidence suggesting that human growth hormone replacement therapy causes any long-term side effects."[23]

Dr. George Merriam of the University of Washington in Seattle, who is conducting one of the National Institute on Aging studies on growth hormone was quoted in the *New York Times*, July 18, 1995, as saying that the preliminary findings of his team includes "a complete absence of side effects."

New products containing growth hormone precursors

Growth hormone can only be obtained with a prescription from your doctor. However, there are many new products appearing in the marketplace that contain precursors to growth hormone or contain ingredients that stimulate the release of HGH by your own body. I suggest you check into the research on any of these products to confirm their efficacy. Ask what research was done and what their results were. Are they using the HGH injection "results" for their selling points?

L-Glutamine and growth hormone

L-glutamine is an amino acid found in protein foods that has been found to increase growth hormone levels. Perhaps the most exciting news for those fighting the aging process is L-glutamine's effect on growth hormone. A recent study at Louisiana State University Medical College gave as little as two grams (2,000 mg) oral dose of L-glutamine to nine healthy athletes in the morning after a light breakfast. The *American Journal of Clinical Nutrition* reported that the blood levels of growth hormone rose 430 percent above initial levels 90 minutes after L-glutamine supplementation.[24]

A study at Oxford University compared the health status of more than 150 runners. Half of the test subjects were given five grams (5,000 mg) of L-glutamine after a strenuous bout of exercise, while the other half took a placebo. Almost twice as many in the group with L-glutamine stayed healthy during the next seven days compared to the placebo group.[25]

I feel L-glutamine is a valuable and affordable product and since it's tasteless, it is easily added to your protein shake or juice. Read the *Let's Put it All Together* chapter for the shake recipe. L-glutamine is available in capsule or powder form.

Nutritional Help for Impotence

It has been estimated that 10 to 20 million American men suffer from impotence. It is thought to affect 25 percent of men over the age of 50, but aging itself is not a cause of erectile dysfunction or impotence. Impotence is considered difficulty achieving or maintaining an erection. Doctors classify impotence as either organic (caused by physical factors) or as psychogenic (caused by psychological problems). In reality, many cases of impotence are a combination of both physical and emotional. Only recently have scientists uncovered the biochemistry that links many organic forms of impotence. This biochemical pathway seems to have a dietary component. This is not to say that a change in diet can cure impotence, but there is a suggestion that diet and nutritional supplements may play an important role.

From a large-scale study of male sexual behavior called *The Massachusetts Male Aging Study of 1984–89,* researchers looked at a cross-sectional random sample of 1,709 men between the ages of 40 and 70 years. Dr. Irwin Goldstein, an organizer of the study, points out that, "Organic factors contribute to impotence in up to 80 percent of men affected." Dr. Goldstein said, "Diabetes, hypertension (medications used), smoking, chronic alcohol use and high cholesterol are major factors in male potency loss."

Drugs that cause erectile dysfunction

Many drugs can lead to erectile dysfunction, including agents used to combat mental depression and high blood pressure. Among the most common drugs associated with impotence are steroids, some appetite

suppressants, opiates, some cholesterol lowering drugs, some antihistamines, acid blockers, antidepressants, tranquilizers and even antifungal
agents. Smoking, marijuana and heroin are also associated with
impotence.[26]

If you suspect a drug is responsible for your impotence, discuss it
with your doctor and see if he can find an effective alternative for you.

The value of DHEA for male impotency

The effects of DHEA on male sexual function was documented in
the same groundbreaking *Massachusetts Male Aging Study*. This study
demonstrated that the risk of severe or total impotency increases
threefold with age. In other words, 5.1 percent of all 40-year-olds
compared to 15 percent of all 70-year-olds complained of complete
impotency. The researchers noted that impotency is often associated
with underlying medical problems as we have just discussed. But of the
17 hormones measured in each of the men only one showed a direct
and consistent correlation with impotency: DHEA. As DHEA levels
declined, the incidence of impotency increased. The Massachusetts
researchers could not explain why DHEA levels were lower in impotent
men. They speculated on many theories.

Dr. Regelson believes that DHEA has a direct effect on sexuality,
saying, "We know that DHEA is converted into testosterone in both
men and women, and that testosterone is known to enhance libido in
both sexes. This would certainly explain why such men when they take
DHEA experience a heightened libido."[27]

Testosterone and impotence

A common symptom of low testosterone is a lack of sexual desire,
and many men who experience this loss of desire assume that they are
impotent. Dr. Regelson, author of *The Superhormone Promise,* says the
fact that a man is low in testosterone does not mean that he is physically unable to maintain an erection and enjoy sex. The problem is that
a man low in testosterone may simply not care enough to pursue it. He
may feel impotent even though he is technically not.

Dr. Regelson went on to say, "Happily, restoring testosterone to
youthful levels can turn this situation around, practically overnight.
Once testosterone levels are replenished, a man will find that he has
recaptured a healthy interest in sex—as well as the capacity to enjoy it."[28]

Nutrients for impotence and increasing sperm co

It is possible to banish impotence, cure frigidity, and even stim fertility, providing real hope of conception, according to Robert Erdmann, Ph.D., in *Amino Revolution*.

HISTIDINE—AN AMINO ACID. Dr. Erdmann reports that histidine needs to be present in good quantity for orgasm to take place. This amino acid is the parent of the active molecule *histamine*. Orgasm is triggered when histamine is released in the body from the mast cells in the genitals. These cells function as part of the immune system, but they also cause the sexual flush experienced during arousal. When there is insufficient histidine in the body, and histamine production is low, both men and women may find it difficult, sometimes even impossible, to achieve orgasm.[29]

MEN AND WOMEN, TAKE NOTE! Dr. Carl Pfeiffer, M.D., Ph.D., a medical researcher, examined the benefit of histidine for women and found that those women with low histamine levels were not able to experience orgasm. When they took extra histidine, they were able to experience orgasm for the first time. Without any psychotherapy, the women who had been given histidine broke the bonds of frigidity, achieving an enormous sense of liberation. They were given 500 mg of histidine before each meal. From Dr. Pfeiffer's research, Dr. Erdmann suggested a balanced nutritional program and a multiple vitamin and mineral formula, which also includes: lysine and arginine with cofactors, vitamin B3 (niacin), vitamin B6 (pyridoxine) and manganese.[30]

IT'S A TWO-EDGED SWORD. Dr. Pfeiffer also examined the benefit of histidine for men, discovering what a two-edged sword it is. Male orgasm is a localized reflex caused by the release of histamine from a large concentration of mast cells in the head of the penis. As expected, the circulating levels of histidine played a significant role, both in the ability of a man to climax and the time it takes him. The higher the levels, the shorter the time needed—so much so that for a few this led to another problem—premature ejaculation, according to Erdmann.

Dr. Erdmann reported how Pfeiffer's studies were then extended to those men suffering from premature ejaculation. He discovered that their high histamine levels could be lowered by methionine (an amino acid), taken with a little calcium as a cofactor. These men are now able to lead more satisfying sex lives.[31]

TYROSINE—AN AMINO ACID. Dr. Richard Passwater states that studies have shown that penile erection is achieved via a complicated pathway involving neurons. A deficiency in the nerve chemical messenger would prevent erection. Animal experiments confirmed that agents that would block or deplete the neurotransmitter (a chemical that affects or modifies the transmission of an impulse across a synapse between nerves or between a nerve and a muscle) did indeed cause impotence. If this is the case, then it is very likely—but to Passwater's knowledge untested—that tyrosine can circulate in the bloodstream to nourish the penile neurons so as to normalize norepinephrine (a hormone secreted by the adrenal medulla and a neurotransmitter released at nerve endings) production and restore penile erectile function. It is certainly worth a try and is a sensible alternative to the alternative, according to Dr. Passwater.[32]

ARGININE AND SPERM PRODUCTION. The importance of the single amino acid arginine for normal sperm production in the human male is well established. There is a relationship between low sperm count and diets deficient in arginine. Human semen is particularly rich in arginine. Studies of men with low sperm counts in which they were given arginine supplements met with mixed results, more having shown benefit than not. In one study, 80 percent of the men had moderate to marked increases in sperm count and motility when given four grams of oral arginine daily—and with clear results. When the study was published, 28 pregnancies were confirmed! Do not take arginine if you have kidney or liver disorders, unless you receive permission of your physician.[33]

These single amino acids may be purchased from your nutrition store, and they are also included in many combination amino acid products in lower potency. Remember, the richest source of all the amino acids is protein foods.

VITAMIN C AND INCREASED SPERM COUNT. Dr. Earl Dawson at the University of Texas Medical Branch in Galveston treated 35 men working in the petroleum industry who were found to have defective sperm—sperm unable to fertilize the female egg cells. After testing the men for vitamin C, the scientists found they were all very deficient in this nutrient. When they were given 1,000 milligrams of vitamin C every day, the condition was corrected and normal sperm appeared after only one week of vitamin therapy.

VITAMIN E AND MALE INFERTILITY. Mild deficiencies of vitamin E allow fewer sperm to be produced, whereas a severe lack of it causes permanent sterility in men. Conversely, when men have increased their vitamin E intake, the quality of their sperm improves markedly, especially if vitamins A and E are taken together, because vitamin A deficiencies drastically lower experimental fertility and damage the sperm-producing cells.[34]

In a study published in the October 1996 issue of *Fertility and Sterility,* the researchers showed that consuming 600 IU per day of vitamin E dramatically improved the function of human sperm. Because spermatozoal disfunction is the most common cause of infertility among men, the authors of the study believe that vitamin E could be an easy and inexpensive means to treat this condition.

Herbal Medicine to the Rescue

There are many herbal sources of help for sexual dysfunction. The brief discussion that follows may provide helpful relief.

Yohimbe—an aphrodisiac?

Twenty years ago a Danish fertility specialist gave his livestock yohimbe *(Corynanthe yohimbe)* and found it to be an instant aphrodisiac. The sexually sluggish bulls and stallions became more active and were able to perform their usual duties. Studies were done on laboratory rats with the same results.[35]

Yohimbe is listed in the *Physicians Desk Reference* as a sensual stimulant. It aids in increasing the sexual desire, but the main function is to increase the blood flow to the erectile tissue. According to Louise Tenney, M.H., in *Today's Herbal Health*, "It has been found to be effective in treating both organic (physiological) and psychogenic (mental) forms of impotence. The aphrodisiac effects associated with yohimbe are related to this dilation. It increases the blood flow and enlarges the vessels in the sexual organs as well as increases reflex excitability in the lower spinal cord."[36]

"Yohimbe has been found to make the erections harder and firmer through the increased circulation to the area. It is also thought to aid in maintaining an erection by causing a compression and preventing the blood from flowing out of the organ. Vascular disease is known to be a major factor in many cases of impotence," according to Louise Tenney.

You can find yohimbe in your nutrition store. Some feel it is a testosterone precursor and is an effective body builder. Yohimbe is a hormone stimulant and is useful as a strong athletic formula herb where increased testosterone is needed.[37] You may find yohimbe alone or in combination with other herbs for men's needs. There needs to be more research on this interesting herb, as not all agree on its use or effectiveness.

Ginkgo Biloba—over 300 million years old

Ginkgo extract is taken from the fan shaped ginkgo leaf. *Ginkgo biloba* is one of the oldest living tree species. Individual trees can live for 1,000 years. Today the ancient ginkgo has sparked renewed interest throughout the world because medical researchers have isolated chemical compounds from ginkgo that show startling effects in humans, including increased sexual energy and longevity.

Because ginkgo is effective on both brain function and blood flow to extremities, including blood to the penis, this compound might be especially useful as a treatment for impotence. An interesting study in the *Journal of Sex Education & Therapy*, 1991, reported that ginkgo biloba extract was effective in helping men regain sexual potency. Some 50 men with proven erectile impotence were provided ginkgo extract for nine months. All had been relying on injectable drugs but found with continued use of ginkgo "they regained spontaneous erections...and demonstrated improved penile flow rates and rigidity." Among 30 men who could not achieve erections even with high-dose drug applications, 19 regained erections with ginkgo.[38]

Ginkgo's effects are more apparent with long-term therapy. Herbalists recommend ginkgo biloba extract in a dosage of 240 mg daily (divided into two or three doses). The product label should state it is standardized to contain 24 percent ginkgo flavoneglycosides.[39] You can read more information on ginkgo in chapter 7, *Anti-Aging Nutrients for Our Brain*.

I was watching a classic program on PBS (Public Broadcasting System) showing an Egyptologist discussing a female mummy found in a temple in Egypt. Since I have traveled to Egypt several times, walked through many of the tombs, and climbed the pyramids, I am always fascinated with these programs. This very prim and proper lady discussing the mummy said they analyzed samples of her hair and found she had been using ginkgo biloba. She said, "Ginkgo is more effective than any Viagra as a sexual stimulant." I couldn't believe what I was hearing. She went on showing the ginkgo plants painted on the temple walls, and discussed the value of ginkgo in ancient times. Sounds like it must be effective!

Korean Ginseng—Used for thousands of years

Korean ginseng *(Panax ginseng)* is an adaptogenic herb, one that has been used for centuries in traditional Chinese medicine as a tonic for impotence. There are no human, double-blind, placebo-controlled studies to prove its effectiveness. Interestingly, we attended a Christmas party at our Korean neighbor's and the host was passing around liquid Korean ginseng to all the men with great glee! He knew it worked and tried to convince the men this was a potent aphrodisiac. You could never have convinced him otherwise, and after thousands of years of use in their culture, they must know!

In studies with animals, sperm formation and testosterone levels increased with ginseng administration. Testes grew and increased sexual activity and mating behavior were observed.[40]

Dr. Donald Brown recommends 100 to 200 mg twice daily (standardized extract containing 4 to 7 percent *ginsenosides*). Use continually for three to four weeks, with a one- to two-week break between rounds.[41]

Damiana's many functions

Those familiar with damiana typically think of it as an aphrodisiac. Damiana *(Turnera aphrodisiaca)* is native to Mexico and the southwestern United States. It has been used as a major herbal remedy in Mexican medical folklore for the treatment of impotence, sterility, diabetes, kidney disease, bladder infections, asthma, bronchitis, chronic fatigue, and anxiety. It is one of the herbs of choice for helping with sexual impotency and infertility with both males and females. It is a relatively safe but bitter-tasting herb.[42]

The Male Prostate Gland

The prostate gland is a male sex gland, and is about the size of a walnut and weighs less than an ounce. It wraps around the upper part of the urethra, a tube that carries urine from the bladder out through the tip of the penis. The prostate gland plays a significant role in the male reproductive system.

Responsible for the production of semen, the prostate adds fluid to the sperm to power it during ejaculation and increases its mobility. It also provides a potassium and enzyme rich fluid that bathes and nourishes the sperm for good health, and serves as its storage area. The prostate needs male hormones to function and the main male hormone is testosterone, which is made mainly by the testicles. Some male hormones are produced in small amounts by the adrenal glands.

Symptoms of prostate enlargement include frequent daytime and nighttime urination, slight pain or a burning sensation, dribbling and difficulty starting or stopping urine flow. When the prostate enlarges, it pinches the urethra and blocks the flow of urine from the bladder, sometimes even causing painful urination. Other symptoms include standing a long time before urination starts, straining to empty your bladder, blood in the urine, with inflammation or swelling, decreased sexual activity or painful intercourse and sometimes back pain.

Prostate problems can be broken down into three categories: prostate infection, prostate enlargement and prostate cancer. Benign prostatic hyperplasia (BPH) is a non-malignant enlargement of the prostate. BPH and prostatitis are the most common prostate problems. Prostate cancer is common among men over 60, strikes about one in eleven men, and is not easily detected in the early stages. Low levels of zinc, vitamin C, bioflavonoids and vitamin E have been shown in those with cancer of the prostate. This disease is also linked to a deficient diet, so it is time to take charge of your health. Prostate cancer is usually treated with surgery or hormone therapy.

The value of zinc

The prostate gland contains the highest concentration of zinc in the body. Zinc levels are significantly lower in men with cancer of the prostate than in men with normal prostates.[43]

In his work at Cook County Hospital in Chicago, Dr. Irving M. Bush found that a zinc deficiency was related to prostate disorders in men. He gave 19 male volunteers 150 mg of zinc daily for two months, followed by 50 to 100 mg a day. This regimen relieved urinary frequency, irritation, and other non-bacterial inflammatory conditions. Fourteen of the 19 men with benign hypertrophy (enlarged prostate) experienced shrinkage of the prostate to normal size, as determined by rectal probing, x-ray, and endoscopy.[44]

If zinc had been taken with vitamin E, selenium, flaxseed oil, and saw palmetto berry extract, would the recovery rate have been much higher? I believe it would have been.

In another study, researcher M. Fahim and colleagues also found that zinc supplementation reduced the size of the prostate and benign prostatic hyperplasia symptoms in the majority of volunteers.[45]

Zinc has numerous relationships with male sexual development and function all through a male's life. Zinc deficiency in childhood leads to impaired development of the male sex organs and secondary sexual characteristics. In adulthood, zinc is vital to the testicles and for testosterone production.

BOTH ZINC AND VITAMIN B6 AFFECT PROLACTIN. The hormone prolactin levels begin to increase when a man reaches his mid-40s. When the prolactin level rises, the body is encouraged to produce more 5-alpha-reductase. That is when the testosterone production begins turning into dihydrotestosterone (DHT), and that is when zinc and vitamin B6 are most needed. Both are effective in reducing prolactin levels, with no side effects. Some researchers believe deficiencies in either zinc or B6 may be a critical factor leading to prostate enlargement.[46]

Even a marginal zinc deficiency can lower a man's libido.[47] Most authorities report that 100 mg zinc should be the maximum dose, and normal amounts would be 30 to 50 mg a day, and vitamin B6 would at least be 50 mg a day, or 50 mg twice a day.

Saw palmetto helps enlarged prostate

Saw palmetto berries *(Serenoa repens)* come from the saw palmetto palm trees that are native to the Atlantic seaboard from South Carolina to Florida. They bear fruit that has a long folk history of use as an aphrodisiac and sexual rejuvenator.

Recent studies on the saw palmetto fruit have shown that the berries have about 15 percent saturated and unsaturated fatty acids and sterols that have been found not only to reduce prostatic swelling, but also to stimulate immune function. Clinical trials have shown repeatedly that saw palmetto extract results in a significant decrease in prostate size, improvement in urinary flow, alleviation of nocturnal voiding, less residual urine, and relief of other prostate symptoms.[48]

An enlarged prostate results from hormone fluctuations that convert testosterone to dihydrotestosterone (DHT). Testosterone by itself isn't the problem; testosterone produces good muscle mass, a lively libido, and a variety of other masculine characteristics. The conversion of testosterone to dihydrotestosterone causes the problem. The extract from the saw palmetto berry blocks that conversion.[49]

Saw palmetto berry extract has had no side effects reported in any of the clinical trials. Detailed toxicology studies on the extract have been carried out on mice, rats, and dogs, and the extract has no toxic effects in these studies.

Other studies of the saw palmetto extract have shown it to be effective in nearly 90 percent of patients, usually within a period of four to six weeks.[50]

Saw palmetto extract has been compared to Proscar, a prescription drug prescribed for BPH. Results showed that saw palmetto may be equivalent or better in its actions, without the side effects associated with Proscar (impotence, loss of sex drive, and abnormal ejaculations), and it was less expensive.[51]

Most men with prostate problems will never hear about saw palmetto berry extract. In 1990, the FDA rejected an application to have saw palmetto approved in the treatment of benign prostatic hyperplasia (BPH). Thus, even though clinical evidence is strongly in support of this natural extract for the treatment of enlarged prostate, manufacturers and distributors of the extract cannot make that claim on their product labels.

DOSAGE FOR SAW PALMETTO. To achieve full benefit from saw palmetto, I believe it is important for men to use the same potency and type of saw palmetto in the clinical studies. The studies used saw palmetto extract, standardized to contain 85–95 percent fatty acids and sterols with a 160 mg potency taken twice a day.[52]

Pygeum has been used for centuries

The powdered bark of pygeum (Pygeum africanus) has also been used for centuries as a treatment for urinary disorders. This herb has been proven in many studies to significantly improve troublesome prostate conditions.

In 1986 at the University of Genova, 20 patients with benign prostatic hyperplasia (BPH) received pygeum orally for two months. Within 30 days, these patients experienced a decrease in nighttime urination, and all the symptoms of BPH had decreased significantly within 60 days. Other human studies have confirmed the benefit of this herb with benign prostatic hyperplasia with no toxic side effects observed, even at large doses and prolonged use.

The scientist in France who isolated its active compound found the herbal preparation did in fact produce anti-inflammatory, anti-edema, and cholesterol lowering properties. Both animal and human clinical trials have shown this herb to promote the regression of symptoms associated with benign prostatic hyperplasia (BPH) with no toxic side effects observed, even at large doses and with prolonged use.

The mode of function of pygeum is that it blocks the entry and breakdown of cholesterol in the prostate. This tends to encourage the production of certain prostaglandins, which exhibit an anti-inflammatory action.[53] At this time there are many research articles on pygeum and prostate function in progress. You should be hearing more about the effectiveness of pygeum in the coming years.

Saw palmetto—pygeum combination

Pygeum can be taken as a preventive (prophylactic), and can be used alone or in combination with saw palmetto extract.

Together they provide several synergistic mechanisms that help prevent or reverse benign prostatic hyperplasia. This combination is considered a safe and effective means of maintaining healthier prostate function into old age. Several combination products are available in your nutrition store.

OTHER SUPPORT FOR THE PROSTATE

Beta Sitosterol: a plant sterol found to improve BPH symptoms. These sterols may even be the actual "prostate active" ingredients in many herbal supplements.

Lycopene: the red-colored carotene has been shown to reduce the growth of prostate cancer cells.

Beta 1,3/1,6 Glucans (yeast): unique polysaccharides extracted from many plants that help stimulate special cells in the immune system. Only yeast of mushroom (fungi) sources seem to have that ability.

Stinging Nettle: a historic Indian herbal treatment for prostatitis and urinary problems in men, and seems to work synergistically with saw palmetto and pygeum. It may work by reducing 5-DHT production. Recent in-vitro studies show effects against prostate cancer cells as well.

Flaxseed has a well-proven protective benefit. There was a study at Duke University in 2001 that showed that ground flaxseed (not just flaxseed oil) may actually slow tumor development in men with prostate cancer. Flaxseed is loaded with fiber and is a rich source of cancer-fighting lignans. Buy them whole and grind in your coffee grinder to use fresh each day. It can be added to cereals, protein shakes, water and juice or even mixed into peanut butter. Be creative. Flaxseed oil should also be added to your protein shake.

Flower Pollen extract: a special rye flower pollen extract that is popular in Europe for treating syptoms of chronic prostatitis or benign prostatic hyperplasia (BPH).

Pumpkin Seed extract: rich in amino acids and zinc, which may help reduce the size of the prostate gland once enlarged. Many men enjoy eating raw pumpkin seeds as a snack.

Hydrangea: used by the Cherokee Indians used this treatment for many urinary disorders, including prostatitis. Hydrangea was introduced to settlers in the 1700s and used traditionally since.

Selenium: the *Journal of the American Medical Association* reported in December 1996 that selenium had the greatest impact on prostate cancer. The study showed that men taking 200 micrograms of selenium a day, for seven years, had a 63 percent reduction of death from prostate cancer. Read the complete story in chapter 3 under the section: The Tremendous Benefits of selenium.

Creatine Monohydrate Increases Strength!

If you have read any of the sports magazines lately, you know creatine is big news. Is it one reason home runs are flying out of the parks, setting new home run records? If your weight training regimen has plateaued, then try creatine. Creatine is a natural substance found in red meat. It regenerates ADP (spent energy) back into ATP (usable energy). It's mode of action is to allow you to work out harder, with more intensity. Consequently, you get stronger, faster.

Creatine is ideal for bodybuilders, football players and other strength sports. However, if you play tennis, volleyball, racquetball, row or swim, plus all the other major sports, creatine can likely enhance your performance, too. Generally speaking, you will find creatine can help you perform at a higher level in any sport requiring short bursts of concentrated power.[54]

Dr. Paul Greenhaff wrote in the *International Journal of Sports Nutrition*, "Creatine should not be viewed as another gimmick supplement. Its ingestion is a means of providing immediate, significant performance improvements to athletes involved in explosive sports. In the long run, creatine may allow athletes to train without fatigue at an intensity higher than that to which they are accustomed. For these reasons alone, creatine supplementation could be viewed as a significant development in sports nutrition."

STUDY OF RESULTS OF CREATINE

- A recent survey of creatine users found that 34 percent experienced BOTH a reduction in their body-fat level and an increase in definition or vascularity.[55]

- A study at the University of Texas Southwestern Medical Center found that when eight weight-trained men took 20 grams of creatine per day for four weeks, their average muscle mass increased by 3.5 pounds.[56]

- In the University of Texas study mentioned earlier, the athletes added 18 pounds to their single-repetition bench press, going from an average of 278 lbs to 296 lbs in just one month. They also went from 11 to 15 repetitions when they lifted a weight that was 70 percent of their one-repetition maximum.[57]

- A separate study found that a week of creatine supplementation boosts mean power output by 6 percent![58]

Dosage of creatine

Typical dosing is to load for 5–7 days with 15–25 grams and then take 5 grams a day of creatine monohydrate thereafter. It is an odorless, virtually tasteless white powder that looks like sugar. If you have trouble finding a high quality, German creatine monohydrate, call Nutrition Express at 1-800-338-7979.

Make sure you read the *Let's Put it All Together* chapter to help you find a balanced program. It is important that you are taking all of the antioxidants, vitamins and minerals. The value of increasing your protein level is very important. That is why I suggest that you drink the Super Energy Protein Shake. (See recipe in chapter 17.)

A New Beginning

It's never too late to start a "health-improvement" program and develop a fresh, new attitude toward life. *Remember, it is your responsibility to take charge of your health, because no one is going to do it for you.* You can do it! You have all this valuable information here at your finger tips, so there are no excuses. So, "just do it." Start taking charge of your own health and enjoy life with increased energy and vitality.

Young Women's Special Needs

Nutrients to Help You Overcome PMS, Fibrocystic Breast, Heavy Periods, and Bladder Infections

When women describe to me their emotional and physical symptoms related to PMS, the first question I ask them is, "What did you have for breakfast?"
—GLADYS LINDBERG

When I counsel with my clients at our store in Torrance, California, I am always interested in the stories I hear. What amazes me the most is how many women have had complete hysterectomies while still in their early 30s or 40s. They tell me it is usually because of very heavy periods or fibroid tumors. One woman told me, "I'm still having hot flashes after a hysterectomy at the age of 32 and I'm falling apart." Still others tell me about their breast cysts, exhaustion, yeast infections, depression, fibroid tumors, bladder infections, heavy menstrual periods and of course, PMS (premenstrual syndrome).

As I reply to those sufferers, the words of Mother keep coming to mind as she would have said, *"Healthy people don't have that, so let's make you healthy."* I suspect you are not much different from these precious women.

When I discuss PMS, it is amazing that the same nutrients are also effective for many other conditions. So if you have heavy periods, menstrual cramps, fibrocystic breast, chronic fatigue or fibromyalgia or feel exhausted, the same nutritional supplements may apply to you.

Although it is impossible to undo damage already done by surgery, it is never too late to start down the path of recovery. For many, there is still time to take the high road of prevention, which is the best defense.

Let's Get Started

In my counseling sessions, I listen to my clients' needs and one of my first questions is usually the same as Mother's, "What did you have for breakfast?" Most people sheepishly answer, "Nothing." Some admit their breakfast was "toast and coffee," or "orange juice." How would you answer this question?

Be sure you read the last chapter about Dr. Stephen Gyland's study of 1,100 patients who had low blood sugar (hypoglycemia). Doesn't nervousness, irritability, exhaustion, weak spells, depression, drowsiness, headaches, crying spells, lack of sex drive, constant worrying and unprovoked anxieties sound familiar? This sounds like "women's problems" but they are just a few of the symptoms Dr. Gyland associated with hypoglycemia. Make sure you read my "Complete Lindberg

Nutrition Program" so you can solve this part of the problem, in the *Let's Put It All Together* chapter.

After I finish explaining the importance of a good breakfast, and how it effects the level of hypoglycemia, they soon understand that my golden rule is: *"You can't leave the house without an adequate breakfast."* The Lindberg Super Energy Protein Shake is an absolute must if you want to feel better! We also need to fortify our bodies with optimum levels of all the vitamins and minerals. There may be some additional herbal products or amino acid supplements that are discussed in other chapters.

After they understand the value of their breakfast and realize the importance of taking all the vitamins and minerals in adequate amounts, I often reach over and hold their hand. If it is cold, I ask: "Are you often cold when everyone else is warm? Are both your hands and feet cold, or do you wear socks to bed? Are you slow getting started in the morning? Do you lack energy?" If the answer is "yes," one of the problems may be an underactive thyroid gland. If you are cold, make sure you take Dr. Broda Barnes Temperature Test described in chapter 10. You can easily check your own thyroid function. This chapter will give you a complete explanation of what you can do to correct this condition. You will find how involved the thyroid gland is in many women's health problems.

Premenstrual Syndrome (PMS)

More than half a century ago, researchers first discovered the wide emotional and psychological swings premenstrual syndrome or PMS can create. PMS refers to a variety of symptoms associated with the menstrual cycle, usually occurring during the 7 to 10 days before menstruation and disappearing a few hours after the onset of menstruation.

Women of childbearing years are the most susceptible. Five or six million women in the United States have PMS severe enough to disrupt their personal and work routines, states material published by Harvard University.[1]

The symptoms and their significance

Authorities report 150 different symptoms caused by PMS, but the most common, according to researchers at the Mayo Clinic and Harvard Medical School are: fatigue, depression, headaches, mood swings, personality changes, crying spells, bloating (especially abdominal), breast swelling and tenderness, skin eruptions, junk food binges, (especially for sugar or salty foods), constipation, clumsiness, irritability, anxiety, hair-trigger temper and hostility.

A small percentage of women have positive changes before their periods, including exhilaration, heightened affection and sexual desire and even more intense concentration. Because I was in good health, I almost never knew when my period would start so I had to watch the calendar. Many women are not as fortunate:

- Up to 50 percent of all suicide attempts by women are made in the premenstrual week.

- Up to 50 percent of all admissions into mental hospitals for women occur in that week.

- Up to 50 percent of the crimes for which women are jailed are committed in that week.[2]

Is caffeine the cause?

The *American Journal of Public Health* notes that the consumption of caffeine in beverages "is strongly related to the presence and severity of PMS." One researcher suggests that caffeine in coffee, tea, colas and cocoa (chocolate) is the actual cause of PMS, linking the beverage to cystic mastitis, or fibrocystic breast disease.[3] Some have shown that just getting off caffeine, even if consumption has been as little as one cup of coffee or one can of cola per day, can have a dramatic effect on PMS for some women.[4]

Effective, natural treatments for PMS

No longer are sufferers from PMS told that they are "emotionally unstable," or that PMS is "all in your head." This syndrome is now finally recognized as a medical problem. However, is it hormonal, biochemical or psychological? No single theory has been totally accepted.

Baylor University Medical School in Texas has listed 237 different drugs to treat PMS and most are not effective.[5] Stephen Berger, M.D., reports that some unfortunate women are given antidepressants, anti-hypertensives, diuretics, Prozac or Valium. Unfortunately, these drugs only mask the symptoms and some may lead to addiction.[6]

There is not enough evidence to say PMS is caused by a single particular physical malfunction or that just one treatment works, because remember—we are all biochemically different. The safest and least invasive method for help should be a change in lifestyle, which includes improving the diet, taking all of the vitamins and minerals in adequate amounts, maybe including a natural progesterone cream and, of course, you must exercise. It is my contention that these changes will be the most effective treatments for all of the special problems women face, especially PMS. As I said, many PMS symptoms resemble hypoglycemia, and the solution may be as easy as changing the diet.

Take a close look at the foods in your cupboard and refrigerator and throw out the ones you know are loaded with white sugar, white flour and hydrogenated vegetable shortening. They will be easier to resist once they are off the shelf and out of the house.

The Importance of Vitamin B$_6$

Alan Gaby, M.D., reported in *B$_6$: The Natural Healer*, "Based on what we know so far about the causes of PMS, vitamin B$_6$ looks like the 'magic bullet' that might possibly be the answer for this monthly suffering." Dr. Gaby describes the research of vitamin B$_6$ for the treatment of PMS in the early 1940s and how this information never became an accepted treatment. He said that the research has already been done that compared the effectiveness of vitamin B$_6$ to that of placebos, and B$_6$ has been found to be of great benefit.[7]

The symptoms of PMS which include depression and other mood changes have been attributed to a decreased synthesis of the neurotransmitter serotonin in the brain. This decreased synthesis may be a result of low vitamin B$_6$ status.

Studies have shown that a B$_6$ deficiency may be caused by the estrogen in the birth control pills. Dr. Gaby explained that a B$_6$ deficiency can be caused by an oversupply of estrogen. One of the possible consequences of estrogen-induced B$_6$ deficiency is depression, a side effect that occurs commonly in women taking the Pill. This adverse psychological change is presumably caused by a deficiency of serotonin, a molecule normally present in the brain, which appears to act as an antidepressant. To sum it up: A vitamin B$_6$ deficiency, caused by excessive estrogen, can result in inadequate production of serotonin, which then could result in depression.[8]

The evidence shows that vitamin B$_6$ (pyridoxine) protects women against metabolic imbalances caused by using oral contraceptives. Women have a greater vitamin B$_6$ requirement, well above the current Recommended Dietary Allowance (RDA) of 1.6 to 2.2 milligrams.[9]

In a study at one of England's prestigious PMS centers, the St. Thomas Hospital and Medical School in London, researchers reported on their seven-year study of 630 PMS patients. Forty percent of the women receiving from 100 mg to 150 mg of vitamin B6 daily experienced reduced PMS symptoms. Sixty percent of those receiving from 160 mg to 200 mg daily showed significant improvements. No side-effects were reported, including no peripheral neuropathy; only less depression, irritability, anxiety, tension, fluid retention, headaches, breast tenderness, cravings and lethargy.[10]

Multiple studies have shown that vitamin B6 can reduce or eliminate depression, fatigue, mild paranoia and can improve concentration.[11] Vitamin B6, being water-soluble, is excreted in the urine eight hours after ingestion, so space it evenly throughout the day. Knowing of the low toxicity of vitamin B6, it seems it should be the first treatment for PMS.[12]

Water retention

Vitamin B6 can also control edema (tissue swelling) of the hands and feet. It may even help with the swelling in the breasts before the menstrual period. It is a natural diuretic for water retention and bloating.[13]

Acne

Some young women who suffer acne before their period have been helped with taking vitamin B6 before and during the period.[14] So gals, if your face breaks out the week before your period, be sure to try vitamin B6. Several authorities suggest between 50 mg to 100 mg a day to solve your problem.

Infertility

Researchers have also reported that women with unexplained infertility experienced a high conception rate after vitamin B6 therapy was started.[15] This is excellent news for those striving to conceive.

Recommended dosage

More vitamin B6 does not necessarily mean better health. Some people are sensitive to excessive supplementation. Researchers have reported nerve damage in seven patients who had been taking 2 grams (2,000 mg) or more of vitamin B6 daily. Four of the seven patients had been taking these doses for two to four months. The first sign of toxic symptoms was numbness in the feet and unstable gait.[16] John Ellis,

M.D., an expert on vitamin B6, rarely prescribes over 150 mg a day of vitamin B6 for carpal tunnel syndrome, edema of pregnancy, rheumatism, etc. He maintains that more is generally not needed.[17]

Many of my clients have great results with a daily supplement between 50 mg to 100 mg a day of vitamin B6, as the research suggests. This should be included in a high potency vitamin B complex, so to keep all the B vitamins in a proper balance. If after one or two cycles you have not improved, increase the B complex (that includes 50 mg B6), to twice a day, for a few monthly cycles. Dividing the dose keeps these water-soluble vitamins in your system longer. Rarely have I known women who need to increase their dose any higher. We are fortunate to have a simple, safe, inexpensive and effective remedy that can relieve so much distress for many young women.

The Significance of Evening Primrose Oil

The pioneering work of Dr. David Horrobin demonstrated the importance of prostaglandin-E1, and thus the need for GLA in restoring a woman's hormone balance.[18] Gamma-linolenic Acid (GLA) is considered an essential fatty acid, which means it cannot be produced by the body, and must be obtained through the diet. The richest sources of GLA are evening primrose oil, black currant oil, and borage oil.

Studies at the Efamol Research Institute in Kentville, Nova Scotia, concluded that evening primrose oil can provide relief for 90 to 95 percent of women's premenstrual tension and cures two-thirds of the women not helped by anything else. Another 20 percent showed great improvement.

"The secret is not to wait until the discomfort begins, but to take 50 mg of vitamin B6 and six 500 mg capsules of evening primrose oil regularly," writes Dr. Richard Passwater. Evening primrose oil is now available in 1000 mg capsules, so you would take three capsules for the same potency. "The oil capsules should be divided into two or three doses during the day. Extremely difficult cases may need nine 500 mg caps and 200 mg of B6 daily. Vitamin E is generally helpful in the 600 IU range," says Dr. Passwater.[19] These nutrients all work synergistically (together).

The *Journal of Reproductive Medicine* reported on 30 patients with severe PMS who received evening primrose oil twice a day or a placebo. After four menstrual cycles, the treated group showed decreased premenstrual symptoms compared with the placebo group.[20] However, remember to add the complete vitamin B complex, including B6. I always recommend the evening primrose oil over black currant oil or borage oil because the major research was with evening primrose oil.

The Magnitude of Magnesium

Magnesium is an important mineral, which plays a role in helping young women with PMS symptoms, including mood changes. A magnesium deficiency is considered an actual causative factor by some.[21]

Magnesium is involved in controlling muscle and nerve function, twitching, cramping, muscular weakness, subduing an excitable nervous system, insomnia, depression, overexcitability of the nervous system, nerve impulses for normal brain function. A deficiency of magnesium may lead to a decreased synthesis of the brain neurotransmitter dopamine, which, in turn, causes an imbalance in other brain chemicals. This and other disruptions are thought to cause symptoms of PMS.[22]

The *American Journal of Clinical Nutrition* reported that levels of magnesium were significantly low in the blood of women with PMS prior to and during their period. This may be due to decreased intake of magnesium, poor absorption or increased excretion of the mineral. Since PMS patients often complain of nervous tension, the magnesium level may be depleted due to stress.[23]

Magnesium deficiency also results in thrombosis, or clotting disorders, and oral contraceptives have been found to lower blood levels of this valuable mineral. This offers a possible clue to the higher incidence of clotting disorders among women on the pill.[24]

A recommended level of magnesium would be 400 mg to 500 mg a day, balanced with twice as much calcium. Be aware that if you take over 500 mg of magnesium, it may cause a loose stool, depending on your individual need. Many people find that extra magnesium eliminates their need for a laxative. Some women with severe PMS can take 1,000 mg with no apparent bowel changes.

The Value of Natural Vitamin E

This vitamin is important for various female-related disorders, including PMS.[25] It is an anti-clotting agent that helps users of the oral contraceptives to avoid clots, strokes and thrombophlebitis (inflammation of the vein in conjunction with a blood clot) that are caused by the "pill." The natural form of vitamin E, d-alpha tocopherol, often helps painful breasts. Women with fibroid tumors of the uterus should also take vitamin E regularly and faithfully to hinder further growth of these tumors.[26]

There is evidence relating vitamin E's protective effects against breast cancer. Studies reported in the *Journal of the American College of Nutrition* have shown that vitamin E reduces the incidence of cancer due to carcinogens. In addition, it even enhances the therapeutic effect of radiation treatment of cancer. One study found that the group of women with the lowest blood serum vitamin E levels had five times the risk of cancer.[27] This is an important reason why natural vitamin E supplements should be an essential part of everyone's nutrition program.

Remember, all of these beneficial effects were the result of the use of natural "d-alpha tocopherol" and not the synthetic "dl-alpha tocopherol," which is made from petrochemicals.[28] Synthetic vitamin E is usually found in discount and drug stores since it is much less expensive, although it may say "natural" on the front label. This is one reason to shop at your health food or nutrition store.

All major categories of PMS symptoms are improved with supplementation of 400 IU of vitamin E daily, according to researchers who conducted a double blind, placebo-controlled study.[29] I have found some young women do better if they take 800 IU to 1,200 IU of vitamin E as other research indicates. It is also one of our best anti-aging vitamins and may even prevent the brown, "age" or "liver spots," that appear on the back of the hands, and sometimes the face.

The Role of the Hormone Progesterone

Progesterone is one of two main hormones, the other being estrogen, which is vital to the life of every woman. These hormones are produced primarily in the ovaries, beginning at puberty and continuing, especially for estrogen, for the rest of our life. Most importantly, there is a delicate balance between these hormones, and when they are out of balance, women begin to have problems. In addition, hormone levels fluctuate: when we age, the time of our monthly cycle, our health in relation to what we eat or don't eat, the vitamins we take, the stress we are under, and the exercise we do or don't do.

Progesterone is a hormone produced by the *corpus luteum* of the ovary, the placenta during pregnancy, and in small amounts by the adrenal cortex. It is the major female reproductive hormone during the latter two weeks of the menstrual cycle. Progesterone is necessary for the survival of the fertilized ovum, the resulting embryo, and the fetus through gestation, when production of progesterone is taken over by the placenta.[30]

From progesterone there are also derived corticosteroids (a group of hormones produced in the adrenal cortex), which are essential for stress response, sugar and electrolyte balance, blood pressure, and not to mention, survival. Progesterone is a precursor to so many other hormones, it is easy to see why a progesterone deficiency can cause such a wide range of problems. Progesterone is beneficial in treating or preventing:

- irregular menstrual flow, cramping, bloating, depression
- irritability, migraine headaches, insomnia, epilepsy
- heart palpitations and other cardiovascular disorders
- miscarriages, infertility, incontinence, endometriosis
- hot flashes, night sweats, vaginal dryness, osteoporosis
- hypoglycemia, chronic fatigue syndrome, yeast infections.[31]

Progesterone and the menstrual cycle

Many young women report this avalanche of symptoms as they approach the week or 10 days before their menstrual period begins and the symptoms disappear when the period starts.

To eliminate PMS symptoms we have discussed the importance of diet, essential vitamin and mineral supplements and exercise, but Dr. John Lee feels the root cause is hormone imbalance. He says, "Progesterone has been wrongly accused of being the hormone responsible for PMS because it's the one that's high just before menstruation. The truth is, however, that women with PMS tend to have lower progesterone than normal at that time in their cycle, when progesterone is supposed to be dominant, so that estrogen is dominant instead."[32]

When a woman's cycle is functioning properly, estrogen is the dominant sex hormone during the first two weeks after the start of her menstrual cycle. Responding to ovulation, estrogen levels drop and progesterone levels rise to assume dominance reaching a peak for the final two weeks during the month. When the progesterone levels drop the menstrual cycle begins in about 48 hours.

Without an adequate supply of progesterone to counterbalance estrogen dominance, many problems begin to surface. Elevated levels of estrogen can lead to: salt and fluid retention; low blood sugar levels; blood clotting; fibroid and tumor development; interference with thyroid hormone function; increased blood fat levels; allergic reactions; copper retention; loss of zinc; increased production of body fat and reduced oxygen levels in the cells.[33]

A deficiency of natural hormones can cause problems.

Just as we have seen that excess estrogen may trigger PMS symptoms, low progesterone levels may be another important cause of PMS in many women.[34] These women are generally deficient in many minerals and nutrients required for progesterone synthesis.[35] This is why I always recommend the nutritional "shotgun" approach to the problem. Supplementation of certain vitamins, minerals and herbs may be helpful for detoxifying estrogen, and in aiding progesterone production in the body. Natural progesterone supplements may be the essential ingredient in your PMS relief.

Many physicians have successfully used natural progesterone supplements, usually in the form of topical creams, to alleviate both the physical and emotional symptoms of PMS. Niels Lauerson, M.D., professor of obstetrics and gynecology at New York Medical College and co-author of *PMS: Premenstrual Syndrome and You*, says of progesterone supplements, "When nothing else works, it is the treatment of choice— in my practice hundreds of women who were severely handicapped by PMS have been completely symptom-free with progesterone." In Dr. Lauerson's practice, more than 90 percent of his patients who have tried it have found relief.[36]

Another example is Dr. Joel T. Hargrove of Vanderbilt University Medical Center who has published results indicating a 90 percent success rate in treating PMS with oral doses of natural progesterone.[37]

Adverse reactions?

Since 1953 in England, Dr. Katharina Dalton, has been the leading investigator of PMS and is its foremost authority. She has published three books and more than 40 articles in leading medical journals. Dr. Dalton has been prescribing progesterone for more than 30 years. She reports no increase in the incidence of cancer with progesterone supplements and believes there is evidence that low progesterone levels may increase the risk of developing breast cancer.[38]

In fact, many say there are only positive results. Dr. Niels Lauerson tells us: "Progesterone is not believed to be cancer causing. No human cancer has been reported during progesterone treatment, quite the reverse, progesterone has been used in treating specific uterine cancer."[39]

With this exciting information about the benefits of progesterone, Dr. John Lee reports, "Because of the great safety of natural progesterone, considerable latitude is allowed." Occasionally, a slight feeling of drowsiness may indicate that you are using more than your body needs.

Synthetic progestins

It is hard to grasp the wonder and safety of using a natural product like progesterone, until you read the side effects of the synthetic progestins. A few of the common side effects of synthetic progestins are nausea, fever, vomiting, erosion and abnormal secretions of the cervix, bleeding irregularities, etc., etc. Some of the most shocking are risk of thrombophlebitis and thromboembolic disorders (blood clots in the lung, brain, or heart); cerebral hemorrhage and other cerebrovascular disorders; mental depression; impaired liver function; and carcinoma (cancer) of the breast. These are just a few. However, when this dear lady showed me the package insert, the one that really got my attention was risk of partial or complete loss of vision and retinal blood clot.[40] The package insert said if you lose your vision, call your doctor immediately!

Before you take any drug, be sure you read the packaged inserts reporting all of the side effects! You can make a better decision if what you have is worse than what the drug can cause.

Dr. Lauerson explains that the synthetic progestins are chemically formulated from progesterone, but rather than duplicating the properties of progesterone, these synthetic hormones react differently. He shows that when a women is treated with synthetic progestins, her body becomes confused and produces less natural progesterone, causing salt build up, fluid retention, and hypoglycemia. Synthetic progestins generally make PMS symptoms worse. So if a woman is about to be treated with progesterone, she should be sure that it is *natural* progesterone.[41]

Michelle Harrison, M.D., researcher at the Western Psychiatric Institute and Clinic at the University of Pittsburgh and the author of *Self-Help for Premenstrual Syndrome,* believes most physicians do not understand the progesterone-PMS connection due to some bad scientific studies on the issue years ago. She explains that when progesterone treatment was first introduced in the United States, many doctors gave women synthetic progestins, instead of progesterone. When the treatment was unsuccessful, they then assumed that progesterone did not work. The problem is, many doctors do not understand this important distinction between natural progesterone and synthetic progestins that are commonly prescribed and found in most oral contraceptives. Oral micronized natural progesterone is now available from your physician on a prescription. They are available from many compounding pharmacies such as "Women's International Pharmacy" or others in your area. They are available by prescription only.

Natural progesterone

Natural progesterone is a cholesterol derivative obtained by extracting specific components from plants (e.g., diosgenin from wild yams or soybeans) and then converting them to actual progesterone in the laboratory. Synthetic progestins are also made from diosgenin, but their molecular structure is not found in nature and as a result has different effects on the body and is metabolized differently than natural progesterone. John Lee, M.D., believes this is the essential reason the synthetic progestins do not work. He also points out that the creams that contain wild yam extract, as a treatment for PMS, may contain diosgenin, but do not contain progesterone. There is no evidence that diosgenin, the laboratory precursor for progesterone, is actually converted in the human body to progesterone or other hormones. The action is unpredictable and the results vary widely from person to person.[42]

NATURAL PROGESTERONE CREAM
THE MOST EFFECTIVE REMEDY AVAILABLE

Natural progesterone cream offers these benefits:

- Protects against fibrocyst formation, especially in the breast
- Keeps the uterine lining healthy, helping to prevent fibroids
- Assists thyroid hormone action
- Normalizes the blood-clotting mechanism
- Restores libido (sex drive)
- Acts as a natural antidepressant[43]

The bottom line is this: clinical studies and experience have shown that application of progesterone creams to the skin can rapidly increase progesterone levels and safely eliminate the symptoms associated with PMS.[44] No prescription is required.

Recommended dosage

This natural progesterone cream is an appropriate method for the absorption of progesterone, and is effective for most immediate symptoms and for long range maintenance therapy. The suggested dose is one-quarter to one-half teaspoon applied to the skin once or twice per day. This has been shown to result in physiological levels of progesterone that match those found in the normal luteal phase. This means to apply on days 12 through 28 of your menstrual cycle, day one being the start of your period. Do not use it during your period. The cream should be applied to the soft areas of your skin.

Natural progesterone creams should contain from 960 mg to 1,000 mg per 2-oz container, and labeled USP (United States Pharmacopoeia) Progesterone. This is the proper amount of added natural progesterone. Natural progesterone cream is found in most nutrition stores.

Dr. John Lee's book, *What Your Doctor May Not Tell You About Pre-Menopause,* would be a great resource if you need more information on these hormones. Also read his newest book, *What Your Doctor May Not Tell You About Breast Cancer.*

Nutrients to Help Depression

The natural progesterone we just discussed also effects mood. Christiane Northrup, M.D., says, "In their capacity as neurotransmitters, estrogen and progesterone clearly affect mood. Estrogen, if unopposed by progesterone, tends to irritate the nervous system. Progesterone, on the other hand, is associated with tranquility and is a central nervous system relaxant. It is possible that the beneficial effects of progesterone for PMS is primarily the result of this relaxing effect on the central nervous system."[45]

L-Tyrosine

The amino acid L-tyrosine is not an essential amino acid since it is synthesized (made) in the body. It has been shown to be intimately involved with the important brain neurotransmitters epinephrine, norepinephrine and dopamine. Anecdotal evidence in the past has reported symptomatic improvement in PMS with L-tyrosine, and now, formal clinical observation has confirmed its effectiveness. L-tyrosine supplements can be quite effective as an antidepressant for some major forms of depression.[46] It is also helpful in reducing the irritation and tiredness associated with PMS.

L-tyrosine capsules of 500 mg should be taken on an empty stomach an hour before each meal for a total of 1,500 mg daily. Some women may need higher amounts to be effective, but they should be under a physician's supervision. Do not take L-tyrosine if you are taking MAO (monoamine oxidase) inhibitor-type anti-depressants or if you have high blood pressure. Then take only under supervision, according to the *American Journal of Psychiatry*.[47] For more information on depression and mood swings be sure to read chapter 7 and discover a list of products that may help you such as 5HTP, SAMe and St. John's word.

Nutrients to Help
Fibrocystic Breast Disease

The symptoms of fibrocystic breast (Cystic Mastitis) are breast tenderness and cystic development, which may recur with each menstrual cycle or become continuous. The breast becomes nodular, with freely movable cysts near the surface of the breast. Cysts are benign but there is a three- to seven-fold increase in the chance of cancer for those women. Over stimulation of the breast by the female hormone estrogen is implicated.

Substances to avoid

Chemicals called methylxanthines are capable of aggravating the condition. These compounds are in coffee, tea, cola and chocolate and strongly linked to cystic mastitis.[48] If you have these problems, it may be wise to removed these beverages and foods from your diet.

Benefits of vitamin E

Dr. Robert London of the John Hopkins University School of Medicine, found that on 600 IU of vitamin E daily, 85 percent of patients in a double-blind placebo-controlled study showed dramatic remission of lumps, and the remaining 15 percent showed clear improvement. In this study, every single person, 100 percent of patients, markedly improved with vitamin E! In other studies he found cystic mastitis manageable with 1,000 to 1,500 IU of the natural vitamin E. The research showed that synthetic vitamin E (dl-alpha tocopherol) was NOT effective. The only vitamin E that produced results was natural vitamin E (d-alpha tocopherol), so read your labels.[49] Many such studies could be cited where vitamin E is very effective in total disappearance of cystic lesions and breast tenderness.[50] Natural vitamin E is safe, effective, inexpensive and should, in my opinion, be supplemented daily by all women, especially those potentially facing this problem.

Importance of iodine

Another nutrient found to help cystic mastitis is iodine. Dr. Bernard Eskin of the Medical College of Pennsylvania found that of 588 cystic mastitis patients, 90 percent had good-to-excellent results with iodine. Complete pain relief was reported by 43 percent of the women.[51] Remember that iodine stimulates the thyroid gland, so thyroid again may be the root problem. Take the Barnes temperature test found in chapter 10 and check yourself. Kelp tablets are a natural form of iodine and may be valuable. Be sure your mineral supplement contains iodine. If you use salt, use only iodized sea salt.

Menstrual Problems

Marie came to see me with her sisters and mother and wanted to lose weight. After discussing her health, she said her periods were extremely heavy. She needed to wear three sanitary pads at a time. These periods would last 7 to 10 days. I told her the most important way I could help her was to slow down her period, then we could discuss her weight. Marie began using our vitamin and mineral program including our protein shake and started taking a "fat burner" (non stimulant) that contained 1,500 mg of choline, 1,000 mg of inositol, and evening primrose oil. She phoned me in about six weeks and was thrilled. Her period was only four days and for the first time she could remember it was light. She felt this was a real answer to prayer. She was so much stronger. Her sisters were also thrilled and they all started the program, including her mother.

Problem of heavy periods

Do you suffer from heavy periods? Heavy periods may be caused by too much natural or synthetic estrogen. This is a problem that needs an answer, because it can lead to anemia, generally poor health, and eventually to a hysterectomy. Even though a woman's body produces natural estrogen, it may still be harmful. According to Dr. Carlton Fredericks, a well-nourished liver will convert the estrogen to estriol which is not carcinogenic (cancer causing) as estrogen can be. The body then excretes this harmless chemical. Many of the women who have called me have had their hysterectomy because of a heavy flow, which is far too radical when it can be treated by nutritional means. Are male doctors forgetting that these are the woman's sex organs?

The liver must be kept healthy for it to carry out its detoxifying duties. Protein intake is important for liver function, particularly the amino acids cystine and methionine. Animal protein is required to do this, according to Dr. Fredericks, who does not believe that soy has the proper amino acid relationships. Soy chelates zinc and takes it out of the body, so you can become zinc deficient. In addition, soy protein doesn't supply vitamin B_{12}, which is vital for liver function.[52]

Evening primrose oil, which we discussed as a treatment for PMS, also aids women who have heavy and prolonged monthly bleeding. Instead of heavy blood loss for 7 to 10 days, their periods normalized to four days.[53]

A menstrual flow that continues to be heavy after three or four days has often been corrected within a single month by taking 600 to 800 IU of vitamin E daily, which prevents excessive clotting and helps maintain a more normal flow.

An excessive flow may also indicate that the thyroid is underactive, in which case protein needs to be increased, and iodine or kelp to support the thyroid. The amino acid, L-tyrosine, we discussed, also supports the thyroid gland. There are natural homeopathic thyroid substances that may also support the thyroid gland. Be sure to take the Barnes easy thyroid test in chapter 10 to see if you fall into this category.

Also include 7,000 IU to 10,000 IU of vitamin A, as it appears to help regulate excessive estrogen levels. Christiane Northrup, M.D., reports that doses of vitamin A as high as 100,000 IU per day can be given, if limited to three months—otherwise there is a risk of toxicity. Do not take a high dose if pregnant or trying to get pregnant. Vitamin A has also been shown to decrease menstrual blood loss.[54] Vitamin C, 500 mg to 1,000 mg with bioflavonoids and pycnogenol, are also important; all of these supplements work synergistically.[55]

Another young lady came into our store after seeing me on a television program where I discussed PMS. She not only had PMS but also very heavy menstrual flow, and she appeared very tired and "washed out." I mapped out a sound nutritional program to build up her body.

When I saw her again, she had faithfully taken all of our vitamins and minerals, plus my recommended protein shake, and followed an excellent diet. Just two months later she came back to see me with her girlfriend. "How are you feeling?" I asked, although I really didn't need to ask because her countenance glowed.

"No more heavy periods," she said enthusiastically. "It now lasts three days, just like when I was a young girl. Could this be normal?"

"Yes!" I told her. "Of course."

"And could the fact that my face has cleared up have something to do with these vitamins?"

"Remember the studies on vitamin B6 and acne I told you about? How just 50 mg one week before and during your period helped 72 percent of the girls. Well you more than fit into the percentage," I told her. "You are receiving enough B6 every day in the vitamin packs I suggested."

She told me she felt so much better she could hardly believe the difference. She was no longer cross and irritable. "Don't get off the program, honey," I said. "Let this be your greatest health insurance! It will pay dividends every day of your life."

Nutrients For Irregular Menstrual Flow

A menstrual flow that is irregular, scanty or nonexistent are signs of general malnutrition or severe hormone imbalance. Usually, these problems are the result of a decrease in the production of the sex hormones.

Various nutrients involved

Either a vitamin B12 or folic acid deficiency may cause irregular and decreased flow or cessation of flow, but normal menstruation usually occurs as soon as the missing vitamins are supplied. Also, the addition of vitamin E along with a diet rich in all the vitamins and minerals will aid the pituitary and sex glands, and menstruation should become normal within a few weeks.

Extremely low-fat diets, with high-complex-carbohydrates, have been the craze for the athletically inclined. Many athletic women will lose their period altogether on this program. Remember, fat makes our hormones and excessive exercise may further reduce body fat stores and disrupt hormone function, which ultimately reduce the estrogen levels in the athlete's body. So if you are too thin, bordering on anorexia, exercise too much and consume no fat, your period may actually stop. Remember, some fats are essential in our diet for life! Deficiencies in essential fatty acids play a role in many female reproductive disorders. So if you want to be fertile, be sure you include these essential oils, and get back on a good diet.

Nutrients for Menstrual Cramps

Millions of dollars a year are spent on aspirin and pain-relieving products for menstrual cramps and bloating. Blood tests show that starting about 10 days prior to menstruation, when the ovaries are the least active, the blood calcium drops steadily. This decrease in calcium results in premenstrual tension, nervousness, headaches, insomnia and mental depression, which are all calcium deficiencies.[56]

The body recognizes this decrease in calcium as a stressor, and produces cortisone and aldosterone. These hormones cause salt and water to be retained in the body. This often results in swelling of the hands, feet, breast and stomach. Your weight increases and headaches may occur because of swelling or pressure on the brain.

When I was 11 years old, a cousin came to visit. I vividly recall the following day, her menstrual period started and she rolled back and forth on my bed with pain, accompanied by moans and sounds of agony. Mother knew exactly what to do. She brought my cousin a glass of milk with calcium gluconate and blackstrap molasses stirred into it. In about 10 minutes she was sitting up, carrying on a normal conversation and her pain was gone. Normally she said she would be in bed for three or four days. After taking the calcium and blackstrap molasses mixture, her muscles relaxed because the drink raised the trace minerals and calcium levels in her blood. She was an instant believer!

That scene is still vivid in my memory. I have never experienced menstrual discomfort but I know many women who have.

Calcium and magnesium

If you have these problems, look to calcium and magnesium for putting an end to cramping. If you are taking your recommended daily amount of 1,000 mg of calcium and 500 mg of magnesium, and you still have cramps, increase the amount to 1,500 mg and 750 mg per day. It is best to take calcium and magnesium with meals so they can be digested with food, spaced out at least twice a day (preferably in capsule form).

During premenstrual syndrome there are significantly fewer problems with mood swings when women received adequate calcium every day instead of 600 mg, according to the U.S. Department of Agriculture. With the high calcium intake, the women reported fewer aches and pains during menstruation. Relief appeared greatest just before and during menstruation when symptoms are most pronounced.

Natural vitamin E

As a mild prostaglandin inhibitor, *vitamin E can relieve pain* in much the same way aspirin does, but without the undesirable side effects. This vitamin has also been effective in eliminating leg muscle cramps and in decreasing breast tenderness before and during menstruation. Some speculate that cramps may be caused by a constriction of the blood supply when the uterine muscle contracts.

Vitamin E promotes a better vascular supply, reducing spasm as it does in other muscle groups throughout the body. It has also been shown to help with exercise cramps and restless legs.[57] Menstrual cramps may be a sign that your nutrition is not adequate, so you need the whole program we have been discussing.

Preventing Bladder Infections

Bladder infections are annoying and painful but usually not fatal. They commonly occur after long usage of antibiotics, which destroy the friendly flora of the genitourinary tract.

Lactobacillus acidophilus and bifidus

A six week series of lactobacillus acidophilus and bifidus is the first line of defense after antibiotics have been taken. Acidophilus will help re-implant and re-establish favorable intestinal bacteria in your large intestine. It helps regulate bowel bacteria.

The unfriendly bacteria in the intestinal tract cannot grow in an acid medium. That is why acidophilus, vitamin C, cranberry juice and apple cider vinegar all help to keep your urine on the slightly acid side.

Cranberry

Cranberry extract capsules are a standard herbal remedy, as the extract has components that prevent bacteria from adhering to the lining of the bladder. Avoid commercial cranberry juice cocktail products as they have high-fructose corn syrup or other sweeteners added.

Apple cider vinegar

Apple cider vinegar also turns the urine slightly acid. I would like to share a dramatic illustration of the effectiveness of this inexpensive product. This occurred in 1979 while Mother and I were traveling to China with a small group of friends. At our first stop in Greece, our friend Sharon related to us the terrible pain she was in because of a bladder infection. After Mother explained the importance of keeping her urine acid by taking apple cider vinegar, Sharon asked our waiter if he had any vinegar available. He returned to our table with a plastic, pint size squeeze bottle, full of cider vinegar. What a stroke of luck!

Others nearby in our group had overheard our conversation about the importance of vinegar and how it even will prevent parasites, so they wanted some, too. Amazingly, the waiter had enough bottles of the cider vinegar for every couple. On to China we went, taking our apple cider vinegar with us. Many of the tourists returning from China were very ill, picking up intestinal parasites; most had diarrhea. This was when China had just opened its doors to the Western traveler. We used the vinegar on all of the cooked greens we were served. We were also taking vitamin C, which helped make our urine acidic. Sharon's bladder infection cleared up right away.

Even visiting in New Delhi, India, where we had the honor of a private meeting with the late Mrs. Indira Gandhi, we all remained totally healthy. Of course, everybody had their vitamin packs, and we were careful what we ate and drank. Nevertheless, it was amazing that nobody in our group became ill during the entire month.

Mother and I also had taken along our protein powder and we used it for breakfast to keep us going, in addition to the traditional Continental breakfast. At that time, Mother was 75 years old, the oldest in the group, but she had a tremendous amount of stamina and energy and not only "kept up" with the group, but surpassed many much younger. She even climbed the Great Wall in China!

Use of the Birth Control Pill

Oral contraceptives, commonly called the "Pill," are probably the most common method of birth control in this country. I want you to be aware that they contain estrogen, which has many potential side effects. There is still a lot of debate over the safety of the Pill for women. If your doctor has prescribed it for you, be sure you read all the contraindications (side effects) in the enclosed package insert, and believe them. Also, be sure to read what I have to say about estrogen in the *Menopause* chapter. Typically, the Pill contains seven times more estrogen and ten times more synthetic progestin than HRT tablets. The reason: Stopping the development and fertilization of an egg requires higher doses of hormones than relieving hot flashes and vaginal dryness.[58]

The Pill has been associated with several health risks, particularly an increased risk of circulatory disorders, such as abnormal blood clotting, heart attacks, and stroke, especially if women smoke. Women who smoke, particularly those over the age of 35, are strongly advised to stop smoking; if they cannot, they should use some other form of birth control.

The birth control pill is not recommended for women who have blood-clotting disorders, such as thrombophlebitis; cancer of the breast, uterus, cervix, ovaries or other reproductive organs; heart disease; liver disorders; gallbladder disease; diabetes; high blood pressure; migraine headaches; or mental depression. The development of visual changes, leg pains that may indicate phlebitis, high blood pressure and other symptoms are among the indications that "the Pill" should be discontinued and a doctor consulted.[59] Some, but not all, studies have also linked the birth control pill to an increased risk of breast cancer in some women. Please make sure you read all the information on estrogen and synthetic progestin in the menopause chapter 15 to make an informed decision on the Pill.

Birth control pills disturb sugar metabolism, and the longer one takes them the more pronounced the disturbance. So if you are on birth control pills and show hypoglycemic symptoms such as anxiety, dizziness, depression, crying spells or exhaustion you must really watch your diet. Be sure to read about the blood sugar levels in the last chapter. Remember, small, frequent feedings of protein foods and complex carbohydrates. Avoid sugar altogether. If you decide you must be on birth control, be sure to increase all your vitamins and minerals.

Estrogen plays havoc with all the nutrients, especially the B complex vitamins, and vitamins C and E. It has been found that women taking oral contraceptives have reduced the tendency of blood platelets to aggregate excessively when they were given just 200 IU of vitamin E.[59] I would suggest a minimum of 400 IU of vitamin E.

Exercise is Also Effective

Exercise is very effective in alleviating the multiple problems of PMS. Take a fast walk for at least a half-hour, four to five times a week. Get your heart rate elevated, breathe deeply to get oxygen to your brain. Increase the time, and the number of days, you exercise. Remember, this is also beneficial to your bones in preventing osteoporosis, as well as help tone your muscles, and exercise can improve your mood to help make you feel better!

I have presented many suggestions to help you along the road toward optimum health.

My prayer is that this information will inspire you to continue to learn how to "take charge of your health."

*N*atural Approaches to Menopause

How to Prevent
Menopausal Difficulties

Many women use synthetic hormone replacement therapy to prevent heart disease and osteoporosis, but I feel they can prevent these conditions without the risk of cancer by adding a combination of vitamins, minerals and herbs to their nutritional program.
—GLADYS LINDBERG

*I*t happens to every woman—every woman, that is, who hits a "certain age." What that age is for you may vary from that of your sister, best friend or even your mother. However, it usually happens between the ages of 45 and 55, with the average age being 50. Menopause is also referred to as "the change of life."

There is a big difference between just surviving menopause and being prepared for it. You need to learn what to expect and most importantly what to do to pass through this phase naturally. Menopausal myths and realities run rampant, and anxiety about this change can put a damper on a woman's happiness in her later years.

The word menopause itself describes what this stage of life is all about—*meno* means "month" and *pausis* is translated as "ending."

By whatever name it is called, most women dread it. Nevertheless, this should be a delightful time of life since the concern about pregnancy is gone and the children are usually grown. It is a time when husbands and wives can enjoy each other with even a revival of romance. You can now do some of the things that you have put off doing for years. It can mean new beginnings or even a new career as you immerse yourself in something you have always wanted to do but were too busy with your family's needs. It can be a beautiful and rewarding phase of your life, especially if you are in good health.

Women facing menopause will experience changes in the patterns of their lives as well. Your children may be leaving for college or setting up their own homes. Your nest becomes empty. I remember how I cried when each of my children left for college. I knew I would miss all their activities—the football, basketball, and soccer games—and I realized they would never return the same.

Menopause may also be a time in our lives when we start caring for our aging parents. Many decisions need to be made on "who" or "how" or with "what finances" we will provide for them. Then we will face their eventual death. If we have had a close relationship with our parents, this can be the most difficult time of all. For me, the loss of my precious Mother was devastating. Not only did I lose Mother's unconditional love, but also one of my best friends and business partner. I always marveled at her wisdom and wise counsel. I was either with her or called her every day for most of my adult life. For years after she was gone I would reach for the phone to tell her some exciting news. My joy is that I know she is in a better place and has the promise of eternal life.

Now We Start to Face Our Own Mortality.

We realize we are the next one in line. We are now the "older genera- tion" or "the old folks" and maybe "grandma" or "grandpa" if we are fortunate!

We are making decisions on what we are going to do with the rest of our lives that will really count. Some of my friends' husbands are retiring, which causes another lifestyle change as they begin to care for their spouses in a different way. And to top it off, as many of these transformations are going on in our lives, we face the enormous hormonal changes in our bodies.

The better a woman feels about herself and her life, the easier a time she will have with the menopausal years. The brilliant researcher Dr. Roger Williams taught us that we are all biochemically different. Some women have more problems with premenstrual syndrome (PMS) and menstrual cramps than do others. I never knew when my period was going to start, so I needed to watch the calendar. It is the same with menopausal symptoms. While many women sail right through these years as I did, others have more of a struggle.

We can master these life challenges. Healthy people can cope with emotional and physical stress, and healthy women can withstand menopause without letting it get them down. The bottom line is, let's make you healthy. That is what this chapter is about, natural and health-building remedies for this unique phase of your life.

Make it happen—by taking charge of your health!

I had the opportunity to discuss health and nutrition at *The International Women's Conference on Possibility Thinking* at the Crystal Cathedral in Garden Grove, California, a few years ago. This is the ministry started by Dr. Robert Schuller, the man who reaches hundreds of thousands of people with his "make-it-happen" philosophy on tele- vision programs around the world.

Women were asked to sign up early so that the conference organ- izers could select an appropriate room size. Neither the seminar planners nor I were quite prepared for the response! The church office called to tell me that they were amazed at the interest in the seminar.

I was assigned to the main cathedral where I made two presentations. The response bore out what Mother and I have said for years—that there is a tremendous hunger for nutritional information, especially as it relates to women's health issues. Menopause and its related challenges are big concerns, and many of these ladies were starting this phase of their life.

Menopause Is Natural

Menopause is the natural cessation of menstrual bleeding. It is the time when the ovaries gradually decrease in size and begin to reduce the production of estrogen and progesterone in preparation for this life transition. This decline in hormone production starts several years before the last period and continues for several years after the actual menstrual flow stops. The median age for the start of menopause is 50 years, which means that half of all women stop menstruating before they turn 50 and the other half stop menstruating afterward.

Not all women passing through menopause have menopausal symptoms. Statistics are hard to prove, but medical authorities estimate that about 50 percent of women in the United States experience some degree of hot flashes during menopause. However, only 15 percent seek medical treatment for them.[1]

Estrogen—made in our adrenal glands

Even after entering menopause, some women make enough female-hormone precursors in their adrenal glands, and enough estrogen from these precursors in their fat deposits and do not experience any symptoms or, at most, have only temporary hot flashes. Also, estrogen is stored in the body's fat cells, so women with a little more weight are usually far less symptomatic than women who have dieted for years and are still a size four at age fifty.

Although adrenal estrogen is not as powerful as ovarian estrogen, at this point in life your body appreciates whatever it can get. In our high stress society where the adrenal glands become exhausted, women have more hormonal problems than we had generations ago. This adrenal stress can also leave many women in a progesterone deficiency, according to my friend Ann Louise Gittleman, M.S.[2]

A progesterone deficiency can cause bone loss, thinning hair and facial whiskers, the latter which may also be due to testosterone dominance. Ms. Gittleman says that this lack of progesterone is particularly common five to eight years before menopause due to the absence of ovulation in many women. An imbalance between progesterone and estrogen levels creates a condition called "estrogen dominance." The less stress you have felt during your life, the healthier your adrenals will be and the less apt you will be to suffer common menopausal complaints. Progesterone is necessary for the production of the adrenal hormones. When the adrenals are overworked and the hormones it produces depleted, progesterone is constantly used to replenish the system.[3]

Hot flashes and other symptoms

When the amount of estrogen begins to decrease, some women develop uncomfortable symptoms. The most common physical effects of menopause are feelings of warmth in the face, neck and chest or sudden intense episodes of heat or sweating called "hot flashes." If experienced during the night they are called "night sweats" and many times result in insomnia.

Others will experience fatigue, depression, mood swings, and even the feeling of apprehension and anxiety with heart palpitations. Interestingly, these are also the symptoms of hypoglycemia or low blood sugar. Be sure to read chapter 17, *Let's Put It All Together.*

Some women find their hair is thinning or very dry. Others will find their muscles and bones ache, almost feeling like arthritis has set in. This may be the beginning sign of osteoporosis. With hormones out of balance, there is a vaginal dryness and thinning, with a decrease in skin elasticity, depending upon the body's ability to continue to make estrogen.

The frequency and severity of the flashes vary widely. Medical literature simply relegates the problem to a defect in thermo-regulation, which means that the temperature control of the body goes wild.

There are differing opinions and theories as to why hot flashes occur, but we know it has to do with changing hormone levels. During these flashes the temperature of the skin rises but the internal temperature of the body does not increase and there is no fever.

There is a wide range of factors that can cause hot flashes, including spicy food, hot drinks, alcohol, sugar, caffeine, stress, hot weather, hot tubs and saunas, tobacco and strong emotions, which further attests to the multi-factorial nature of flashes.

Dr. Carlton Fredericks would tell Mother and me that these hot flashes were once believed by the medical profession to be the "psychosomatic imaginings of neurotic middle-aged women." This condition is very real for women who experience it, but the flashes are not life-threatening, and they go away once the body becomes accustomed to the reduced estrogen levels.

Vitamin E to the rescue

Drs. Evan and Wilfrid Shute reported 50 years ago that natural vitamin E helps with hot flashes and menopausal headaches. The Shute brothers found that some women responded to 400 IU of natural vitamin E per day, while others needed 800 IU. In some instances the doctors found that they had to increase the daily supplements of natural vitamin E to 1,000 IU or even 1,400 IU. You should increase your intake slowly. Do not take these high doses if you have hypertension. According to the Shute doctors, in one month you should be over your hot flashes.[4]

Make sure you take *natural* vitamin E (*d*-alpha tocopherol), the form your body uses. *Synthetic* vitamin E (*dl*-alpha) is made from less costly raw materials and studies show it is not utilized by the body as well. The natural form is more expensive because it must be extracted from soybean oil which contains only about one-tenth of one percent d-alpha-tocopherol. Make sure you shop at your nutrition store for natural E and not the drug store or discount houses which are cheaper and most always synthetic.

Bioflavonoids

The white part of citrus fruit contains bioflavonoids, which improve capillary fragility and make the blood vessels more permeable.[5] They are also helpful in relieving hot flashes. Therefore, we recommend that you peel the rind from an orange or grapefruit and eat the white pulp along with the fruit. Processing removes much of the bioflavonoids from frozen or reconstituted citrus juice. Many natural vitamin C supplements contain the bioflavonoids. Grape seed extract, pycnogenol and alpha lipoic acid are all forms of the flavonoid family and may also be helpful for hot flashes.

Studies have shown that menopausal women tend to have lower levels of vitamin C. Vitamin C strengthens the blood vessel membrane, acts as a potent antioxidant, and is also considered an essential nutrient for optimal function of the adrenal glands.

Herbal remedies

There are many effective herbal remedies and herbal combinations which usually contain black cohosh, licorice, ginseng, dong quai, red clover, and vitex. Be sure to read about the *phytoestrogens*, such as black cohosh and red clover found later in this chapter.

The isoflavones in soy may minimize hot flashes and actually help protect against excessive estrogen. In addition to having an anti-cancer effect on cells, soybeans manipulate estrogen by blocking its ability to stimulate malignant changes in breast tissue. Thus, soybeans could help prevent both the occurrence and spread of breast cancer in both premenopausal and postmenopausal women.[6] This is why some women use soy protein for their protein shake.

DHEA is an estrogen precursor

This means that DHEA (dehydroepiandrosterone) is converted to estrogen in the body. After menopause, when the ovaries stop making as much estrogen, small amounts of estrogen continue to be manufactured in the adrenal glands from hormones, including DHEA. As we age, DHEA levels fall and we may be prone to many forms of degenerative diseases including cancer, heart disease, diabetes, obesity, high blood pressure, and Parkinson's disease, to name a few. Raising DHEA in postmenopausal women to more youthful levels through supplementation appears to be a way of increasing estrogen levels naturally, and we may forestall the occurrence of these ailments.[7] Read more on DHEA in chapter 12, *Anti-Aging Therapies*.

Natural progesterone cream

Natural progesterone cream may provide significant relief from hot flashes. Using natural progesterone in a topical cream form is an excellent way to accomplish this. For effectiveness, a transdermal (through the skin) cream should contain a minimum of 400 mg to 500 mg USP progesterone per ounce. The usual dosage of these standardized progesterone creams is one-quarter to one-half teaspoon on the skin one or two times per day. Christiane Northrup, M.D., reports there is virtually no danger of overdose, and many women use 400 mg or the equivalent of an entire tube or jar per week with no ill effects.[8] I will explain more about this cream later in the chapter.

Hysterectomy and Menopause

Hysterectomy is the surgical removal of the uterus, usually done to remove tumors or to treat hemorrhages or severe pelvic inflammatory disease or a cancerous or pre-cancerous condition. There are three different ways in which hysterectomy may be performed. A *total hysterectomy* is where the cervix is removed along with the uterus. In a *partial hysterectomy,* the uterus is removed but the cervix and other female reproductive organs remain intact. A *pan hysterectomy* is the most extensive form of hysterectomy where the ovaries, fallopian tubes, and the uterus are removed.[9]

Menopause is not clearly age-related today. More than one third (37 percent) of the women in the United States have hysterectomies. The majority of these women had their surgeries between the ages of 25 and 44. Over 30 percent of the hysterectomies performed in the U.S. are done to remove fibroids. Other conditions for which a hysterectomy is performed include endometriosis (20 percent) and prolapse of the uterus (16 to 18 percent).[10] Our country led the world in the number of hysterectomies, with twice as many as in Great Britain. The Medical Boards finally changed the rules and before a hysterectomy can be performed, a board must agree upon it.[11]

If you are considering having both of your ovaries removed, you should be warned that there will be an abrupt and total shutting down of hormone production which can be devastating. This is actually castration, equal to a man having his testicles removed. It may also reduce sexual responsiveness and actually double the risk of osteoporosis.[12]

Women who have had these surgeries must follow the advice of their physician on the use of estrogen. Be sure to read about estriol (a form of estrogen) on the following pages, which may be an acceptable estrogen replacement.

Estrogen (ERT) Prescribed for Women

The *Dictionary of Medical Terms* defines estrogen as "a general term for the female hormones (*estradiol, estrone, estriol*) produced in the ovaries (and in small amounts in the testes and adrenals). In women, estrogen functions in the menstrual cycle and in the development of secondary sex characteristics (i.e., breast development in adolescence).

"As a synthetic preparation sold under many trade names, estrogen drugs are used to treat menstrual irregularities, to relieve symptoms of menopause, to treat cancer of the prostate and in oral contraceptives."[13]

You should use these estrogen drugs with caution because estrogen has side effects, some of which are hotly debated and recently questioned in new scientific research. These side effects include stroke, blood clots, gallbladder disease, liver tumors and enlargement, fluid retention and weight gain, headaches, endometrial cancer and fibroids. Estrogen is not recommended for patients with uterine or breast cancer, a strong family history of cancer, obesity, phlebitis, varicose veins, diabetes, hypertension, edema, fibroids or fibrocystic breast.[14]

These warnings vividly demonstrate the controversy surrounding the use of one of the most prescribed and researched hormones of this century. Are the benefits so great that untold numbers of women should be using the therapy? I feel that if these women knew all the risks, their answer would be "no." At least more attention is now being given to these negative side effects.

The following is a serious and honest look at the benefits versus the downside of synthetic estrogen. Indeed, new revelations about the efficacy of natural estrogen and natural progesterone have caused many authorities to reconsider their past beliefs, which has led to new thinking on this controversial subject. I have cast my vote with the "natural" side and I'll explain why in the next few pages.

Cautions with premarin

Premarin is a form of conjugated estrogen that is called "naturally occurring" because it is extracted from the urine of pregnant horses. That's how it got its name: Pre (pregnant), mar (mare's), in (urine).

Wyeth-Ayerst Labs, the makers of Premarin, include a summary of prescribing information about the drug for the patient. It examines the risk of cancer of the uterus and cancer of the breast.

PART OF THE REPORT STATES: "The risk of cancer of the uterus increases the longer estrogens are used and when larger doses are taken. One study showed that when estrogens are discontinued, this increased risk of cancer seems to fall off quickly. In another study, the persistence of (cancer) risk was demonstrated for ten years after stopping estrogen treatment. Because of this risk, it is important to take the lowest effective dose of estrogen and to take it only as long as you need it. There is a higher risk of cancer of the uterus if you are overweight, diabetic or have high blood pressure."[15] Remember, this is from the people who make the product for you. The risk may last for up to ten years after you stop using the drug! If you are taking this product, be sure to read the complete product information insert.

Cancer: an unacceptable side effect

According to the medical journal *Primary Care and Cancer,*

published by M.D. Anderson Cancer Center in Houston, Texas, the latent period from exposure to hormones and the development of an overt malignancy may be as long as 15 to 30 years. As with most substances known to cause cancer, risk is related to both the intensity and duration of exposure, and these variables are hard to quantify. The journal also reported that the development of any cancer is an unacceptable side effect for an elective therapy unless an overriding benefit can be demonstrated.[16]

In 1995, Emory University and the National Cancer Society published a report of an eight-year study of over 240,000 women. A research article entitled, "Estrogen Replacement Therapy and Fatal Ovarian Cancer" found that those women who were given unopposed estrogen therapy (estrogen without progesterone) had a 72 percent higher risk of fatal cancer of the ovaries.[17]

There are numerous studies going back to the 1960s on estrogen's involvement as a suspected cancer-causing agent. *The latest medical reports tell us that cancer of the breast will affect one in every nine women.* Of course, this is just breast cancer. The American Cancer Society also reported that *cancer will affect one in three people in this country* sometime during their lives.[18] This statistic is startling! One person in every three is going to get cancer? What is causing this response in our bodies?

Breast cancer death

An excellent television program on breast cancer was presented on PBS (Public Broadcasting System—October 1993) by Susan Love, M.D., who was a cancer surgeon at the University of California at Los Angeles (UCLA). She reported that more women have died of breast cancer in this country than all of the American lives that were lost fighting all of this country's wars, including the Civil War. This is amazing considering all our wars: Civil War, World War I, World War II, the Korean War and Vietnam. One woman dies every 12 minutes from breast cancer alone. Dr. Love stated that it takes eight to ten years before you can feel a lump, so you should get several medical opinions before you make a final decision on the type of treatment for your condition.[19]

Estrogen could stimulate the growth of an already existing cancer, and women with a personal or family history of breast cancer are often advised to avoid estrogen altogether.[20] In addition, if you discover that you have cancer, one of the first treatments to be administered is often an estrogen-blocking substance.

Estrogen and heart disease!

We were also told to take estrogen because it is a preventive for heart attacks and because more women die of heart disease than cancer. Now studies are verifying the truth about the warning of side effects printed by Wyeth-Ayerst Labs on the insert inside of the Premarin package:

> Abnormal blood clotting: Taking estrogens may increase the risk of blood clots. These clots can cause a stroke, heart attack or pulmonary embolism, any of which may be fatal.[21]

We have been told to take a hormone to prevent heart disease, yet in the pharmaceutical literature they report that it may actually cause a stroke, heart attack or pulmonary embolism! Another warning in the package insert reads:

> Gallbladder disease: Women who use estrogens after menopause are more likely to develop gallbladder disease needing surgery than women who do not use estrogen.[22]

FDA warnings on package inserts

In 1976 Senate hearings, the FDA stated they would see that users of estrogen products, including the pill, would have detailed product inserts warning of health risks associated with the product. Then women would be free to make up their own minds. The *Pharmaceutical Manufacturers Association* fought this regulation, claiming it would reduce sales. They were joined by other medical groups, the *American College of Obstetricians and Gynecologists* and the *American Society of Internal Medicine*, who were not happy about such patient warnings. They argued that women will not read them anyway.

Some physicians seemed concerned that a class of patients, the menopausal female, would be more susceptible to adverse psychological reaction. In other words they were arguing on the premise, "what you don't know won't hurt you," but in this case it does. Despite the efforts of the drug manufacturers and the medical establishment, and after a year of debate in Congress, the package inserts are in place. Congress won! Be sure to read them!

As you will see in the rest of this chapter and throughout the book, you can protect your heart and bones and also improve your quality of life with natural products. Moreover, you won't have the fear of creating other conditions by taking synthetic hormones!

Natural ways to prevent heart disease

There are other things we can do. Exciting news presented at the American Heart Association's 65th Scientific Session was reported to doctors in the *Medical Tribune*, with front page headlines that read, *"Vitamin E May Cut Heart Risk."* In two studies of over 130,000 people with no history of cardiovascular problems, the use of vitamin E for at least two years reduced the risk in women for heart attacks by 46 percent and by 26 percent in men. It was thrilling to see the story picked up in the *New York Times* and *Chicago Tribune*, and by the media across the country. The protective effect of vitamin E appeared to be independent of beta carotene or vitamin C.[23]

Another important study was published in the *Lancet*, March 23, 1996, and evaluated approximately 2,002 patients with a history of heart disease in a randomized, controlled trial. Half received 400 to 800 IU's of vitamin E daily; the others received a placebo. They were followed for a total of 17 months and the researchers noted a *75 percent reduction in heart attacks in the vitamin E group*, compared to the placebo group. These research studies go on to explain that the benefits of vitamin E were from supplements, not foods.

There is a tremendous amount of valuable information on how vitamin E protects against cardiovascular disease, including heart attacks and stroke. Be sure to read chapter 8, *Protecting Your Heart*.

CoEnzyme Q_{10} for our heart

The use of CoQ_{10} to treat heart disease has become well established in Japan, where researchers began testing CoQ_{10} for heart disease in the 1960s. By 1987, more than ten million Japanese were estimated to be taking CoQ_{10} as a prescription drug for cardiac problems.[24]

Here in the United States, CoQ_{10} is not a prescription drug and is available in your nutrition store. CoQ_{10}'s anti-aging benefits potentially include treatment of cardiac conditions by giving your heart a stronger pumping action, helping to prevent congestive heart disease and treating high blood pressure. It also is valuable in helping protect against carcinogens, improving recovery time after surgery, increasing the function of the immune system, enhancing vitality and increasing life span.[25] Wow! I hope we all consider taking CoQ_{10}. Read more about CoQ_{10} and other valuable nutrients in the *Heart* and *Blood Pressure* chapters.

Hormone Replacement Therapy?

Estrogen Replacement Therapy (ERT) had been the way of treating menopausal symptoms in women for years. Now the more common treatment is Hormone Replacement Therapy (HRT), which is a combination of estrogen and progestin, a synthetic form of progesterone.

"The Truth About Hormones": the Women's Health Initiative

The cover of *Time* magazine July 22, 2002 read, "The Truth About Hormones: Hormone Replacement Therapy is riskier than advertised." The inside article was "What's a Woman to Do? Women are mystified and confused." In the same week, the cover of *Newsweek* read, "Beyond Hormone Therapy" and the inside article was, "The end of the age of estrogen."

Time magazine reported:

> A large federally funded clinical trial, part of a group of studies called the Women's Health Initiative has definitively shown for the first time that hormones in question—estrogen and progestin—are not the age-defying wonder drugs that everyone thought they were. As if that weren't bad enough, the results, made public last week, proved that taking these hormones actually increases a woman's risk of developing potentially deadly cardiovascular problems and invasive breast cancer, among other things.

This has obviously caused great concern and confusion for women who have been taking these hormones for years.

The article went on, "But the principal message is this; taking estrogen and progestin for years in hope of preventing a heart attack or stroke can no longer be considered a valid medical strategy."

Last year, U.S. pharmacists filled some 45 million prescriptions for Premarin and an additional 22 million for Prempro, which consists of estrogen and progestin.[26] Hormone therapy was also believed to prevent fractures due to osteoporosis, but the new study raises questions about that, too. *Women in the trial who were on hormones had a slightly higher rate of hip fractures than those taking a placebo, the opposite of what was expected.*

Newsweek reported, "Federal health officials announced last Tuesday that the jury was finally in—and that Prempro does significantly more harm than good when taken for long periods. Women had been told for decades that estrogen taken with progestin would not only ease hot flashes and insomnia but help preserve bone strength, mental acuity and, most important, heart health. There's no question that HRT can ease the acute symptoms of menopause and the claim about bone strength has held up to scrutiny. *But after observing more than 16,000 women for roughly five years, researchers found conclusively that the hormones in Prempro raise the risk of heart attack, stroke, blood clots, and breast cancer"* (emphasis added).

These findings were so striking that the study was stopped three years short of its scheduled completion. The formal scientific report will be published in the *Journal of the American Medical Association,* but this information was released early at a press conference in Washington.

COMBINING ESTROGEN AND SYNTHETIC PROGESTIN = CANCER

Even years ago, a very important study reported in the *New England Journal of Medicine* in 1989 and also in *Science* examined the risks of breast cancer when the regimen of estrogen replacement therapy includes progestin along with estrogen. "Physicians have suspected that this combination could be more natural, and because therapy with estrogen alone has been linked to uterine cancer, this treatment might reduce the risks. *However, the latest findings for combined treatment suggest that it may actually increase the risk of breast cancer over the risk of treatment by estrogen alone."*[27] "Many in the scientific community are not surprised by this finding, in part because it stimulates the growth of epithelial cells such as those found in the glands and ducts of the breast."[28]

Natural Estrogen: The Value of Estriol

As I noted earlier, estrogen is not a single substance. It exists in the body in at least three forms including *estradiol, estrone* and *estriol.*

Dr. Marcus Laux, in his wonderful book, *Natural Woman, Natural Menopause,* reports, "Estrogens, in general, tend to promote cell division, particularly in hormone-sensitive tissue such as the breast and the uterine lining. Of the three estrogens, estradiol is the most stimulating to the breast and estriol the least. Estradiol is 1,000 times more potent in its effects on breast tissue than estriol. Studies conducted two decades ago clearly found that over exposure to estradiol (and estrone, to a lesser extent) increases one's risk of breast cancer, whereas estriol is protective."[29]

Estriol and cancer protection

In fact, estriol has been used as a treatment for breast cancer. Alvin M. Follingstad, M.D., presented results of a study in the *New England Journal of Medicine* in which small doses of estriol were given to a group of post-menopausal women with spreading breast cancer, and 37 percent of them experienced remission or arrest of their metastatic lesions. There have been recent reports that it is better than Tamoxifen for women with breast cancer.

Dr. Follingstad also reported in an article called, "Estriol, the Forgotten Estrogen," in the *Journal of the American Medical Association*, that estriol should be given to women who need estrogen therapy but who are at high risk for developing cancer or who have had a hysterectomy. The role of estriol in postmenopausal hormone replacement therapy should, therefore, be given a closer look.

ESTRIOL IS CONSIDERED A WEAK ESTROGEN. Consequently, more estriol is required to relieve menopausal symptom. But if a proper dosage is given, symptoms do improve. A dose of 2 mg to 4 mg of estriol is as effective as 0.6 to 1.25 mg of conjugated estrogens or estrone.[30] You need your doctor to write a prescription for estriol.

Dr. Alan Gaby reported in his book, *Preventing and Reversing Osteoporosis*, "The standard estrogen preparations frequently cause a potentially precancerous proliferation of the uterine lining, known as endometrial hyperplasia. In contrast, most investigators have found that estriol does not cause *endometrial hyperplasia*, even when given in doses as high as 8 mg per day. In one study, for example, 52 women with severe menopausal symptoms were given estriol continuously for six months in doses of 2 mg to 8 mg per day."

"Improvements in symptoms occurred within one month and persisted as long as estriol therapy was continued. The degree of symptom improvement was related to the dose—moderate at 2 mg per day, but marked at a dose of 8 mg per day. Estriol therapy also produces an improvement in vaginal atrophy and in the quality of the cervical mucus. However, endometrial biopsies failed to show hyperplasia in any case, regardless of the dosage of estriol used. Breakthrough bleeding also was not a problem."[31]

Watch out for environmental estrogens

According to Dr. Michael Murray, "Harmful chemicals, including pesticides, can enter the body and become lodged in our fat cells. These chemicals—known as environmental estrogens (xenoestrogens)—mimic the activity of estrogen in the body and may be a major factor in the growing epidemic of estrogen-related health problems such as PMS and cancer."[32] But we can break down these harmful substances if we are healthy...read on.

CONVERTING ESTROGEN TO ESTRIOL. Carlton Fredericks, Ph.D., stated in his book *Breast Cancer: A Nutritional Approach* that, "the body breaks down estrogen, degrading it into the much less active and thereby less threatening hormone estriol. In converting estrogen into estriol, the body actually turns a carcinogenic (cancer-producing) compound into a harmless chemical that is ultimately excreted." Dr. Fredericks writes, "This isn't theory—in population groups where the women tend toward higher estriol and lower estrogen levels, breast cancer is always less frequent."[33] These studies found that the liver is the essential organ in converting the most active form of estrogen, estradiol, to the much less active form, estriol.

YOU NEED A HEALTHY LIVER. For optimal conversion to estriol, your liver requires several nutrients in the diet. A number of nutritional factors are critical to support this liver function, including the B-complex vitamins. Protein has also proven to be a critical nutrient in the support of liver function.[34]

It was found that "well-fed" women with estrogen-dependent disorders, ranging from premenstrual tension and prolonged menstruation to excessive hemorrhaging and cystic mastitis, lessened their symptoms when they supplied their bodies with more generous amounts of the entire vitamin B-complex (at least 50 mg of each, a day) and protein.

Other important nutritional compounds include the lipotropic factors, such as choline and inositol, which are nutrients needed in sufficient amounts to promote ideal fat metabolism. Because estrogens are fat-soluble hormones, both nutrients have long been known to have beneficial effects on the liver.

You should include choline (1,500 mg) and inositol (1,000 mg) per day as part of your nutritional program. *Soy Lecithin* is one of the richest natural sources of choline and inositol, also called lipotropic factors. Lecithin is easy to add to your protein shakes, cereals, salads or juice. Take one tablespoon a day of soy lecithin granules, which should contain phosphatidyl choline (1,725 mg); phosphatidyl inositol (1,050 mg); plus essential fatty acids such as linoleic acid (2,195 mg.) I suggest you use the granulated form of lecithin because you'd have to take 10 large softgel capsules to equal the same potency as 1 tablespoon of lecithin granules.

What else is needed?

Besides the vitamin-B complex and choline and inositol, I think it is also very important to take an antioxidant formula containing a natural (d-alpha) vitamin E, at least 400 IU to 1,000 IU daily. The *British Journal of Cancer* reported a study of over 5,000 women where the risk of breast cancer was found to be 5.2 times higher for women with the lowest levels of vitamin E than for those with the highest.[35]

Vitamin C is another important antioxidant and a daily dose of 1,000 to 2,000 mg or more would be beneficial. Most authorities would also suggest evening primrose oil (GLA), three 500 IU (1,500 IU) capsules twice a day. Evening primrose oil is particularly beneficial for anyone with PMS, as it is a valuable source of prostaglandin-E1. Read chapter 14 for more information on PMS.

It is important to include a complete mineral formula, containing calcium, magnesium, zinc, boron, chromium and selenium plus the others, in adequate amounts. The herb milk thistle *(silymarin)* extract, known for helping to regenerate the liver, would be an important addition to this nutrition program. Read the benefits of these nutrients in chapters 3 and 4, especially about selenium's ability to prevent 50 percent of cancer deaths.

Phytoestrogens:
Natural Hormone Replacement

There are many proven plant and herbal options that women may consider in place of synthetic estrogen. The *phytoestrogens* (*phyto* is Greek for plant) are common dietary compounds, and are capable of producing estrogenic effects, although their activity compared to synthetic estrogen is low. Phytoestrogens have been present in the human diet for thousands of years. However, they are much weaker than steroid estrogens, having an estrogenic potency between about 1/20,000th to 1/50th as much as estradiol.[36]

Phytoestrogens: How do they work?

Phytoestrogens are similar to estriol (the good estrogen) in structure which enables the phytoestrogens to mimic the effect of estriol in the body. They bind to estrogen receptor sites in the breast and protect against free-floating estradiol (the form of estrogen we don't want). They also protect the breasts from invasion of *xenoestrogens* (environmental estrogens). We discussed earlier that these are estrogen-like substances found in our environment in the form of pesticides, DDT, the breakdown of plastics, etc. They bind to estrogen receptor sites in the breasts and elsewhere and can become carcinogenic (cancer causing).

According to our friend Dr. Shari Leiberman, author of *Get Off the Menopause Roller Coaster*, "People who consume large quantities of phytoestrogens keep those receptor sites busy with healthy, protective substances. The estriol-like phytohormones bind to the receptor sites, rendering them unavailable for the invading xenoestrogens, and also for any free-floating estradiol that the liver has not managed to convert into estriol."[37]

Dr. Leiberman goes on to say, "An equally important function of phytoestrogens is in the actual conversion of estradiol into estriol. The liver uses phytoestrogens extensively in its conversion process. Phytoestrogens facilitate the healthy functioning of the liver, and therefore increase the amount of estriol in the body." This is why it's important we have a healthy liver. We should take all these essential nutrients for the liver, to make sure this conversion process is possible.

The most popular phytoestrogen: isoflavones

Recently, *isoflavones* have emerged as one of the most popular of the phyto-estrogens because they have the most potent estrogenic activity of all the common phytoestrogens.[38] They also have an extensive range of biological activity in the body. There are over 1,000 different isoflavones in the plant kingdom and are distinguished by being almost exclusively in legumes. These legumes include plants such as chickpeas, soy, clover, lentils, and beans.

Natural Herbal Support

I strongly recommend these isoflavones and herbal formulas, but we must give them a chance to work, as they are not overnight remedies.

Black Cohosh *(Cimicifuga racemosa)*

Those of you who remember Lydia Pinkham's *Vegetable Compound* may be interested to know that black cohosh was one of its main ingredients. Black cohosh is a tonic for the central nervous system, and Dr. Michael Murray has reported that black cohosh is the most thoroughly researched, natural approach to menopause. The clinical documentation is exceptional, particularly where hormone replacement therapy is contraindicated, i.e., women with a history of estrogen-dependent cancer, unexplained uterine bleeding, liver and gallbladder disease, pancreatitis, endometriosis, uterine fibroids or fibrocystic breast disease. It is effective for hot flashes, night sweats, headaches, heart palpitations and vaginal atrophy. Psychological problems such as depression, anxiety, nervousness, sleep disturbances and decreased libido can also be alleviated with black cohosh.[39]

Dr. Murray reported in the *Encyclopedia of Natural Medicine,* 2nd Edition, that a large open study involving over 629 female patients, *cimicifuga* extract (black cohosh) produced clear improvements in menopausal symptoms in over 80 percent of patients within six to eight weeks. Improvement was experienced in both physical and psychological symptoms.

"Most patients reported noticeable benefits within four weeks after the initiation of *cimicifuga* therapy. After six to eight weeks, complete resolution of symptoms was achieved in a large percentage of patients. *Cimicifuga* was well tolerated; there was no discontinuation of therapy, and only seven percent of patients reported mild transitory stomach complaints," according to Dr. Murray.[40]

Red clover extract

It has more than a decade of scientific research and trials among menopausal women. Red clover extract *(Trifolium pratense)* provides all four of the major estrogenic isoflavones: *genistein, biochanin, daidzein* and *formononetin*. Red clover, is also the world's richest source of isoflavones.

It can protect our bones from osteoporosis, prevent heart disease and even Alzheimer's disease. New reports indicate it may even help in diabetes. The recommended dosage is only 40 mg a day. It is available from your nutrition store under different brand names.

Valuable herbal remedies

There will be many new herbs and phytoestrogen combination

products coming to your nutrition store soon, as many women are opting to go through their change of life using safer, more natural products than synthetic, pharmaceutical drugs.

"Tonic" herbs have long been recognized for their benefits to the female glandular system. Here are some examples of the benefits of just a few of these herbs: Black cohosh used in the German studies, as well as Dong Quai, *(Angelica sinensis)*, known as the "queen of all female herbs" which exerts a natural effect on the vascular system that is extremely useful in dealing with the frequency and intensity of hot flashes and night sweats.[41] It has been used in China and Japan since 588 B.C. for dysmenorrhea (painful menstruation). Its principal use has been for female problems, especially for ailments affecting the female organs and the smooth muscles of the uterus.[42] Chaste Tree Berry or Vitex *(Vitex agnus-castus)* has been used for centuries and has been reputed to be a hormone balancer.[43] These natural plant estrogens may help fill the gap for those with low estrogen levels. Chaste berry may also help reduce some of the undesirable symptoms that can occur during menopause, such as vaginal dryness, hot flashes, dizziness and depression, according to herbalist Christopher Hobbs.[44] "Licorice *(Glycyrrhiza glabra)* exhibits alternative (tending to restore normal health) action upon estrogen metabolism, i.e., when estrogen levels are too high, it inhibits estrogen action, and when estrogen levels are too low, it potentiates estrogen action when used in greater amounts. The estrogen action of licorice is a result of its isoflavone content, as well as its *glycyrrhetinic acid* content," according to Michael Murray, N.D.[45]

False unicorn *(Helonias opulus)* and Red raspberry *(Rubys idaeus)* are plants primarily used to lessen the symptoms of menopause, although they have also been used to improve menstrual function and many other physical and mental functions.[46]

There are three different herbs that fall under the label ginseng: American ginseng *(Panax quinquefolium)*, and Korean or Chinese ginsengs *(Panax ginseng)*. Earl Mindell, R.Ph., Ph.D., reports that Chinese ginseng is believed to increase estrogen levels in women and is therefore often recommended for menopausal symptoms caused by a drop in estrogen production.[47] Siberian ginseng *(Eleutherococcus senticosus)* is technically not ginseng at all, but has many of the same properties of ginseng and is therefore used the same way.

These herbals are usually used in combination for a more synergistic effect, so look for these in your nutrition store.

Risks of Synthetic Progestin

Synthetic progesterone is called *progestin* (and sold by prescription as Provera). It mimics the action of progesterone, but the body does not respond in the same way.[48]

If you are taking progestins, you may bleed every month even if you have passed menopause. *The Worst Pills, Best Pills* 1999 edition also reports, "Because progestins have potentially significant risks, you should only use them (or progestin and estrogen combinations) to treat serious symptoms, and then for as short a time as possible."[49] We now know it is not advisable to take these synthetic hormones for long periods of time.

Worst Pills, Best Pills goes on to report, "Progestin use has been associated with blood clots, strokes, and blindness in women. What? Blindness in Women?! This drug causes breast and uterine cancers when administered to laboratory mammals, and researchers are investigating whether it causes breast cancer in women by itself or further increases the risk of breast cancer when used with estrogen."

The *Physician's Desk Reference* 1995 edition lists numerous contraindications, and some of the progestin side effects are toxic. Women who take progestin sometimes complain of bloating, headaches, moodiness or other side effects.[50] Obviously, I do not recommend taking synthetic progesterone.

Benefits of Natural Progesterone

Progesterone is a hormone that in many cases can safely and effectively relieve menopausal symptoms, protect against cancer, act as a natural tranquilizer, prevent osteoporosis and may even stimulate new bone formation. There is only one progesterone, the specific molecule made by the adrenal glands or by the ovaries as a consequence of ovulation. The name was derived from "pro" meaning *in support of*, and "gestation" meaning *pregnancy*. Natural progesterone is necessary for the survival and development of the embryo and throughout pregnancy.[51]

There seems to be confusion as to what natural progesterone really is. Progesterone was first crystallized in 1934, and today it is available from plant sources. Natural micronized progesterone is an exact chemical duplicate of the progesterone that is normally produced by the ovaries. Women using natural progesterone experience a mild tranquilizing effect and an enhanced feeling of well-being.

Progesterone is produced in large amounts by the placenta during pregnancy. If a woman does not produce enough progesterone, she will have a miscarriage. Progesterone is given to women who have trouble carrying their pregnancy to term. In fact, the so-called French abortion pill, RU-486, works by blocking the action of progesterone, resulting in a spontaneous abortion of the fetus.[52]

My dear friend, Frank Varese, M.D., encouraged me to attend a presentation by Ray Peat, Ph.D., from Oregon. He was lecturing on the subject of natural progesterone, its many roles in human health and why the medical profession had not yet recognized this important hormone. I was able to discuss this subject with Dr. Peat, and was very impressed with his research.

John R. Lee, M.D., was first inspired to learn about progesterone at a similar presentation given by Dr. Peat. After 30 years, Dr. Lee retired from private practice in California, and he now teaches professionals and lay audiences about the importance of hormone balance and the use of natural progesterone.

Dr. Lee sent me an article on the benefits of natural progesterone. In it he states, "As women approach menopause, they find themselves losing energy, retaining fluids, fighting fat, developing wrinkles and facial hairs, being prone to headaches and depression, and less interested in sex. Common wisdom assigns these symptoms simply to the aging process."

"They see their doctors, take their diuretics and, occasionally, thyroid medication, and face their future with fading enthusiasm. They seek out cosmeticians for their wrinkles, see their beauticians more often for their thinning hair, and take more calcium for their thinning bones. What they are unaware of is the importance of proper hormonal balance, particularly the lack of this singularly important hormone, progesterone."[53]

Dr. John Lee wrote an excellent book on the subject—*What Your Doctor May Not Tell You About Menopause: The Breakthrough Book on Natural Progesterone*. He wrote, "Our present preoccupation with supplemental estrogen and our neglect of natural progesterone is a medical oddity peculiar to the past three to four decades. The reasons for this are complex, but include incomplete knowledge and the pressures driven by pharmaceutical profits. At this time it is important to understand and know the effects of these two important hormones." The following chart lists the benefits Dr. Lee cites.

PHYSIOLOGICAL EFFECTS OF ESTROGEN
AND PROGESTERONE

ESTROGEN EFFECTS

- causes breast stimulation
- creates proliferative endometrium
- salt and fluid retention
- increases fat in body
- depression and headaches
- interferes with thyroid hormone
- increases blood clotting
- decreases libido, sex drive
- impairs blood sugar control
- loss of zinc and holding of copper
- reduces oxygen levels in all cells
- increases risk of breast cancer
- slightly restrains osteoclast or rate of bone loss
- increases risk of gallbladder disease
- increases risk of endometrial cancer
- increases risk of autoimmune disorders

PROGESTERONE EFFECTS

- protects against fibrocysts in breast
- maintains secretory endometrium
- natural diuretic
- helps use fat for energy
- natural anti-depressant
- facilitates thyroid hormone action
- normalizes blood clotting
- restores sex drive
- normalizes blood sugar levels
- normalizes zinc, copper levels
- restores proper cell oxygen levels
- helps prevent breast cancer
- stimulates osteoblast bone building
- restores normal vascular tone
- restores proper cell oxygen level
- precursor of cortisone synthesis
- prevents endometrial cancer
- precursor of corticosteroids
- necessary for survival of embryo

While estrogen levels drop only 40 to 60 percent at menopause, progesterone levels can drop even lower. Progesterone has an opposing, or balancing, effect on estrogen. When progesterone levels drop very low we have estrogen dominance which causes a long list of unpleasant symptoms just mentioned. Estrogen dominance does not necessarily mean that a woman has too much estrogen; it simply indicates that estrogen levels are relatively higher than progesterone levels, creating a hormonal imbalance with its estrogenic side effects.[54]

A bone–building hormone

A growing body of evidence indicates that progesterone is a powerful bone-building hormone and that progesterone replacement therapy could be the next major advance in the battle against osteoporosis.

Jerilynn C. Prior, M.D., of the Division of Endocrinology and Metabolism, University of British Columbia in Vancouver, has written a comprehensive review of the evidence that progesterone stimulates bone formation. *Research found that progesterone binds to osteoblast cells that build new bone.* This research suggests that progesterone acts directly on osteoblasts and may promote bone formation.[55]

In a study by Dr. Lee, 100 postmenopausal women with osteoporosis were treated with transdermal (through the skin) natural progesterone cream plus a calcium-magnesium supplement and were followed for at least six years. They improved not only in maintaining their height and reducing bone fractures, but of the 63 women who also had bone mineral density scans, an average 15.4 percent increase in bone mass was recorded. This is remarkable, since this group of women would be expected to lose at least 4.5 percent of their bone density over this period.[56]

Why use a progesterone cream?

This natural progesterone product is not offered by the major pharmaceutical firms. Being a natural substance, progesterone is not patentable and therefore the profit motive for major scientific research on it is absent, as well as the marketing dollars to promote it.

Dr. Lee, who is a leading authority on the subject, says, "My preference among the various available forms of progesterone supplements remains the transdermal (through the skin) route. My reasons have to do with the appropriateness of hormone supplementation. Remember that the goal is physiologic hormone balance. By physiologic, I mean that the dosages approximate (and not exceed) normal hormone needs and responses. When intervening in a system of biofeedback controls, it is unwise to exceed the normal responses of the healthy gland. In the case of hypothyroidism or adrenal deficiency, supplemental dosages greater than normal will suppress normal function of the target gland. I try to follow the same principle concerning estrogen and progesterone...I do not wish to suppress whatever function still remains in the ovary."[57]

The full benefits may not become apparent for several weeks or even several menstrual cycles if using it for PMS, and for several months if you are using it for menopause. This time variation is due to individual differences in body fat content and the extent of your progesterone deficiency.

Progesterone cream is absorbed through the skin into the underlying fat layer, from which it diffuses into the capillaries permeating the fat, where it can be taken up in the blood as needed. The cream is very easily and quickly absorbed.[58]

WHERE DO I APPLY THE CREAM? If you have hot flashes, vaginal dryness or other menopausal symptoms, you can take a little of this cream and apply it to any soft tissues like your face and neck, the upper chest and breast, inside your arms, and behind your knees. You should rotate the areas where you use the cream.

Skin areas to which progesterone cream has been applied become less dry and more youthful in texture. This is why I use it on my face and neck several times a week. Skin aging may be prevented more effectively with a progesterone cream than with estrogen creams.

IT MAY HELP PREVENT BREAST CANCER. I found a very interesting study in *Dr. Susan Love's Hormone Book*. Researchers discovered that breast cell proliferation is higher in the second half of the menstrual cycle when progesterone levels are higher, so they assumed that progesterone may stimulate breast tissue to cause cancer. To investigate this further, a study was done on women who were about to undergo breast-reduction surgery. The breast tissue could then be examined after the surgery. Each woman applied progesterone cream to one breast every day for two weeks before the operation. After the reduction surgery, the pathologist examined the breast tissue to see if the progesterone had stimulated the tissues to multiply. They found that the progesterone cream had decreased cell division, or there was less cell division. This has been interpreted as demonstrating that progesterone prevents breast cancer. The researchers conclusion was that progesterone directly applied to the breast might even help prevent breast cancer. [59]

HOW MUCH PROGESTERONE CREAM SHOULD I USE? Make sure that the cream you buy contains enough progesterone. Each two-ounce jar or tube should contain 950 or 1,000 milligrams. This two-ounce jar or tube would be enough to maintain adequate progesterone needs in a postmenopausal woman for two months. This would amount to 20 to 30 milligrams of progesterone per day, or about ¼ to ½ teaspoon of cream twice a day. I suggest that you use it in the morning and before bed. I keep a tube next to my bed on my night stand, and before I go to sleep I rub it on. I also have a tube in my bathroom, and I use it again before dressing in the morning.

The best way to tell if you are using enough is whether your symptoms are relieved. Because we are all biochemically unique and the ability to absorb the cream varies, your actual dose may be more or less than these recommendations.

IF YOU STILL HAVE A MENSTRUAL PERIOD. Use progesterone cream approximately two weeks per month as long as you are having a menstrual period. Count the onset of bleeding as day one. Since normal progesterone production can reach 20 mg per day between days 12 to 26 of the cycle, Dr. Lee recommends using the cream between days 12 to 26 of the cycle. Some women whose cycles are naturally longer will use it from day 10 to 28. Do not use the cream during the week of your period. If bleeding starts before day 26 (or before it would normally begin), stop the progesterone, start counting up to day 12, and then start the progesterone again. Menstrual periods may be irregular due to progesterone deficiency, so it may take three cycles of cream use before regularity is restored.

FOR MENOPAUSE. Because many postmenopausal women are deficient in progesterone to start with, and since much of this fat-soluble hormone will be initially "lost" in the body fat stores, it is wise to use the full two-ounce dose each month for three months or so to overcome the deficiency state and relieve the symptoms. After that, the dosage can be reduced. Dr. Lee recommends that you take a week off each month in order to maintain receptor sensitivity.[60]

ARE YOU TAKING ESTROGEN HORMONES? William Regelson, M.D., feels if you are using the progesterone cream just referred to, along with estrogen (such as Premarin), be sure that you are being monitored by your physician to keep watch for signs of uterine hyperplasia. Some doctors feel you are better off if you find a doctor who will write a prescription for the weakest natural estrogen like estriol, and make sure you are getting the proper dosage along with using natural progesterone.[61]

Progesterone capsules

Dr. John Lee reports that the disadvantage of taking oral capsules (by prescription only) is that they need to be given in very large doses—100 to 200 mg per day—to compensate for the 85 to 90 percent that will be excreted almost immediately through the liver. This is 10 to 20 times greater than transdermal doses just to get the 20 to 24 mg needed daily. The doctor feels there is no need to put our liver to all this work.

Progesterone for a lifetime

Dr. John Lee feels that most women should take natural progesterone cream for the rest of their lives. I have discussed many of the benefits of progesterone in this chapter, which includes building bones to protecting against osteoporosis, all the way to helping protect against breast cancer and endometrial cancer. It restores the sex drive, normalizes blood clotting, helps thyroid hormone action, and the list goes on and on. Therefore, you can see why it would be valuable for us women to take it for the rest of our lives.

In 2001, I had the privilege of hearing Dr. John Lee speak on "Hormone Therapy" at an International Anti-Aging Conference held in Monte Carlo, Monaco. I have always taught and referenced Dr. Lee in my counseling with my customers. He has been "right on target" with his natural approach to menopause and his lecture confirmed how valuable progesterone cream is, and that we can use it for the rest of our lives.

Preventing vaginal dryness—The big V.D.

Years ago when I appeared on a television program with host Jim McClellan, we were talking about the symptoms of menopause. Jim made a comment, "When we come back we'll talk about the big V.D." He then whispered to the TV audience, *"Vaginal dryness."* We all laughed because of the way he said it. Later I received a letter from an older lady who said, "You tell Jim that vaginal dryness is not funny. I have it and it hurts." Indeed, it is not funny at all.

Reduced estrogen levels may cause the mucous membranes of the vagina to change. The vaginal walls begin to lose their elasticity and become drier and thinner. The vaginal secretions and the secretions from the cervix become less acidic, and the risk of vaginal infection increases. The vagina itself shrinks, becoming shorter and narrower. This can cause increased frequency of urination and may result in increased urinary tract infections, and leaking of urine upon coughing, laughing, or sneezing. These changes may result in discomfort during intercourse for some women.

It would be especially important to use the progesterone cream on the vaginal area since proper lubrication is essential. You should also buy a good quality vitamin E oil and apply it to the general area every day. In chapter 5, I discuss vitamin E and vitamin A mixed in jojoba oil, which would also help you. When used externally, vitamin E is excellent for dry skin, burns, wounds, cuts, etc. You could try using an unscented lubricating cream, A & D ointment, or pure Aloe Gel for healing as well.

Years ago we were taught the Kegel exercises which we used in high school to prevent menstrual cramps. This set of exercises is now used to help increase vaginal blood flow and improve muscle tone. Dr. Kegel, a gynecologist who developed these exercises, states they can be done anytime. All you do is imagine that you need to stop urinating, which tightens muscles around the anus, urethra, and vagina. Hold for a few seconds, then relax. Repeated often, this helps strengthen the whole vaginal area.

Remember that antihistamines, diuretics, and cold pills designed to dry up the nasal tissues can also dry other tissues. Avoid douches and even colored or scented toilet paper, which can irritate sensitive vaginal tissue. Also, drink plenty of clean water that can help the dryness and itching.

Conclusion

There is a tremendous amount of information in this chapter to give you many options on how to help you through this time of your life. There are other chapters you should read to give you more information on how to "take charge of your health."

My special prayer for you is that you will be able to sail right through this phase of your life.

Osteoporosis Can Be Prevented and Reversed

Supplements to Help
Rebuild Bone

*Many elderly people who think they have broken a
bone as a result of a fall have actually done just the
opposite; a bone gave way, causing them to fall.
This can and should be prevented.*
—GLADYS LINDBERG

Nearly half of the women between the ages of 45 and 75 show signs of some degree of osteoporosis, and over a third suffer from serious bone deterioration. It was reported that the current National Health Care Cost in this country could be reduced by $16 billion dollars if women would take a supplement of just 1,000 milligrams of calcium a day. This may prevent 25 percent of broken hips! More than one million hip fractures occur in women over the age of only 45, and many older patients die of complications. One's bone density today determines their skeletal strength tomorrow.

It is very common for women to be completely unaware of having osteoporosis. The word osteoporosis is derived from Latin, and means "porous bones." Bones gradually become weaker and weaker, causing changes in posture and making the individual extremely susceptible to chronic lower back pain and bone fractures in this progressive disease. Bone mass, which is the amount of minerals in the bone, reaches its peak with woman between the ages of 30 and 35. After that, it begins to decline. Women must realize that significant bone loss occurs during the 10 to 15 years before menopause. A good percentage of women arrive at menopause with osteoporosis well under way.

Anyone with osteoporosis or disc problems may definitely benefit from following a good vitamin and mineral program containing calcium, magnesium, boron and vitamin D. Studies have shown that over a long period of time, as much as 40 percent of the calcium may be lost from bones before it is confirmed by x-ray. However, as much as 50 percent of a woman's bone loss over a life span is lost before the onset of menopause.

Chronic lower back pain is also one of the first symptoms of osteoporosis. When a person becomes immobilized by the pain of arthritis or back pain, bones quickly lose calcium and other minerals that provide strength. Calcium and magnesium are vital supplements, along with the other trace minerals, especially boron, which help us "hang on" to our calcium, according to a U.S. Department of Agriculture study.

We Can Build Our Bones and Prevent Osteoporosis

This condition is preventable. Recently there has been an incredible push for supplementing calcium in an effort to halt bone loss. We will be reporting some of the information here, because there is a lot of medical evidence. But, while it appears to be sound medical advice, osteoporosis is much more than a lack of dietary calcium. As Mother would always say, "there is no magic bullet in preventing these diseases, it takes a shotgun approach." That is what we are going to discuss, the bullets for the shotgun.

The importance of calcium

The National Institutes of Health and a panel of medical experts announced that most women in the United States are not getting enough calcium in their diets. Their recommendation was from 1,000 to 1,500 mg per day to stem osteoporosis, an affliction of 20 million Americans. Most Americans are getting only a third to a half of the calcium needed for the maintenance of good health.[1]

Our bones and teeth contain about 99 percent of our body's calcium and one percent is circulating in our blood, body fluids, and the soft tissue. Calcium is essential for human life and for the functioning of every cell in our body.[2] There is a complex system designed to keep this calcium in the blood and tissues, no matter what our diet consists of. If our diet becomes low in calcium, to compensate for this lack, the body begins taking calcium from our bones, thinning them and making them brittle in the process. This is the start of osteoporosis or brittle bones that can fracture easily. Our bones are sacrificed for the balance of blood calcium.

Calcium is involved in many activities of the body including blood clotting, cell division, the production of energy and maintenance of immune function. Calcium is crucial for nerve conduction and muscle contractions. It works in our brain, as we all know that a glass of warm milk can have a sedative effect and calm the nerves. Calcium helps to alleviate cramps in the legs and back aches. Many find it helps lower blood pressure and even prevents high blood pressure, and new evidence states that it prevents colon cancer. Severe calcium deficiency may lead to abnormal heartbeat, dementia, muscle spasms and convulsions.

Bone is more than just a collection of calcium crystals. Bone is active, living tissue, like the rest of your body. Although it generally turns over a little more slowly than other tissues, it is continually remodeling itself. Osteoblastic cells (bone forming) build up the framework of bone tissue along with calcium, magnesium, manganese, boron and other minerals, and osteoclastic cells breakdown bone. Like any living tissue, bone has diverse nutritional needs. Failure to meet these needs could presumably compromise the strength and integrity of bone tissue.[3]

When calcium is reabsorbed or removed from bone by the body, new calcium must be deposited in order for your skeleton to remain in a constant state of balance. The control of this process of bone breakdown and bone reformation is one of the most complex areas of human biochemistry. There is perhaps no more sensitive a regulator of cellular activity than the calcium ion. It is so sensitive that even a slight change in its concentration can cause a biologic event, such as a heartbeat, to occur, or maybe not occur. This all requires very fine regulations, for if the calcium ion in the cells exceeds certain levels, those cells can be destroyed. Magnesium appears to be the prime regulator of calcium flow within cells. It is this delicate collaboration that may well be the major determinant of the rate at which the cellular flame burns.[4]

Bone consists of a complex mineral called *hydroxyapatite*, which is made up of calcium and phosphorous. Your body cannot manufacture calcium and phosphorous; these minerals can only be obtained through your foods or supplements. Calcium is poorly absorbed from the diet and needs to be transported into the blood from the intestinal tract by way of specific calcium-binding proteins that are stimulated by vitamin D. One can get vitamin D either directly from the diet or manufactured in the skin when exposed to natural sunlight. Once calcium is in the bloodstream, it is deposited in the bone by the control of a hormone released by the thyroid gland called *calcitonin*. The *parathyroid hormone*, secreted by the parathyroid gland, controls calcium resorption from bones. When these processes are in balance, your skeleton is neither growing nor diminishing, your bone density is staying constant. When the resorption process exceeds the depositing, however, you are now losing bone and over time will slowly, progressively have weaker bones which are more susceptible to spontaneous fracture.[5]

In five years we can have new bones

Each year 20 percent of the minerals in your bones leave your system. They can actually be urinated away. In five years you have a complete calcium turnover. Bone loss of smokers after menopause occurs 50 percent faster. Excessive coffee drinking interferes with calcium absorption causing an additional increase in bone loss. Drugs such as aspirin, tetracycline, diuretics, aluminum containing antacids interfere with absorption and availability of calcium.

Tums and other antacids neutralize the acid in the stomach, making it difficult to absorb calcium and other minerals. Isn't it amazing that Tums are recommended as a source of calcium because they contain calcium carbonate, with no thought of the assimilation. The hydrochloric acid our stomach naturally produces helps with calcium absorption, and the antacids block absorption. As reported in the *Lancet*, one thousand men and women had less hip fractures when taking calcium with added hydrochloric acid (HCl).[6]

Reporting in the *Journal of Clinical Nutrition,* the authors concluded that normal postmenopausal women within ten years of menopause whose calcium intake was below 1,000 mg, and who increased the amount to 1,400 mg, reduced the rate of bone loss.[7]

Other studies shown anywhere from 1,000 to 2,500 mg of calcium daily was needed to reduced the incidence of vertebrae fractures by 50 percent.[8]

With that amount of calcium they experienced only a 50 percent improvement, but if magnesium, vitamin D and the mineral boron plus hydrochloric acid had been added to this research program, I'd wager the improvement would have been much greater. The average American woman consumes only 450 to 550 mg of calcium each day. This is below the daily minimum requirement.

It's never too late to prevent hip fractures

Some 200,000 people are hospitalized each year for hip fractures alone. Half of the women who suffer hip fractures are unable to resume independent existence, with one-forth of them requiring continuous care in nursing institutions. About 10 percent of these women will die within the first year following the fracture from the complications. Our government is finally realizing the importance of prevention, and their answer is just 1,000 mg of calcium.[9] This sounds like an easy answer but of course there is more to it.

As we age, we have increasing difficulty absorbing calcium from our intestines. Our body begins leaching calcium from our bones, thinning them and making them brittle.

In a 1992 study reported in the *New England Journal of Medicine,* French researchers stated that, among the women who completed the 18-month study, the number of hip fractures was 43 percent lower and the total number of nonvertebral fractures was 32 percent lower in the volunteers who were given vitamin D and calcium, compared with those receiving a placebo. Their ages ranged from 69 to 106, and they lived in nursing homes or apartment houses.[10] To be accepted for the study, the women had to be ambulatory, that is, they could walk about with the aid of a cane or a walker, and they had no serious medical problems.

In the supplemented women, it was noted that calcium and vitamin D supplementation increased cortical bone density. This is not surprising, as I pointed out that bone is living tissue and is constantly undergoing changes.

The researchers concluded that, "18 months of daily supplementation with 1,200 mg of elemental calcium and 800 IU of vitamin D3 was safe and decreased the incidence of hip fractures and other nonvertebral fractures among elderly women. As these results demonstrate, it may never be too late to prevent hip fractures."[11]

One of the preventable deformities we all want to avoid is getting a *dowager hump*, the hump that develops at the base of the neck on top of the shoulders. Again, this problem may be one of calcium being stripped out of the bones, causing height loss and the resulting hump. Recent studies indicate that at least 26 percent of all women over 60 have osteoporosis severe enough to cause deformity, height loss and pain.[12]

What is causing this bone loss?

Some of the reported reasons for bone loss are stringent, weight-reducing diets which may induce loss of bone as well as soft tissue; calcium losses during pregnancies not compensated for adequately by prescribed prenatal supplements (especially in women with pre-pregnancy calcium deficiencies); failure of mothers who breast feed their babies to continue calcium supplements; and calcium and bone losses associated with hormonal changes in menopause and a high-phosphorous diet, which includes a lot of soft drinks.[13]

Other factors that contribute to bone loss in the elderly are: physical inactivity; abstaining from dairy products, especially milk; decreased exposure to sunlight; increased dependency upon highly processed foods which are low in calcium and high in phosphorous; a diet high in refined sugars. Many authorities believe that both osteo-porosis and arthritis could be avoided if proper diet and supplementation were followed.[14] Another factor is changing hormone levels (decreased estrogen) that comes with aging.

Symptoms to look for

If bone loss is occurring, look for a few of these signs: nighttime leg cramps; heavy plaque or calculus formation around the teeth; pyorrhea, which allows the support structure to degenerate and the gums recede and teeth look longer and may start to loosen. A tendency toward kidney stone formation and osteoarthritic changes in the joints that lead to pain and tenderness and low back pain are also involved. As people become older, they tend to have less minerals responsible for bone re-formation. They also have lower levels of hydrochloric acid in their stomach so assimilation becomes an essential factor.[15]

Periodontal disease: One of the first signs of osteoporosis

Dentists are usually the first to recognize the beginnings of osteo-porosis, as it initially appears in the jawbone. It actually looks like your teeth are growing (getting longer). Check your dental x-rays and discuss how the structure around your teeth looks with your dentist.

Bone loss from the jaw produces pockets around your teeth, promoting bacterial infection. The result is periodontal disease, called pyorrhea. It may begin at an early age and progresses for many years before teeth are loosened and finally lost.[16]

Nearly 80 percent of Americans have some degree of periodontal disease, and half have lost teeth to this disease by the age of 60. Periodontal disease is influenced by many other factors, but the loss of jawbone and tooth loss are associated with calcium and mineral defi-ciency or imbalance in other areas of the body.[17]

Understanding the Calcium/Phosphorous Ratio

The levels of calcium and phosphorous in the diet play a big role in controlling bone loss. As the diet becomes higher in phosphorous and lower in calcium, it encourages bone breakdown and calcium loss from bones. The reason for this is that phosphorous stimulates the secretion of parathyroid hormone which increases calcium resorption, whereas dietary calcium increases the secretion of calcitonin which causes bone reformation.[18]

For the calcium in your body to be effectively utilized, you ideally need to take in equal amounts of calcium and phosphorous. If the diet is equal in calcium and phosphorous, the blood calcium will be two and a half times higher than phosphorous, which is optimal. The normal blood test analysis should read Calcium 10, Phosphorous 4. It is interesting to note that mother's milk is also two and a half times higher in calcium than phosphorous (the same as our blood calcium ratio), another important reason for breast-feeding a baby.

Why should we be concerned about all this? Because the average American diet, including many of the foods nutritionists recommend, is very high in phosphorous in proportion to calcium. This chart should inspire you to take a calcium supplement, especially without phosphorous added.

CALCIUM/PHOSPHORUS RATIO
FOR COMMON FOODS

An example of the calcium-phosphorous ratios in 100 grams or a little less than half a cup, would be:

rice bran	76 mg cal—1386 mg phos
wheat bran	119 mg cal—1276 mg phos
wheat germ	72 mg cal—1118 mg phos
flour—100% wheat	45 mg cal—423 mg phos
beef or most red meat	11 mg cal—207 mg phos
cottage cheese	94 mg cal—152 mg phos
oatmeal/rolled oats cooked	21 mg cal—138 mg phos
cracked wheat bread	88 mg cal—128 mg phos
rice-cooked brown	18 mg cal—110 mg phos
milk-whole, nonfat	118 mg cal—93 mg phos
blackstrap molasses	684 mg cal—84 mg phos
dark greens: broccoli, mustard, kale, collard, watercress	184 mg cal—37 mg phos

(U.S. Government Composition of Foods Handbook.)
One hundred grams is the unit of measure for each food listed
(28 grams=one ounce, so 100 grams is a little less than half a cup).[19]

The use of phosphate food additives (a binding agent that stops microbe growth), should be carefully controlled in our food supply because they can lead to net calcium loss. Be sure you read labels of processed foods because words like *pyrophosphate*, *polyphosphate*, *sodium phosphate*, *phosphoric acid* and others increase our dietary intake of phosphorous with no balancing of calcium.

Soft drinks use phosphorous to reduce the acidity that would actually dissolve our teeth. One average 8 oz can contains 136 mg of phosphorous, with no calcium. This adds up fast, especially if you are "super sizing" your order and consuming 62 or 84 oz of soda! We can begin to see reasons for wide spread calcium deficiencies.

Remember, your intake of the two nutrients should be approximately equal. If you don't have enough calcium in your diet, or if you have too much phosphorous, your body will actually pull calcium right out of your bones and teeth. There are many misleading articles that say people who eat meat will get osteoporosis. They do not explain that meat is high in phosphorous, so you need to balance the calcium. But what about those people who consume a lot of wheat or rice bran? It is like pulling the calcium out of your bones.[20]

The changes in our dietary habits during the last 50 years have brought with it profound changes in our skeletal system. The use of processed foods, the extremely high consumption of carbonated beverages, the excessive use of beef which is not balanced with fish or chicken, and almost the elimination of dairy products and milk—one of our richest sources of calcium—have gotten us in trouble. The calcium-phosphorous ratio in the blood must stay constant, even at the expense of your bones.

Magnesium—The Amazing Mineral

All human cells contain magnesium, totaling about 25,000 mg in an adult. About 60 to 70 percent of the body's magnesium is found in the bones, the rest is located in the soft tissues and blood. It plays a role in the prevention and treatment of osteoporosis. Magnesium is necessary for efficient calcium utilization. To balance this mineral, you should take twice as much calcium as magnesium, approximately 2:1. Some authorities feel this ratio should be equal 1:1. Alcohol causes a very high urinary loss of magnesium. The more protein you eat, the more magnesium you need.[21]

One of the important functions of magnesium is it is necessary for the contraction of the muscles and is considered a key element in the regulation of the heartbeat. As a nerve soother, magnesium is necessary for the sending of nerve impulses, for normal brain function, and for sleeping.[22]

Deficiencies of magnesium

When you see the symptoms of magnesium deficiencies you can see the emotional and physical ramifications of this mineral. The first symptoms are usually apathy, depression, apprehensiveness, confusion, disorientation, vertigo (a condition in which the room seems to spin around), muscular weakness and twitching, and over-excitability of the nervous system, which may lead to muscle spasms or cramps. Other possible symptoms of magnesium deficiency may include insomnia, jumpiness, sensitivity to noise, irritability, and a poor memory.[23] More serious deficiencies result in tremors and convulsions. So many of these symptoms sound like menopause, PMS, psychological problems, and just plain aging.[24]

Magnesium protects against the accumulation of calcium deposits in the urinary tract. Such deposits may otherwise lead to bladder or kidney stones. Magnesium seems to be important in controlling the manner in which electrical charges are utilized to induce the passage of minerals in and out of cells. It may be associated with the regulation of body temperature.[25] Could this include hot flashes?

It is magnesium, not calcium, that forms the kind of hard tooth enamel that resists decay.[26]

The following list offers the approximate percentages of magnesium that Dr. Lewis E. Barnet found in various bone materials. These percentages reveal the vital role magnesium plays in bone hardness.

☙	Bones of patients with osteoporosis	.62 %
☙	Bones of healthy people	1.26 %
☙	Teeth of healthy people	1.50 %
☙	Elephant tusks (from which almost indestructible billiard balls are made)	2.00 %
☙	Teeth of carnivorous animals (which crush and grind the bones of their prey)	5.00 %[27]

Vitamin D

It is one of the most important regulators of calcium. It enhances intestinal calcium absorption in the intestine and decreases the excretion of calcium in the kidneys, thereby contributing to a favorable calcium balance.

Those who lack adequate exposure to the sun's ultraviolet rays do not get the sterols within the skin converted into vitamin D. Therefore, many of us must obtain our vitamin D from foods, including vitamin D-fortified dairy products, fish, eggs, and liver. Also, of course include vitamin D supplements. The RDA is 200 IU, but many authorities feel this is too low and it should be increased to 400 IU to 800 IU.

In a 1997 study published in the *New England Journal of Medicine*, researchers evaluated the effect of calcium and vitamin D on bone density in both men and women sixty-five years old or older. After three years, the people who took 700 IU of vitamin D and only 500 mg of calcium every day had significant increases in bone density. In general, 400 IU to 800 IU is considered effective, and dosages exceeding over 1,000 IU may not impart any greater benefit.

Boron—an exciting trace mineral

There were headlines in the *Chemical Marketing Reporter*, "Boron Found to Have Role in Hardening Bones." It was repeated in several others like *Business Week*, "A New Recruit in the Battle Against Bone Loss."[28]

Boron apparently plays an important role in hardening bones. US Department of Agriculture scientists reported, this trace mineral has been found to reduce excretion of the minerals calcium, magnesium and phosphorous, which are necessary to keep bones hard. It also increases blood levels of active forms of estrogen and testosterone, steroid hormones thought to be important for maintaining calcium levels and healthy bones.

A six-month study points up the possible new role for boron in preventing osteoporosis, says nutritionist Forrest H. Nielsen and anatomist Curtis D. Hunt of USDA's Agricultural Research Service. During the study, the researchers were using just 3 milligrams of boron and within eight days, the scientists discovered they lost 40 percent less calcium, one-third less magnesium, and slightly less phosphorous through the urine. The women's calcium and magnesium losses were lower than pre-study levels when they were on a normal diet.[29]

Mr. Hunt said, "These elements are important in maintaining the integrity of the bone. Boron had a remarkable effect on indicators that the body was conserving calcium or preventing bone demineralization, but we really became excited when we saw its effect on steroid hormones." Blood levels of the most active form of estrogen—estradiol 17B—doubled to "levels found in women on estrogen replacement therapy," he said. They were also higher than pre-study levels. The blood levels of testosterone—the precursor of estradiol—more than doubled.

Mr. Hunt said he suspects that the body needs boron to synthesize estrogen, vitamin D and other steroid hormones, and it may also protect these hormones against rapid breakdown.[30]

Additional studies confirm that boron enhances and mimics some effects of estrogen ingestion in postmenopausal women.[31]

Boron is hard to get in our foods because excessive use of soluble chemical fertilizers has damaged the soil, and low concentrations of minerals affect several aspects of mineral metabolism. Levels of boron in this country have dropped considerably in the last 50 years.[32]

RECOMMENDED DOSAGE. Most adults would benefit with 3 mg daily to help increase the absorption of calcium. Excellent sources of boron include alfalfa and kelp (also high in silicon), spinach, snap beans, cabbage, leafy vegetables, legumes, apples, pears and grapes.[33] Also take calcium, magnesium, vitamin D3, zinc, manganese, copper and betaine hydrochloric acid.

Ipriflavone: The New Bone Builder

This is a newer dietary nutrient that has been shown in clinical studies to result in greater bone mineral density and inhibit bone loss in individuals that have experienced a loss in bone mass. Like other isoflavones (plant phytoestrogens), the chemical structure of ipriflavone resembles that of estrogen, likely explaining why it mimics the hormone in certain ways.

Despite its ability to augment the activity of naturally occurring or administered estrogens, ipriflavone does not appear to have any classical "estrogenic" effects such as stimulating breast or uterine tissue growth.[34]

Carl Germano, R.D., C.N.S., L.D.N., in his book, *The Osteoporosis Solution* states, "Ipriflavone seems to be the best bet yet for preventing and treating osteoporosis. Estrogen and other drugs may be effective, but who wants to take on the risk of cancer and other serious side effects? Ipriflavone is a safe and effective alternative to prescription drugs. Used in conjunction with diet, exercise, and lifestyle changes, and other supplements, ipriflavone is one of the most important elements in a comprehensive prevention and treatment plan for osteoporosis."[35]

Several studies suggest that ipriflavone and its metabolites exert their osteoprotective effects in a similar manner, by inhibiting bone resorption.[36] Ipriflavone's ability to reduce bone loss is the estrogen-like effect researchers find most intriguing. Estrogens inhibit bone-degrading osteoclast activity, a process also called bone resorption. Several studies suggest that ipriflavone and its metabolites exert their osteo-protective effects in a similar manner—by inhibiting bone resorption.[37]

Research also indicates that ipriflavone may help prevent high blood cholesterol associated with estrogen deficiency, reduce bone pain and increase immunity. It may even prove helpful to older men who also are at risk of osteoporosis. Before such claims can be substantiated, however more clinical trials must be conducted.[38]

Ostivone is one of the brand names for ipriflavone that has been the subject of over 60 extensive clinical studies conducted by doctors internationally. Over 2,700 individuals have participated in these controlled trials. The recommended dose is two, 300 mg capsules a day (total 600 mg) to be taken with at least 1,000 mg of calcium. This was the recommend dosage used in the clinical studies. You will find several brands at your nutrition store.

Ostivone is the product promoted by the famous actress, Linda Evans, who spoke at the Natural Products Expo in Anaheim, California, which I attended. You can read more about Linda's testimony and how my Mother, Gladys Lindberg, helped her regain her health in chapter 1.

Progesterone Builds Bones and Prevents Osteoporosis

A growing body of evidence indicates that progesterone is a powerful bone-building hormone and that progesterone replacement therapy could be the next major advance in the battle against osteoporosis.

Jerilynn C. Prior, M.D., of the Division of Endocrinology and Metabolism, University of British Columbia in Vancouver, has written a comprehensive review of the evidence that progesterone stimulates bone formation. It was found that progesterone binds to osteoblast cells, which build new bone. This research suggests that progesterone acts directly on osteoblasts and may promote bone formation.[39]

According to John Lee, M.D., a lack of progesterone causes a decrease in new bone formation. Adding natural progesterone will actively increase bone mass and density and can reverse osteoporosis.[40]

Make sure you read all of this important research in the *Young Women's* and the *Menopause* chapters. They both go into great detail on the value of progesterone and how the cream can be used topically.

DHEA: The Who's Who in Osteoporosis Prevention

Alan Gaby, M.D., author of *Preventing and Reversing Osteoporosis*, explains that DHEA reads like the "who's who in osteoporosis prevention." DHEA functions as a precursor hormone that plays a role in bone loss. Preliminary results suggest DHEA is the only hormone that appears capable of both inhibiting bone loss and stimulating bone formation.[41] Dr. Regelson has shown that DHEA is an estrogen precursor, which means that DHEA is converted to estrogen in the body. Supplementing with DHEA in postmenopausal women appears to be a way to increase estrogen naturally.[42]

The Importance of Exercise

Exercise is one of the most important things we can do to keep our bones strong. You must do weight-bearing exercises. There is something about the gravity of weight that must occur. So, make certain that you get up and move around, walk, run, lift weights or bike ride! What ever we do, we need to keep moving.

Walking 20 to 30 minutes a day at least three times a week, getting your heart rate up to 60 to 70 percent of your maximum heart rate, is excellent. The maximum heart rate can be calculated by subtracting your age from 220. Since it's easy and doesn't require expensive clothes or gear, walking is an exercise you will most likely stick with.

Exercise improves the quality of life, enhances blood circulation and permits greater food intake, thus increasing each cell's nourishment while helping to prevent obesity. Exercise enables your body to maintain a vital reserve, which has a protective effect during stress. At a three-day conference on aging and the role of exercise in prevention of physical decline, researchers offered incontrovertible evidence that physical activity can retard factors that have always been considered the inevitable consequences of the aging process. *They emphasized that the body is the one machine that breaks down when it is not used; in fact it works better the more it is used.*[43] *Just Do It!*

Let's Put It All Together

The Complete Lindberg Nutrition Program

You must learn how to "take charge of your own health" because nobody is going to do it for you! This nutrition program will pay great dividends for the rest of your healthy life.

—GLADYS LINDBERG

*T*his chapter represents a comprehensive, balanced program incorporating the latest scientific and nutritional information. It has truly stood the test of time. I recommend it to you today as a program originated by my Mother, Gladys Lindberg, one of the true pioneers of applied nutrition. It is a beginning point from which to develop your own personal nutritional program to stay on for the rest of your life. Remember, it is never too late to get started. Let's make today your first day toward more vibrant health!

The *Lindberg Nutrition Program* emphasizes the value of protein-rich foods, fresh fruit and vegetables (organic if possible), the essential fatty acids, and complex carbohydrates that are natural and without man-made additives. This program is not a diet, per se, but rather a program designed for better overall nutrition so that you can enjoy vibrant health the rest of your life.

Many people who come into our store bring with them a long list of health problems and symptoms. Nearly always, their list includes feeling run down, irritable, and exhausted. They complain of having no energy. You probably have a list, too!

I recently received a wonderful letter from one of our customers. She came to our home with her mother, before we opened our first store in 1949. She has been on the Lindberg Nutrition Program, taking our famous vitamin and mineral packs, the protein shakes, and our other supplements for well over 50 years. Her handwriting was beautiful, not the least bit shaky. She lives alone, takes care of herself and amazingly, still drives her own car. I could hardly believe it when she wrote that she was 97 years old! I just had to call her and amazingly, she is very sharp and alert! Pauline is a great example that our program works! She is just one of the many, many people I hear from that have been on the Lindberg Nutrition program for twenty, thirty, even fifty years!

This program is designed to help you eat right and stresses the value of taking nutritional supplements to build sound health. It emphasizes the importance of proper digestion, assimilation, regular elimination, the need for sound rest at night, and adopting a positive mental attitude!

Understanding Hypoglycemia

Many years ago Mother counseled with individuals suffering from what was later classified as hypoglycemia. Hearing their complaints and learning of their dietary habits, she was prompted to study the problem. Mother found an original paper on the discovery of low blood sugar and its symptoms, published in the *Journal of the American Medical Association* in 1934 by Seal Harris, M.D., professor of medicine at the University of Alabama.[1] He wrote that a person whose blood sugar drops rapidly is suffering from hypoglycemia, meaning "below normal blood sugar." Dr. Harris was a pioneer in the treatment of diabetes and in the recognition of low blood sugar as a disease entity. He wrote that, "the hypoglycemic of today is the diabetic of tomorrow." Mother agreed and reached the same conclusion that there was too much sugar and devitalized, refined carbohydrates (white rice, white flour products, white sugar) in their diets...and she was correct.

Hypoglycemia is not an incurable or even a debilitating disease, but a problem of epidemic proportions nevertheless. It is a metabolic dysfunction related to sugar intake.

In the form of glucose, sugar is a normal and necessary blood constituent. The body converts it from carbohydrates, protein, fats, and sugar into energy. Maintaining the proper level of sugar in your blood is crucial for the efficient operation of the body. The right level is moderated by insulin, a hormone produced in the pancreas, which takes extra sugar out of the blood and stores it (in the form of glycogen) in the liver and muscles. Then, when additional energy is needed, adrenaline releases this stored glycogen back into the blood.

Protein is the best nutrient to eat in order to maintain an even blood sugar level, because it is metabolized over a long period of time. An impressive 58 percent of protein can be converted to glucose if need be. Carbohydrates, on the other hand—particularly refined carbohydrates which contain sugar such as cake, cookies, soft drinks, ice cream or white flour products—are quickly metabolized, causing a rapid rise in blood sugar level. When refined sugar enters the bloodstream, insulin must flood to the rescue to keep the glucose at its proper level.

Both of these extreme conditions can develop from *overconsumption of sugar.* When the pancreas is constantly bombarded by requests for insulin, it can become desensitized and respond with too much or too little insulin. Too little insulin results in diabetes. In the case of too much insulin (too much sugar gets stored in the liver) you're likely to feel tired. To feel energetic your body must produce adrenaline which stimulates the adrenal cortex to manufacture cortisone that can call the sugar back out of storage in the liver. But if the adrenal glands have been overtaxed by stress and stimulants, they too may become desensitized and fail to produce adequate adrenaline.

What stimulates the adrenal glands?

They are stimulated when anything toxic enters the body. Fear, worry, anxiety, coffee, caffeine, nicotine, alcohol, drugs and medications, stimulate the production of adrenaline, which triggers the alarm reaction in the body. This alarm reaction stimulates the central nervous system through the thalamus and the hypothalamus to the pituitary gland, which manufactures a hormone called ACTH. The ACTH works on the outside core (adrenal cortex) of the adrenal gland to produce cortisone and about 55 other hormones.

Cortisone raises the blood sugar by pulling glycogen out of the liver, calcium out of the bones, and protein out of the muscles. In effect you "cannibalize" yourself. When this alarm reaction becomes exhausted by years of overuse and runs out of material to make cortical hormones, then we may suffer from arthritis, asthma, and other degenerative conditions.[2]

What causes hypoglycemia?

The hypoglycemic's problem can be caused by inborn errors of metabolism (babies can be born with exhausted adrenals); acquired as a result of overindulgence in refined carbohydrates, alcohol, stimulants, and drugs; or may be triggered by stresses that exhaust the adrenal glands. In addition, the physical problems have psychological manifestations.

The problem has not changed through the years. Almost everyone I counsel with shows several symptoms commonly associated with low blood sugar.

Our friend, Dr. Carlton Fredericks, described a doctor's experience in his book *Psycho-Nutrition*. "His symptoms were so multiple that Dr. Stephen Gyland vainly visited fourteen specialists and three diagnostic centers, including Mayo Clinic, in a effort to find an explanation for the blackouts which had already involved him in two automobile accidents, and for his nervousness, fatigue, irritability and difficulties in concentration. He emerged from the seventeen diagnostic consultations with a number of verdicts: he was constitutionally inadequate, too frail to stand the stresses of practicing medicine; he was a neurotic; he had (Mayo Clinic said) a brain tumor; his blood vessels were occluded, and circulation to the brain was impaired."

"He finally arrived at a correct diagnosis, which he made himself, after reading and acting upon Dr. Seal Harris' paper on hypoglycemia (the same paper Mother had read). When a simple change in Dr. Gyland's diet had wiped out his symptoms, he went back into medicine and began to specialize in hypoglycemia, treating more than a thousand patients with the disorder."[3]

Is it any wonder that low blood sugar is considered by many doctors and nutritionists to be one of the most difficult and thought-provoking problems known? It has been nicknamed "the great impersonator." And no wonder, since its symptoms include just about every imaginable complaint.

Hypoglycemic symptoms are so multiple that Dr. Gyland, a recovered victim of low blood sugar, treated 1,100 patients and compiled a long list of symptoms, along with the percentages of his hypoglycemic patients in which each of the symptoms occurred.

The chart below shows Dr. Stephen Gyland's list.[4]

HYPOGLYCEMIA SYMPTOMS

Symptom	Percentage
❏ Nervousness	94
❏ Irritability	89
❏ Exhaustion	87
❏ Faintness, dizziness, tremor, cold sweats, and/or weak spells	86
❏ Depression	77
❏ Vertigo, dizziness	73
❏ Drowsiness	72
❏ Headaches	71
❏ Digestive disturbances	69
❏ Forgetfulness	67
❏ Insomnia	62
❏ Constant worrying, unprovoked anxieties	62
❏ Mental confusion	57
❏ Internal trembling	57
❏ Palpitation of heart and/or rapid pulse	54

- ❏ Muscle pains   53
- ❏ Numbness   51
- ❏ Indecisiveness   50
- ❏ Unsocial, asocial, or antisocial behavior   47
- ❏ Crying spells   46
- ❏ Lack of sex drive in females   44
- ❏ Allergies   43
- ❏ Lack of coordination   43
- ❏ Leg cramps   43
- ❏ Lack of concentration   42
- ❏ Blurred vision   40
- ❏ Twitching and jerking of muscles   40
- ❏ Itching and crawling sensations
  of the skin   39
- ❏ Gasping for breath   37
- ❏ Smothering spells   34
- ❏ Staggering   34
- ❏ Sighing and yawning   30
- ❏ Impotence in males   29
- ❏ Unconsciousness   27
- ❏ Night terrors, nightmares   27
- ❏ Rheumatoid arthritis   24
- ❏ Phobias, fears   23
- ❏ Neurodermatitis   21
- ❏ Suicidal intent   20*
- ❏ Nervous breakdown   17
- ❏ Convulsions   2

***Suicidal Intent:** *A disorder in which 220 patients out of 1,100 were thinking about suicide.*

Now, go back through this list and put a check mark next to any symptoms you may have.

Notice that nervousness, irritability, and exhaustion tend to be the most common symptoms. It is alarming how many symptoms are primarily mental: depression, forgetfulness, constant worrying, unprovoked anxieties, mental confusion, even suicidal intent, to name a few. Not only do you feel run down, but mentally you fall apart. We must always keep in mind that we cannot "separate" our minds from our bodies. They are part of the same chemical system!

A glucose tolerance test will reveal if a person's problems are due to low blood sugar. The test must be administered by a physician specially trained to interpret the glucose tolerance curve. It is a long procedure that takes five to six hours. For this test to be accurate, the blood should be drawn and analyzed every half hour, which frightens some people, although some of the trauma can be alleviated by a machine that tests the blood by a prick of the finger. I do not recommend you go through this procedure unless your symptoms are severe. It is unnatural to take the large glass of sugar syrup—100 grams of glucose—which is required.[5] I feel that if you have these symptoms of low blood sugar, you can assume you have it and change your diet. However, ask your physician and follow his advice.

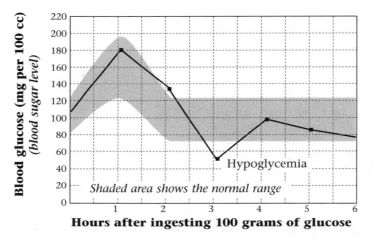

Typical hypoglycemic curve. This curve is almost normal, except for at the three hour mark, where the blood sugar level drops sharply to about 55. This is the point at which the symptoms of hypoglycemia occur, and the body loses sodium, glucose, and oxygen.

What Happens When Blood Sugar Level (Glucose) Falls?

Your blood sugar drops when the adrenal glands become exhausted. They run out of the material needed to make the cortical hormones that prevent this from happening.

A "normal" range is often cited as from 80 to 120 mg per 100 cc (cubic centimeter). During active periods of the day, however, our blood sugar level is actually about 140 on the same scale.

When your blood sugar falls to 60 or 70 milligrams, your symptoms are comparatively mild and may consist of slight headaches, faintness, muscular weakness, hunger, irritability, and perhaps a feeling of nervousness or tension. If it falls still lower, the symptoms become more severe including headaches (even migraines), dizziness, fatigue, sweating, tremors, heart palpitations, marked irritability, and general nervousness. If your blood sugar continues to fall to 40 milligrams or lower, you can experience palpitations of the heart (a feeble but rapid pulse), and pallor will be more pronounced, until unconsciousness and convulsions occur.

Calcium drops.

Not only does your blood sugar level drop as your adrenals become exhausted, but the amount of calcium in the blood is affected as well. When the adrenals are stimulated by stress, drugs, other stimulants and low blood sugar, they go into high gear and pull calcium out of your bones. The big muscles at the sides of your neck and head go into contractions, fluid gathers in the brain, and you may feel as if the top of your head is going to come off. You might feel shaky and tremble inside, or have "restless legs" and back aches.

Oxygen decreases.

When your blood sugar level drops, so does your supply of oxygen. You yawn (gasping for oxygen). You cannot concentrate. You doze off at meetings and find it hard to stay alert. Your blood carries oxygen to every cell in your body. Glucose is almost the only fuel used by the brain and central nervous system. The combination of glucose with oxygen keeps the brain functioning. A drop of glucose in the blood stream will cause profound mental changes, according to Broda Barnes, M.D.[6]

Salt is lost.

When blood glucose drops, salt is lost in the urine. It is salt that keeps the plasma in the blood vessels. When this salt is lost, the plasma becomes thinner and enters tissues it should not enter. Here is Mother's classic way of describing these conditions:

> When fluid goes into the brain, the condition is called a migraine headache...When the fluid goes into the eyes, the condition is called glaucoma...when the fluid goes into the nose, you have a stuffy nose and the condition is called hay fever, sinus problems, post-nasal drip, or allergies...when the fluid goes into the middle ear, the

condition is called Meniere's syndrome, and you experience ringing and noises in the ear, loss of hearing, and dizziness...when the fluid goes into the lungs, the condition is called asthma.

Such conditions as these may respond to a half-teaspoon each of salt and baking soda in an eight-ounce glass of warm water. You might want to add a teaspoon of honey. I suggest you use "iodized" sea salt which is made from evaporated sea water. This salt and soda mixture raises not only the sodium, but also your blood sugar level. It brings the adrenals out of shock and stimulates the thymus, which in turn will stimulate the tonsils, adenoids, and lymph glands and make antibodies. A child who suffers from asthma attacks in the early morning may find relief by taking the salt and soda drink before taking other measures. Giving the child some protein food a half hour later should help keep the blood sugar level up.

Your Lowest Ebb

If you have low blood sugar problems, your lowest ebb will probably be at three or four o'clock in the morning. Some people wake up at these times and cannot go back to sleep. The usual hypoglycemia symptoms are often compounded at night by irrational fears and nightmares. If this has been happening to you, then you might want to take a protein shake before you go to bed at night. Do the same when you wake up.

This early morning low ebb can actually become very serious. When the blood sugar, blood calcium, and blood oxygen levels drop, you may experience palpitations of the heart, rapid pulse, muscle pains, and numbness (go back over the list). If you start to think this is a heart attack and fear sets in, then adrenaline may flood into the body and the heart could begin to pound harder still. A blood vessel can spring a leak as a result, causing a thrombosis (a blood clot within the vessel). If this condition progresses, it may even cause a heart attack. A small feeding of protein or a protein shake before you go to bed could help maintain your blood sugar level throughout the night. The statement, "don't eat before you go to bed," is wrong in my opinion, especially for older people who don't eat very much. But do not eat ice cream, cake or cookies...eat protein. If you are waking up in the middle of the night, it shows you need this extra feeding. These feedings also help keep your adrenals healthy and the pancreas functioning properly. Make sure your diet is low in refined carbohydrates and sugars, and your lifestyle free of unnecessary stimulants. This same low ebb can be at three or four in the afternoon. That is why I suggest a mid-afternoon protein feeding.

Hypoglycemia in Children

Children who overeat, or who do not want to eat at all, are likely hypo-glycemics. They may have impaired memory, so when they state that they did not say or do something, they probably don't remember what they did. Low blood sugar children frequently have trouble learning, or they may fail in a particular subject. You will often find that the class in which the child is failing occurs around ten or eleven o'clock in the morning. Such a child may be mischievous and restless. However, children manifest different symptoms—another child might be consid-ered lazy and show signs of mental fatigue, dullness, indifference, lack of initiative, and a severe inability to make decisions.[7]

It may come as a surprise that low blood sugar problems can be far more serious for children than for adults. My friend's child suffered from severe headaches that regularly awoke her at night. After being misdiagnosed as having a brain tumor, I described the symptoms of low blood sugar and she changed her daughter's diet. This change of diet (eliminating refined sugar and refined carbohydrates) and a protein drink before bed and another one around midnight relieved her of these headaches and allowed her to sleep peacefully. As long as the program was followed, she never had another headache.

Diabetes: The Refined Carbohydrate Disease

I have spoken several times to the Diabetic Support Group at the Torrance Memorial Hospital in Torrance, CA. In attendance were people who wanted to be informed and learn new ways to improve their diabetic condition.

According to figures published by the American Diabetes Association (ADA), 15.7 million people in America now have diabetes. This disease is the sixth leading cause of death in America. If diabetes is not properly controlled, it can lead to damaged blood vessels, which in turn, may cause eye disease, heart disease, peripheral and autonomic neuropathy (nerve damage in the limbs and internal organs), and diabetic nephropathy (kidney disease).[8]

Diabetes is divided into two major categories: Type I (insulin dependent diabetes mellitus) and Type II (non-insulin dependent diabetes mellitus). Ninety percent of diabetics are Type II and are not dependent upon insulin. Although genetic factors appear important in susceptibility to diabetes, environmental factors are required to trigger it. Obesity is another significant environmental factor, as 90 percent of diabetics are obese. This excessive weight, particularly in the abdominal area, is part and parcel of Type II diabetes. When you see people carrying excessive weight and a protruding stomach, their chance of being diabetic is great, but they may not know it.

In Type II diabetes, the pancreas does not produce enough insulin to fuel the cells. The cells may also become resistant to the effects of what little insulin there is in the bloodstream. The classic symptoms of Type II diabetes are frequent urination, excessive thirst, excessive appetite and obesity. Because these symptoms are not deemed serious, many people may actually have this type of diabetes, and don't know it. They therefore do not seek medical care.

The nutritional needs are high.

The dietary requirements of a diabetic are undoubtedly many times greater than those of a healthy individual. In the 1950's Dr. Walter Mertz, of the U.S. Department of Agriculture, isolated a substance secreted from the liver that allows body cells to process insulin. He termed this substance the glucose tolerance factor (GTF). Since the GTF is involved somehow in the entry of glucose into the cells from the blood, its absence can cause diabetes. According to Dr. Jeffrey Bland in *Your Health Under Seige*, "The glucose tolerance factor has been found to depend upon the essential trace mineral chromium. And chromium is a mineral that is easily lost in the milling of grains and the processing of foods and may be commonly deficient in the 'average, well-nourished' American."

Chromium picolinate

The mineral chromium helps to increase the efficiency of insulin, the hormone that controls blood glucose (blood sugar) levels. Picolinate is an amino acid derivative that allows the body to use chromium much more readily. When chromium is combined with picolinate, a truly effective means of providing supplemental chromium is developed. Through a complex chemical process, once chromium and picolinate are joined together, the body's cells are then able to accept the chromium.

I find the addition of chromium picolinate supplements valuable for all diabetics. Its effect on insulin requirements are very real. Blood sugar levels must be monitored carefully and the appropriate dosages of insulin and/or other drugs adjusted as needed in response. So watch your insulin levels as chromium picolinate may do its job and stabilize your blood sugar level. Suggested dosage is 400-600 mcg daily.

Vitamin B complex

Each one of the B vitamins is important for the diabetic to take in a high enough dose to do some good. The suggested range would be 50 mg of each, maybe even two times a day. The B vitamins work best when taken together.

Natural vitamin E

Adelle Davis wrote that "diabetic patients have improved remarkably and many have been taken entirely off insulin when 300 units to 600 units of natural vitamin E have been given daily. Furthermore, this vitamin has been particularly helpful in persons with diabetic gangrene and other complications arising from atherosclerosis. Results have been especially striking when three tablespoons or more of granulated soy lecithin were taken daily with the vitamin E."

Hypothyroidism or low thyroid

According to Stephen Langer, M.D., in his excellent book on the thyroid, *Solved: The Riddle of Illness,* he feels that Dr. Broda Barnes is worthy of a Nobel prize in medicine for many solid reasons. One of his most important discoveries was that thyroid supplementation for diabetics, who are hypothyroids, can stop diabetic complications and, in some instances, even reversing them. He said, "I know this is true from my own practice and from that of other doctors who follow Dr. Barnes' methods."

On two occasions, Dr. Barnes told Dr. Langer, "All diabetic and hypothyroid complications arise from the same basic cause; clogged arteries, which prevent the blood from bringing in food and oxygen, and carrying off wastes." Dr. Barnes had noticed that various neuropathies (nerve deterioration which often limits leg, arm or eye function), together with other diabetic complications, such as diabetic arteriosclerosis which is gangrene, disappeared when thyroid hormone was administered. Gangrene occurs mainly in the legs because their circulation is less efficient. Be sure you go back and read the discussion of the thyroid in chapter 10, and Dr. Broda Barnes' valuable information on all aspects of the thyroid. Take your temperature test while you are there.

The big four—chromium, zinc, manganese and magnesium

Diabetes is one condition where the scientific literature is showing increasingly the importance of minerals in preventing degenerative changes in the pancreas. Dr. Robert Atkins calls chromium, zinc, manganese and magnesium the "Big Four." They are essential minerals that have key roles in metabolic pathways and are so frequently deficient in our overly refined Western diet.

Nutritionally, we know that the cells of the pancreas that secrete insulin must have calcium in the intercellular fluid before they can respond to the stimulation from glucose. Manganese, chromium and zinc have each been shown to be vital in helping to remedy carbohydrate metabolism problems. Chromium works closely with insulin, and insulin's effectiveness is greatly decreased when there is chromium insufficiency. Zinc is a crucial trace mineral that speeds wound healing and is involved in the granulation and storage of insulin. Diabetics lose more zinc in the urine than do non-diabetics.[9]

Vitamin C

Since ascorbic acid assists the action of insulin, it is important that your body maintain optimum levels of this valuable vitamin at all times. Moreover, since ascorbic acid is a potent detoxifier that counteracts and neutralizes the harmful effects of many poisons in the body, and since it increases the therapeutic effect of different drugs and medicines by making them more effective, it may be that many diabetics could reduce their insulin requirements if they were supplied with sufficient amounts of vitamin C.

Alpha lipoic acid

I also suggest taking this valuable nutrient, alpha lipoic acid. The amount a diabetic should take to prevent the many side effects of diabetes is discussed in the *Building Immunity* chapter. Be sure to read this information and take this essential nutrient.

Small feedings often

If you are one of the many people who suffer from diabetes, be sure to have five to six small feedings spaced evenly throughout the day. This schedule will give you a pickup each time your blood sugar starts to drop after not eating for three or four hours. Stay away from all sugar and refined carbohydrates, and be sure you get protein with every feeding.

Since protein is metabolized slowly, it will help you maintain your blood glucose level. Read about the *Super Energy Protein Shake* under

Breakfast #1. I feel this is the way a diabetic should start the day, and I would suggest a protein shake to be taken mid-afternoon to help keep the blood sugar stable, and even before bed if you had an early dinner. Or at least have some form of protein like cottage cheese or yogurt.

Over-consumption of sugar

It is hard to believe that the average person in the United States consumes about 170 pounds of sugar a year, or more than 3¼ pounds a week. That's more than one-third pound of sugar a day for every man, woman, and child! In reality, the average is much higher than that because infants and some adults don't eat as much sugar.

To demonstrate how quickly sugar adds up to equal one-half pound a day, my daughter Laura and I presented on a Trinity Broadcasting Network television program the quantity of hidden sugar in desserts. Laura counted out the teaspoons of white refined sugar into a bowl for each food as I relayed foods traditionally served at a child's birthday party:

Piece of chocolate cake (or cherry pie) =		15 tsp
Large scoop of ice cream	=	6 tsp
Glass of chocolate milk or cola drink	=	9 tsp
Total		30 tsp of sugar

With just these three "foodless" foods, we had a bowl full of 30 teaspoons of sugar! Would you give this bowl of sugar to your child or grandchild or even eat it yourself? Hardly. Yet we do so as a way of saying "I love you." But do you really? That is why diabetes, obesity and hypoglycemia conditions are so common and can be so severe.

Carbohydrates—particularly refined carbohydrates such as cake, candy, soft drinks, white flour and sugar—are quickly metabolized, causing a rapid rise in blood sugar level. When refined sugar enters the bloodstream, insulin must flood to the rescue to keep glucose levels from going too high.

The Value of Protein

Before we discuss a complete nutrition program, we need to understand the value of protein in our diet. Proteins are necessary for tissue repair and for the construction of new tissue. Every cell needs protein to maintain its life. Protein is also the primary substance used to "replace" worn out or dead cells. Your muscles, hair, nails, skin, and eyes are made of protein. Those with thinning hair and too many wrinkles for your age may lack protein. The basis for neurotransmitters in your brain, and the substances that form the body's immune response against infection, is made from protein. The most active protein users of the body are all of the hormones.

Next to water, protein is the most plentiful substance in your body. In fact, if all the water was squeezed out of you, half of your dry weight would be protein. One third of this protein would be in your muscles, a fifth in your bones and cartilage, a tenth in your skin, and the rest in your other tissues and body fluids. Even 95 percent of your hemoglobin is protein.

Protein is the best nutrient to eat in order to maintain an even blood sugar level, because it is metabolized over a long period of time. Protein can be converted to glucose if need be. Now you have a better understanding of why I keep emphasizing the value of protein. A quick and easy way to get more protein into your diet is to use a protein powder supplement.

Suggestions for choosing a protein powder

Not all protein powders are alike, so it's important that you read labels. There are several types of powders dominant today. These protein powders may be used alone or in combination with other powders. Look for a powder formula that contains NO refined sugar such as white sugar, sucrose, dextrose, maltose, corn sweeteners or the artificial sweetener, aspartame.

These are the four sources for protein powder that I recommend. You can find these types at your nutrition store.

WHEY PROTEIN—CONCENTRATES AND ISOLATES. Whey concentrates and isolates have gone through a manufacturing process to remove most of the carbohydrates, fat and lactose from regular whey or sweet whey. The process is called "ion exchanged" or "filtered," both of which result in almost a pure protein. It also removes the majority of lactose for those who are intolerant to milk.

The protein content is about 80 percent in the whey concentrates and 90 percent in the whey isolates. One method to rate the quality of one protein versus another is called Biological Value (BV). Proteins with the highest biological value promote the most lean muscle gains. Whey concentrates and isolates have higher biological values than regular whey, milk, egg or soy.

CASEIN (MILK PROTEIN). Casein is the predominant protein in milk.

For example, the protein in cheese and cottage cheese is casein. Sometimes called calcium-caseinate, or sodium or potassium-caseinate. It contains all the essential amino acids and is a good source of protein. It is very low in lactose. This slow digesting protein keeps you full longer since it must form a gel during digestion before it is absorbed. This slower transit time may extend the exposure to the protein in the intestines and may help increase absorption.

EGG PROTEIN (EGG WHITE OR EGG ALBUMEN). This protein used to be the "gold standard" against which all other proteins were measured, until whey protein became available. Egg white protein provides all twenty-two of the amino acids with a proper balance of essential amino acids. It is an excellent protein source, but not very tasty compared to the milky taste of whey or casein. Some manufacturers add egg white powder to their protein powder to boost the quality of the protein. Egg white protein powder contains no cholesterol.

SOY PROTEIN. Soy protein is processed from the soybean plant and most of the fat, fiber and carbohydrate has been removed. Since it is a vegetable product, it has no cholesterol. The amino acid profile is not quite as good as the other protein sources. Do not attempt to substitute soy flour for soy protein powder. The two are very different products. Soy flour must be heated for it to be assimilated by the body.

Soy is a nutritionally significant dietary source of isoflavones. These naturally occurring isoflavones are *genistein*, *daidzein* and *glycitein*. Recent human research suggests that these isoflavones are ideal for people of all ages, especially women concerned about bone health, those looking for an alternative to hormone replacement therapy and women experiencing menopausal symptoms. However there are differing opinions on soy and relief of menopausal symptoms. These isoflavones also work in conjunction with soy protein to lower cholesterol. Research has shown that 25 grams of soy protein a day, used as part of a diet low in saturated fat and cholesterol, may reduce the risk of heart disease.

Some brands use GMO soy, meaning it is from genetically modified soybeans. Most brands are switching to the more expensive non-GMO (non genetically modified) soy for this reason. Check your label and use the non-GMO brands.

In summary, different proteins offer varying advantages. I suggest you consume a variety of proteins and be sure to get adequate amounts for optimal health.

Lindberg Super Energy
Protein Shake

Using a good protein powder as the base to make your own *Lindberg Super Energy Protein Shake*, I suggest that you add the following ingredients to boost its nutritional value.

Soy lecithin granules

The word *lecithin* comes from the Greek word for "egg yolk." It helps keep the arteries free of cholesterol deposits, and also stimulates the transportation of cholesterol to the liver, before the cholesterol has a chance to accumulate or settle as plaque.[10] Its primary role in cardiovascular health is its ability to lower cholesterol levels. Adelle Davis explained how many physicians have successfully reduced cholesterol levels with lecithin. For example, within 3 months of taking four to six tablespoons of lecithin daily, levels of blood cholesterol dropped markedly.[11] (See the discussion of soy lecithin granules in chapter 8.)

Lecithin is a rich source of choline. Clinical studies have shown that choline is valuable for improving various mental functions, particularly memory. It is also a constituent of our brain and nervous system. Soy lecithin is a natural phosphatide, an essential constituent of all living cells of the human body. We have used lecithin as part of our nutrition program for well over 50 years with great success! Add two tablespoonfuls to your shake. (See benefits of lecithin for your brain in chaper 7.)

MSM powder

This natural form of dietary sulfur can be helpful for most types of musculoskeletal pain and inflammation, including rheumatoid arthritis, osteoarthritis, tendonitis and gout. Dr. Stanley Jacobs, author of *The Miracle of MSM: The Natural Solution of Pain*, reported, "MSM may be the new 'miracle cure' for arthritis. Sulfur is necessary for the manufacture of collagen, which helps to form bones, tendons, and connective tissue, and promotes smooth skin, lustrous hair and strong nails. It also helps to build the body's natural barriers against toxins, allergens and parasites."[12] It has a slightly bitter taste and is completely non-toxic. Add 1 teaspoon (4,000 mg) of MSM powder to your shake. Read the *Arthritis* chapter for all of its other benefits.

Organic flaxseed oil

Organic flaxseed oil is a rich and valuable source of the omega-3 unsaturated fatty acid, alpha-linoleic acid, as well as the omega-6 and omega-9s. Omega-3s are crucial for the production of many hormone-like substances called prostaglandins, which control thousands of different, important functions in the body. Probably the most important and widely studied benefit of the omega-3 fatty acids involves the cardiovascular system. It is also used in the fight against arthritis and other diseases. Dieters have found it is a powerful aid in weight management and appetite control as well. Add one tablespoon to your shake. (See index for more references to flaxseed oil.)

L-glutamine

L-glutamine is a single amino acid. It has great benefits for those under stress. Trauma, burns, infections, prolonged exercise and other stressors can deplete the glutamine stores in your body. The more stress you are under, the quicker you can deplete your L-glutamine supply. In addition, during calorie restriction your body might not synthesize L-glutamine as quickly as you need it. Consequently, researchers speculate that your body will use L-glutamine to fuel the brain and other body systems first. If any is left over, it will then be used to build muscle and maintain a strong immune system. The *American Journal of Clinical Nutrition* reported that a 2-gram oral dose of L-glutamine increased growth hormone levels by 430 percent.[13] Increasingly, growth hormone has been directly correlated with increased lean body mass, increased fat burning and improved strength. Powdered L-glutamine is available from several manufacturers. Add one teaspoon to your shake. (See index for more references to L-glutamine.)

L-carnitine liquid

L-carnitine is an amino-acid like compound found in all animal and human tissues, with the highest concentrations found in the adrenal glands and heart muscle. L-Carnitine has been shown to support the heart and cardiovascular system, helps athletes optimize performance, may allow fat to burn more easily, promotes healthy sperm function and helps rejuvenate our aging brain. It is valuable for the lowering of elevated triglycerides and is excellent for a weight loss program, in a dosage of 2–4 tablespoons (1 Tbsp. = 1,000 mg).

Nutritional yeast (Brewer's Yeast)

Brewer's yeast has generous quantities of all the major B-vitamins (except B12), 16 amino acids (which makes it a complete protein), and

18 or more minerals, including selenium and a rich source of chromium, which is not found in many foods. Brewer's yeast was originally made as a by-product of beer manufacturing, but now is made from food sources like sugar beets. It greatly enhances the nutritional value of any food to which it is added! One of the best known properties of nutritional yeast is its ability to increase energy. Nutritional yeast is dried and is a different strain than the live yeast used in baking. *It does not cause "yeast" infections or candida problems.* Add one tablespoon to your shake.

Dr. Pat Robertson's Age Defying Protein Shake

Dr. Pat Robertson's "Age Defying Protein Shake" from *The 700 Club* on CBN and TBN is very similar to my *Super Energy Protein Shake* that we have used for years. There are only slight variations in what we both recommend. I was thrilled one morning while I was watching *The 700 Club* and Dr. Pat Robertson started to make his famous protein shake. He began quoting me saying, "Judy Lindberg McFarland told me about soy lecithin and how valuable it is for you. Judy Lindberg McFarland also taught me about the importance of MSM for our joints." The biggest surprise was after he had made his shake and was discussing how these shakes kept him so healthy, he stated, "You can get these products wholesale by calling Judy Lindberg McFarland's company, Nutrition Express at 1-800-338-7979." Of course, we had thousands of calls. I understand *The 700 Club* has had over 445,000 responses for this recipe, and I am sure now there are many more. What an incredible blessing!

Beginning the Lindberg Nutrition Program

To get started I always believe it is best to "start fresh." We need to establish an internal environment that allows for full assimilation of nutrients, and we need to have proper elimination.

Before breakfast and before bed

A number of serious conditions can be related to infrequent or inadequate elimination. If you have elimination problems or have been on a series of antibiotics, I feel it is vitally important that you take the following:

ACIDOPHILUS (*LACTOBACILLUS* AND *BIFIDUS*). Acidophilus and bifidus will help reimplant and reestablish favorable intestinal bacteria in your large intestine. It is beneficial and soothing to the intestinal tract and helps to regulate bowel bacteria.

ALFALFA TABLETS (*MEDICAGO SATIVA*). Alfalfa is an excellent source of raw, green dietary fiber and chlorophyll, sometimes called "nature's broom and deodorizer." The alfalfa plant sends its tap root extremely deep into the soil to draw out a wide spectrum of nutrients and trace minerals. Read more detail about these two products under the *Elimination* heading at the end of this chapter.

The Importance of Breakfast

Breakfast is undoubtedly the most important meal of the day. How you "break the fast" from the night before actually determines the way you will feel the rest of the day. Your energy level in the afternoon hours in determined by what you had for breakfast. Without a high quality source of protein to start your day, your body has a hard time maintaining healthy muscle, thick hair, strong nails, elastic skin and adequate energy levels. Remember, there is NO excuse for leaving home without an adequate breakfast!

I will never forget our son, Douglas, saying to me when he was only in junior high school, "I can't think all the way to noon if I don't have my protein shake." Douglas recognized early in his life that he had a better attention span, could think more clearly, and was a better student if he had his protein shake. As a medical doctor today, he is still drinking protein shakes for breakfast and now is giving them to his four children.

I sent each of my children to college with a small refrigerator and a blender so they could make these drinks for breakfast and snacks. I knew they wouldn't eat the dorm breakfast or have time to go to the dining hall for breakfast. Our oldest son, Gary, once said to me about the food at his college, "I don't know if this education is worth ruining my health." He played college soccer and it was an intensely competitive and demanding sport. The protein shakes were just what he needed to provide the extra nourishment his body required.

Breakfast Suggestions

Now that my family has grown, and has established their own homes, my husband's and my choice for breakfast is usually a protein shake! We have found these to be the most beneficial and "live-able" breakfast on a consistent daily basis. We usually have larger, more traditional breakfasts on weekends, but during the week, fortified protein shakes keep us going and actually give us more energy. Through the years my children had a protein shake along with their normal breakfast.

Breakfast #1: Lindberg's Super Energy Protein Shake

Here is the *Super Energy Protein Shake* recipe that I have recommended to my customers for years. These are all excellent products I
discussed earlier in the chapter and I highly suggest following our
recipe below. More information on all the following nutrients can be
found on previous pages of this chapter.

LINDBERG'S SUPER ENERGY PROTEIN SHAKE RECIPE

- **8 oz. Organic Milk** (non-homogenized if possible or low fat)
  diluted fresh fruit juice, pure water or soy milk.
- **3 Tbsp.** (or scoop) **Protein Powder**
- **2 Tbsp. Soy Lecithin Granules**
- **Fresh Fruit**—fresh or frozen banana, strawberries, blueberries, or other fresh or frozen fruit.
- **Natural sweetener** (optional)

Blend all ingredients together and enjoy!

To make this drink even more power packed

Add several of the following ingredients. I personally use all these additional nutrients:

- **1 tsp.** (or more) **MSM powder** (1 tsp. = 4,000 mg)
- **1 Tbsp. Organic Flaxseed Oil**
- **1 tsp. L-Glutamine powder**
- **1–2 Tbsp. L-Carnitine liquid** (1 Tbsp. = 1,000 mg)
- **1 scoop Vitamin/Mineral Powder**

You can see how power-packed this shake can be! Use a variety of
these excellent products according to your special needs. Most of these
products are available from your local nutrition store or order them by
mail at: www.NutritionExpress.com

Sweetening your protein shake

Add one of the following natural sweeteners if necessary:

- frozen concentrated orange or apple juice
- unsweetened frozen strawberries (or other dark berries)
- fresh or frozen banana, apple or other fresh fruit (always peel your fruit unless it is organic)
- honey or Stevia *(Stevia rebandiana)*.

I recommend you avoid refined white sugar, corn syrup, or the artificial sweetener aspartame (Equal or Nutrasweet).

If you try this program for a few months, you will be amazed at the change in the level of vitality and health you will experience. Many of our clients have reported a tremendous increase in their sense of well being, energy levels, and peace of mind, knowing they are practicing the best kind of preventative health care.

If you want just the basics

For those of you who want to get started on a basic protein shake, my suggestion is to choose one of the protein powders and follow the instructions under *Lindberg's Super Energy Shake Recipe*, on the previous page. This includes just the protein powder and the granulated soy lecithin for a very basic shake recipe. Blend in the fresh fruit, and have it for your breakfast. Take your vitamins and minerals with your shake. As you become more confident with this "start up" program, you can slowly add the other ingredients I have discussed. If you try this basic program for a while, I am sure you will realize how great you'll be feeling.

Breakfast #2: Consider eggs for breakfast

Eggs are an excellent nutritional food and may be included in your nutritional program as often as you like. In 1999, the *Journal of the American Medical Association* reported that one or more eggs a day did not show any increased risk in cardiovascular disease. Eggs have received a lot of negative press in recent years, but they contain the highest quality protein available. Plus, they contain natural lecithin to emulsify the cholesterol in the yolk. Remember your hormones are made out of cholesterol. Eggs are a superior, complete food.

USE FERTILE EGGS IF POSSIBLE. A fertile egg results when a rooster mates with the chicken and the egg can then hatch. With most grocery store eggs the chickens have never seen a rooster! The DNA and RNA is different in fertile eggs since they are "live" foods. Grocery store eggs are next best if fertile are not available. You may scramble them, make an omelet or quiche, or eat them poached, soft boiled, or hard boiled. (Don't fry in shortening or margarine!)

If you're not overweight, add whole-grain toast, bagel, corn bread, or oat bran muffins for carbohydrates to burn as energy. Use real butter and not margarine. Add fresh fruit and a beverage.

NOTE: NO BACON, HAM, SAUSAGE, OR HOT DOGS! I suggest you avoid bacon, ham, and sausage for two reasons—their high fat content and the chemicals which are added in the curing process (nitrates and nitrites), which many believe to be cancer-causing. Nitrates and nitrites are also found in most cured and "smoked" meats: hot dogs, bologna, pepperoni, corned beef, pastrami, salami, smoked turkey and luncheon meats.

Researchers at the University of North Carolina at Chapel Hill discovered that *youngsters who ate hot dogs once a week or more had twice the risk of brain tumors compared with non-hot dog eating kids. Moreover, youngsters eating most other cured meats, such as ham, bacon, and sausage, had an 80 percent higher risk of brain cancer.* Children taking vitamins were less vulnerable to the brain cancer, suggesting that antioxidants countered the carcinogens in the cured meats.[14]

Hot dogs have also been linked to childhood leukemia, according to researchers at the University of Southern California School of Medicine in Los Angeles. *Youngsters eating more than 12 hot dogs a month had nearly ten times the risk of leukemia* when compared to children who ate no hot dogs. The most likely culprits are the nitrites and nitrates which are used to cure the meat. *Eating sausage was linked to colon cancer* risk in a Dutch research study.[15]

Recommended breakfast fruit

Less than ten percent of Americans eat five or more servings of fruit and vegetables a day. And more than half of Americans do not eat a single serving of fruit, vegetables or fruit juice on any given day. Breakfast is a good place to start.

To any of the breakfasts I discuss, add a variety of fresh fruit rather than canned. Eat the dark colored berries, such as blueberries, blackberries, raspberries, strawberries, dark cherries, and Concord grapes. The dark-colored fruit contains antioxidants and phytonutrients—*phyto* for plant. These substances contain anti-cancer compounds.

Also enjoy oranges and grapefruit and eat all of the white pulp of the citrus fruit to take advantage of the bioflavonoids naturally found there.

RECOMMENDED BEVERAGES

Beverages at meals may include any of the following:

- Pure water—filtered, spring, bottled, but not tap water in most cities. Remember: eight to ten glasses a day.

- Organic milk—no hormones, certified raw if possible, or non-homogenized milk, whole goat milk, acidophilus milk or buttermilk.

- Soy milk—soy milk is a good alternative but don't overdo it. Read the ingredients and avoid added sweeteners.

- Herbal teas of all varieties.

- Fruit juices should be diluted—a full glass of juice is very high in natural sugar. I recommend you eat whole fresh fruit instead of juice, as chewing the fruit helps digestion and you receive all the pulp and associated fiber.

- Green drinks, such as wheat grass, chlorella, Green Magma by Green Foods and Kyo-Green by Wakunaga.

- Regular, organically-grown coffee, water-processed decaffeinated coffee, or coffee substitutes, depending on your general health condition.

Some people truly enjoy a cup of coffee and feel a need for this pick-up in the morning, as long as this coffee is not considered "breakfast." This program needs to be one that is "livable" so I don't recommend a complete denial of coffee for some people, but rather moderation. Most of the negative reports are usually associated with the amount of coffee that is consumed.

Breakfast #3: Cereal or fortified pancakes

This breakfast is for those who can afford the high carbohydrates. These are good choices for those who have their weight under control, for active children or teens, but not for those wishing to lose weight.

NATURAL CEREAL: Grains by themselves do not contain all of the essential amino acids and thus are not a complete protein. To complete and increase the protein content of the cereal, I recommend adding a scoop of whey protein to your cereal or make a fortified milk mixture (shown below). Oatmeal can be topped with oat bran, raisins, seeds, raw nuts, banana slices or berries. In a study at the University of Kentucky, people with high cholesterol added 3¼ ounces of oat bran to their daily diet and lowered their cholesterol as much as 30 percent. Use fruit and beverages from the recommended list.

Fortified milk for cereals

I recommend the following for healthier milk sources:

- 2 cups organic milk—non-homogenized, low-fat or soy milk
- 2 or 3 scoops whey protein powder or powdered skim milk

Blend together, chill and use as a cereal topping.

HEALTHY PANCAKES OR WAFFLES. Make sure these are fortified with soy flour or powdered skim milk and made with whole grains and fresh eggs. Try yogurt with fresh berries or sliced bananas as a topping. My family has enjoyed pancakes and waffles topped with raw applesauce.

HIGH PROTEIN PANCAKES. Mix 1 scoop of protein powder in place of one scoop of the dry pancake mix. This will make the pancakes much more nutritious and higher in protein!

LOW-CARBOHYDRATE PANCAKES. Use ½ cup cottage cheese, 2 eggs, 1 scoop whey protein powder (strawberry is delicious), plus sweetener (if needed) into a blender. Blend and pour onto pan or griddle. Top with butter and non-carbohydrate syrup. These pancakes are a great low-carb alternative.

RAW APPLESAUCE TOPPING. Peel and cut up raw apples and put them in the blender with a little apple juice. Crush and add several vitamin C tablets or capsules to prevent the apples from oxidizing (turning brown). You can also add other fresh fruit, such as strawberries or yogurt to this mixture. Blend well. A delicious topping.

You might also top your pancakes or waffles with pure maple syrup diluted with water (so it is not as sweet). Don't use commercially marketed syrups that are loaded with sucrose and corn syrup. You may want to try sorghum, or use pure fruit jam sweetened with fruit juice. Be sure to read the labels closely.

Cook up the extra batter and have cold pancakes as a "snack food." Children love these topped with peanut butter and honey.

After Breakfast: Take your Vitamin and Mineral Supplements

Vitamins and minerals should always be taken with foods or a protein shake for better digestion and assimilation. You can divide your supplements among your meals, or take them all after breakfast, depending how many you are taking. Suggestions about vitamins and minerals are given later in this chapter.

Mid-Morning Feeding (About 9:00–10:00 A.M.)

If you eat a very early breakfast, say at 5:00 or 6:00 A.M., you may need to eat mid-morning. Too many hours between an early breakfast and lunch can cause symptoms of low blood sugar (hypoglycemia). Several snack suggestions are given under the mid-afternoon heading.

If you have a late breakfast, of course, you won't need this feeding. Try to space your feedings about three hours apart, throughout the day, going no more than four hours without a feeding.

Luncheon Suggestions

It is very important that you eat a well-balanced lunch. Your serving size will depend on your weight and activity level. We always stress small feedings often.

- A protein food—salmon, water-packed tuna, chicken, cottage cheese, yogurt, hard boiled eggs, cheddar or other natural cheese, turkey, tofu or soy product, and so forth.

- A raw, dark green and yellow vegetable salad—dark green lettuce, a variety of fresh vegetables including cruciferous vegetables such as broccoli, cauliflower, and cabbage; tomatoes, avocados, carrots, sprouts, green or red bell peppers. Use an oil and vinegar salad dressing (extra virgin olive oil or flaxseed oil are the best).

- A piece of fresh fruit, organic if possible.

- A whole grain product—a slice of multi-grain bread, a rice cake, a piece of corn bread, a bran muffin, or cooked brown rice, if your weight permits.

- A beverage—herb iced tea, mineral water, etc.

Note: *If you have a protein shake as a mid-morning snack, eat a smaller lunch.*

Mid-Afternoon Feeding (About 3:00 P.M.)

A feeding at this time of the day staves off your lowest nutritional ebb, which is near four o'clock. Be sure to have this feeding before your blood sugar level gets too low. It is an important key to feeling your best.

I always carry whey protein powder with me, especially when I travel. Recently, I was in New York and visited the *Live with Regis* show. Regis Philbin has used our *Lindberg Varsity Pack 2* vitamin and mineral supplement for about 20 years. After the show, we had lunch together and were discussing his incredibly busy schedule. He was going to be taping two other shows later that afternoon. I asked him, "Regis, are you taking your protein shakes?" He replied, "No, I just haven't been able to do that." The waiter had just served us coffee, so I took out of my purse the baggie of whey protein powder. I showed him how he could add it to his coffee, instead of cream. I explained that it is an easy way to increase his daily intake of protein. We each mixed it into our coffee and Regis thought it was delicious. He remarked, "Now I can do that!" Note: make sure the coffee is not too hot!

SUGGESTIONS FOR MID-MORNING AND MID-AFTERNOON FEEDINGS

The following make excellent snacks:

- Natural whey shake—add 1 scoop of whey protein powder to nonfat milk, diluted juice or bottled water
- High protein bar (found at nutrition stores)
- Cottage cheese with fresh fruit
- Half a tuna sandwich on whole grain bread or rice cake
- Apple with cheddar or string cheese
- Turkey jerky or beef jerky—nitrate/nitrite-free
- Sunflower seeds, pumpkin seeds, cashews, or other nuts
- Plain yogurt (unsweetened) with fresh fruit
- Whole-grain cereals – granola with no added sugar
- A "green" drink made with spirulina, wheat or barley grass, chlorella or combination

Dinner Suggestions (5:00 to 7:00 P.M.)

Enjoy a leisurely dinner served in a calm, pleasant atmosphere, which aids in the digestion of foods. Be sure to eat a well-rounded meal, including a variety of fresh foods.

Many ethnic dishes are very nourishing and have lasted through the centuries. Some of these ancestral dishes would be considered "health foods" today. Yogurt and cultured products such as goat's milk cheese, a wide variety of unprocessed grains, legumes (such as a hearty lentil soup), sea vegetables (including kelp for the thyroid), fish soup, tofu, and many other dishes have high nutrient value. Learn about your ancestral dishes and incorporate them into your diet, but be sure to leave out the heavy white processed fat and refined sugars.

The following are some menu suggestions to stimulate your creativity.

A large fresh, raw salad

Make a large fresh, raw salad, using dark green lettuce or spinach, to which you add broccoli, cauliflower, carrots, grated raw beets, chopped purple or green cabbage, green or red bell peppers, cucumbers, zucchini squash, snow peas, radishes, celery, fresh mushrooms, cherry tomatoes, and alfalfa or bean sprouts. These vegetables are a rich source of carotenes and phytonutrients.

JUDY'S SALAD DRESSING TIP

Since I am usually busy, I purchase the already made Italian with Cheese type dressing which is deliciously seasoned and most of the oil (usually canola) is separated at the top. I take it home, pour off all the oil, let it stand a little longer and then pour off the rest of the oil. Then I replace the canola oil with organic flaxseed oil, an excellent vegetarian source of the omega-3 fatty acids. It tastes great! Enjoy using generous amounts of this healthy salad dressing. Use it up quickly so it stays fresh and refrigerate after opening. Flaxseed oil has a short shelf life.

Select a protein food

Choose chicken, fish, salmon, turkey, eggs, moderate amounts of lean beef or lamb. Bake, broil, steam, or saute them. Be careful not to burn or blacken any of your meat or fish on the barbecue grill. The

Chinese method of cooking with a wok is quick and efficient. You can also combine protein foods and vegetables to make soups or stews, even adding whole-grain rice or lentils to the broth mixture.

Include complex carbohydrates

Choose a serving of natural brown rice, baked potatoes, yams, lentils, beans, legumes, or moderate amounts of whole-grain pastas or multigrain bread or muffins. If your fresh vegetables are not in your salad, have them for your complex carbohydrate such as carrots, broccoli, string beans, zucchini, etc.

Fresh fruit—the perfect dessert

Pineapple and papaya are great for digestion and wonderful to serve after a meal. We sometimes freeze fresh blueberries, strawberries, watermelon or bananas, then put them through our juicer or blender to make a wonderful after dinner natural sorbet.

Include essential oils

Use extra virgin olive oil and flaxseed oil. Use real butter and avoid hydrogenated vegetable shortening and margarine.

Before Bedtime (9:00 to 10:00 P.M.)

If you eat your evening meal at around 5:00 or 6:00 P.M., and don't retire until 10:00 or 11:00 P.M., your stomach will be empty by bedtime. If you don't eat breakfast until the following morning, say about seven o'clock, you will have fasted for almost 14 hours! That's a long time, nutritionally speaking, for many people, especially those who are older, who are very thin, and those who have low blood sugar or diabetes and other health problems.

If you have trouble sleeping, wake up exhausted, have nightmares or night terrors, wake up with palpitations of the heart or a rapid pulse rate, you may be suffering the effects of night time low blood sugar. Go back and read the list of symptoms for hypoglycemia. Do some of these symptoms sound like yours? Try adding an extra feeding around 9:00 P.M. or an hour before bed. I never believed in the statement of, "don't eat before going to bed." It's wrong in my opinion.

Young children and older people especially need this small extra feeding to help them sleep through the night, and to keep their bodies replenished with nutrients.

Teenagers who want to build muscle, or those who just want to feel better, can also benefit from a protein shake at this time or eat a snack, such as granola, yogurt, or cottage cheese with fresh fruit.

This before-bedtime feeding is not the time for sweets. Please: NO ice cream, cake, pie, sugared cereals, or other sugary foods before bedtime. They will only cause a greater drop in nighttime blood sugar and you may wake up feeling worse than if you hadn't eaten at all. Remember this "rule of thumb": *Small feedings often.*

Vitamin and Mineral Supplements for Optimal Health

I want to give you an idea of what potency to look for in a formula. Since we each have a great variance in size and weight, as well as differing medical histories, environments, and stress factors, your needs may be more or less for the nutrients listed below.

Mother never believed in the one-a-day or even three-a-day formulas because the potencies were too low. I agreed with her. These suggested ranges are what my husband and I take and most all of my family. I recommend an all capsule formula for ease in digestion and assimilation. A larger person with more weight would take the higher range of vitamins and minerals. A woman with her menstrual period would include the natural form of iron. Extra nutrients can always be added for special health conditions.

SUGGESTED VITAMIN AND MINERAL SUPPLEMENTS

VITAMINS	Men's Formula	Women's Formula
Vitamin A (dry fish liver oil)	7,500 IU	7,500 IU
Beta-Carotene (natural D. salina)	17,500 IU	17,500 IU
Vitamin B_1 (thiamin)	50 mg	20 mg
Vitamin B_2 (riboflavin)	50 mg	20 mg
Vitamin B_3 (niacin, niacinamide)	100 mg	100 mg
Vitamin B_5 (pantothenic acid)	200 mg	200 mg
Vitamin B_6 (pyridoxine)	50 mg	30 mg
Vitamin B_{12} (cobalamin)	100 mcg	100 mcg
Biotin	50 mcg	50 mcg
Choline Bitartrate	50 mg	50 mg
Inositol	50 mg	50 mg
Folic Acid (folate)	400 mcg	400 mcg

PABA (Para-Amino Benzoic Acid)	50 mg	50 mg
Vitamin C (ascorbic acid)	1,000 mg	500 mg
Vitamin D3 (dry fish liver oil)	400 IU	400 IU
Vitamin E (d-alpha-tocopherol)	400 IU	400 IU
MINERALS		
Boron	3 mg	3 mg
Calcium*	1,000 mg	1,000 mg
Chromium		
(polynicotinate or picolinate)	200 mcg	200 mcg
Copper	1 mg	1 mg
Iodine (atlantic kelp)	150 mcg	150 mcg
Iron (men and menopausal women		
rarely need iron)	0 mg	18 mg
Magnesium	400 mg	400 mg
Manganese	5 mg	5 mg
Molybdenum	75 mcg	75 mcg
Phosphorus	(not recommended—high in our foods)	
Potassium (maximum allowed by law)	99 mg	99 mg
Selenium	200 mcg	200 mcg
Zinc	15 mg	15 mg

Women at risk of osteoporosis should take 1,000 to 1,500 mg

Abbreviations: 1,000 mcg=1 mg 1,000 mg=1 g
mcg=microgram mg=milligram g=gram IU=International Unit

As you read through this book, you will see the value of other very important products. Here are a few you should consider adding to your program:

- Pycnogenol or Grape Seed Extract   50–300 mg
- CoEnzyme Q10   90–300 mg
- Alpha-Lipoic Acid   100–600 mg

As you read all the chapters you will find additional supplements and hormones that can be added to your nutritional program.

If You Have Digestive Problems

Proper digestion, good assimilation of food, and regular elimination are requirements for good health. These three functions are interdependent; one cannot proceed smoothly unless the others do.

Our mouths are the first step in the digestive process. Chewing food well breaks it down into particles that can be readily acted upon by the digestive enzymes, decreasing the likelihood of indigestion.

The salivary secretions in the mouth begin the digestive process. Human saliva contains the enzyme *pytalin*, which is important in the digestion of sugar and starch. There are no sugar and starch digesting enzymes in the stomach, so not until sugar and starch reach the small intestines is an enzyme from the pancreas added to complete the digestive work on these nutrients. Proteins must be broken down into amino acids (poly-peptides), large sugar molecules must be changed into simple sugars, and fats must be reduced to fatty acids before they can be absorbed into the blood or lymph vessels.

Food leaves the stomach in a semifluid state and passes on through the pyloric valve, which is the gateway to the first section of the small intestine, known as the duodenum. This valve opens and if there has been enough hydrochloric acid in the stomach, the pancreatic enzymes and bile from the liver are triggered to flow and start acting upon the food.

The pancreas

The pancreas is an endocrine gland lying below and behind the stomach and it controls blood sugar levels and also takes part in the digestion of proteins, starches, and fats. In a normal person, as much as two quarts of pancreatic juice enters the small intestines daily, largely after meals. It contains water, alkaline-forming materials which can neutralize the hydrochloric acid from the stomach, one fat-splitting, four carbohydrate-splitting and eight protein-splitting enzymes.[16]

As food passes gradually into the small intestines, bile from the liver finishes the digestion process. If no food is being digested, the bile is stored in the gall bladder. Bile is especially important in the digestion and assimilation of such foods as cream, butter, oils, and other fats. If an insufficient amount of bile is available, the result will be gas and indigestion. Bile breaks up fat into tiny droplets that are then surrounded by the fat splitting enzymes and then are quickly digested. Undigested fat makes it impossible for the protein and carbohydrate–splitting enzymes in the intestine to do their job. Thus, a lack of bile interferes with the digestion of proteins and carbohydrates.

Symptoms of a poorly functioning digestive system could be food allergies, bloating, chronic indigestion, foul-smelling gas, heartburn, acid reflux, pancreatitis, gastritis and other intestinal disorders.

The saying "you are what you eat" should actually be, "you are what you digest and assimilate." Even if you eat the best foods and take all the right vitamins, if you do not digest, assimilate and absorb your foods properly, then your striving for optimum health may be impaired. As we age the level of digestive secretions begins to slow. Vital nutrients may not be absorbed the way they should be.

Acid reflux, heartburn or hiatal hernia

When digestive disturbances occur, food often gets blamed. People will complain of "heartburn" or a "sour" or "acid" stomach and say that they "have had to put up with this for years." Many take antacid tablets and alkalizers to neutralize their stomach acidity. This is not the answer.

When the stomach lacks hydrochloric acid, another problem common among older people can result. The stomach balloons up through the diaphragm, forming what is called a *hiatal hernia*. The valve at the end of the stomach does not open when there is a lack of hydrochloric acid, so food remains in the stomach and ferments. It is the gas from this fermenting food that balloons the stomach.

With *heartburn*, many people feel like they have too much acid in their stomach. Instead, the burning sensation results when the acidic contents of the stomach flow back up (reflux) into the esophagus. The esophagus doesn't contain the protective layering like the stomach does, so it will sense pain and burning easily. The medical term to label heartburn is *reflux esophagitis*. Heartburn can also result from a stomach that is too full or it can be due to a weakness of the muscular valve (sphincter) that normally prevents the stomach contents from entering the esophagus. The problem tends to occur when you are lying down, so it is more likely to happen at night.[17]

Mother described how she handled all these problems: "If I did not have hydrochloric acid tablets and pancreatic enzymes, I would have a difficult time helping most people. Actually, taking antacids is exactly the opposite of what they should be doing. *Their problem is that they do not have enough hydrochloric acid,* or if they have too much, they are not keeping the right kind of food in their stomach to take care of it. Most people past 40 years of age do not have enough hydrochloric acid in their stomach." I find the exact same problem with people that come to see me. Giving them the hydrochloric acid and pancreatic enzymes helps them digest their food at the next meal.

When I attended an International Anti-Aging Conference in Monte

Carlo, Monaco, one of the young doctors made this same statement, "Most people past 40 do not have enough hydrochloric acid in their stomach." I wondered if he had heard Mother!

You need acid in your stomach.

Alan Gaby, M.D., explains one of the other major factors that influences nutrient absorption is stomach secretions. Gastric juice contains a protein-digesting enzyme called *pepsin* and a vitamin B$_{12}$ binding substance known as the *intrinsic factor*. In addition he said, "a healthy stomach is capable of secreting hydrochloric acid at a concentration so strong that it could corrode a copper penny."

Dr. Gaby said, "Acidity is measured in units called pH. The lower the pH, the more acidic the solution. The pH scale is logarithmic, which means that a one-point drop in pH is equivalent to a ten-fold increase in acidity, and a two point drop is equivalent to a one hundred-fold increase. The normal pH of stomach juice is about 1.5 compared to about 7.4 for blood."

"What that means is stomach secretions are nearly one million times more acidic than blood. Producing such a highly concentrated acid requires an enormous amount of metabolic energy, and one must assume that nature has a good reason of endowing the stomach with such extraordinary acidifying capabilities."

It is wonderful to know hydrochloric acid is a protective barrier against millions of bacteria and microorganisms from the outside. Bacteria, viruses, and fungi inhaled or ingested would normally be destroyed by the strong acid secreted by the stomach. As a result, the stomach and small bowel are normally sterile, or free of microorganisms. People who lack hydrochloric acid are frequently found to have any number of different organisms growing in their stomach or small intestines.

Foods can cause allergic reactions

Those who are allergic to foods such as milk, eggs, or whole grains usually react with skin and respiratory problems because food allergies are linked to digestion. There are always millions of bacteria in the large intestine. The more food left undigested, the greater the number of bacteria that can grow on this undigested food and the fewer particles of digested food that are brought into contact with the absorbing surfaces of the intestinal walls. This condition may create an immunological response in our bodies that may be an allergic reaction. Gas is formed in the bacterial breakdown of undigested food, and the result can be distention and pain.

As Mother would say, "You are never allergic to the foods you digest." Bloating, burping hours after a meal, and flatulence are most likely signs of poor digestion. Supplemental hydrochloric acid and pancreatic enzymes may be necessary to support your own digestive process.

Hydrochloric acid in the stomach also determines an individual's ability to tolerate bacteria-laden food. For example, the concentration of normal gastric juice in a human being is about 2 to 3 parts per 1,000, while in a healthy dog, the concentration is almost twice as strong—about 5 parts per 1,000. That is why a dog can eat tainted meat with no ill effects, while if man ate that same meat, he could develop a severe reaction and may even die.

Increasing hydrochloric acid in the stomach helps prevent "tourista," an acute diarrhea that often afflicts visitors to foreign countries because of bacterial invasion from food and water.

Helpful Enzyme Supplements

I also recommend taking digestive enzymes with each meal when traveling, and of course, it is prudent to exercise caution in choosing food and drink.

BETAINE HYDROCHLORIDE WITH PEPSIN

It provides your stomach with the necessary enzyme (pepsin) and hydrochloric acid for protein digestion. The stomach lining of a healthy person secretes adequate amounts of gastric juices containing two factors necessary for the initial stages of digestion. They are hydrochloric acid and pepsin enzyme.

Pepsin hydrolyzes (breaks down) protein molecules into certain amino acids. The partially digested protein is then finally broken down among all the other amino acids in the small intestine, as the result of other enzymes secreted by the pancreas. The hydrochloric acid converts pepsin to its active form.

How to take: Take two to four tablets with each meal that includes protein. You may increase the dosage as needed or follow the label suggestions. Take with pancreatic enzymes as they work together.

PANCREATIC ENZYMES

Pancreatic enzymes help support your own digestive process by providing additional enzymes to help you digest and absorb important nutrients. Iron Ox Bile acts like the bile produced by the liver and secreted by the gall-bladder into the small intestine. Bile helps emulsify and solubilize fats so they can be broken down by the enzyme lipase and finally absorbed into the lymphatic system.

There are three principal digestive enzymes:

- **Proteolytic enzymes**, or **Protease**, digests protein.
- **Amylolytic enzymes**, or **Amylase**, breaks down carbohydrates or starch.
- **Lipolytic enzymes,** or **Lipase**, breaks down lipids or fats for absorption into the lymphatic system. The combination of lipase and bile is especially important for the proper absorption of the fat-soluble vitamins A, D, and E.

These pancreatic enzymes are similar to the ones produced by a normal healthy pancreas. They assist in the digestion of protein, carbohydrates and fats in the small intestine.

How to take. Take two to four tablets after each meal that includes protein, fat and carbohydrate. Take along with Betaine Hydrochloride with Pepsin or follow the label suggestions.

Help for Elimination Problems

I usually ask my clients if they have a normal bowel movement. One of my clients responded with, "Well, it's normal for me." I wondered what she meant and asked her if she had one or two bowel movements a day. She said, "Oh no, I go every six days, but the doctor said it is normal for me." I have never forgotten that statement. Can you believe how toxic that would be to her system?

A number of serious problems are related to infrequent or inadequate elimination. Cancer of the colon and rectum is the second most common form of cancer in the United States, with approximately 150,000 new cases reported each year and upwards of 60,000 related deaths per year.[18]

Diverticulitis, hemorrhoids (occurring in half of all people over the age of 50), irritable bowel syndrome, spastic colon, ulcerative colitis, and Crohn's disease are all colon-related problems.

Generally, constipation is quickly relieved when adequate amounts of raw fruit and vegetables are added to one's diet. Also, remember to drink pure water, six to eight glasses a day at the minimum. Most authorities feel these colon problems may be helped with good nutrition, including plenty of fiber, hydrochloric acid and pancreatic enzymes (for digestion), and proper bowel habits.

Dr. Ilya Metchnikoff, who received the Nobel Prize for his research, studied Bulgarian people who were more than 100 years old. He found that they all had one thing in common: their bowels were acidic, just like those of a nursed baby. These people had been given no antibiotics, ate only natural foods, and had all been nursed as babies for their first two or three years. For the rest of their lives, they drank a quart of unsweetened yogurt nearly every day. Yogurt got the credit for the people's longevity and amazing good health, and soon, everyone in Europe started eating yogurt. Later investigation proved that the yogurt was simply providing the real hero, the friendly bacteria *acidophilus* that had been first established in nursing.[19]

Lactobacillus acidophilus and bifidus

My clients usually begin their nutrition program with a series of Lactobacillus Acidophilus and Bifidus capsules for at least six weeks. The large intestine normally contains this "friendly" bacteria and secretes acids that prevent the growth of "harmful" bacteria. Taking acidophilus in freeze-dried capsule form will help reimplant and reestablish the favorable intestinal bacteria in your large intestine (colon). This bacteria is established originally in the intestines when a baby is nursed, and a person needs to maintain sufficient friendly bacteria in order for nutrients to be properly assimilated by the body. Remember, antibiotics destroy friendly bacteria. Begin a series of acidophilus for at least 6 weeks.

HOW TO TAKE. Take one or two capsules of Lactobacillus Acidophilus and Bifidus or other various strains of the culture with a glass of water 20 minutes before breakfast and again before bedtime. Or follow the label directions. We carry a form of acidophilus which has a special polysaccharide matrix that attaches to the bacteria which makes it heat and acid resistant. After the capsules are swallowed, it bypasses the stomach acid and the matrix of healthy bacteria then releases into the intestines. Those with candida or other "yeast" associated problems should probably stay on acidophilus and bifidus until the condition clears up. Feel free to change the brand, because various manufacturers offer different strains of bacteria.

Alfalfa tablets

The name alfalfa *(Medicago sativa)* is from the Arabic language that means the "father of all foods." It is a legume which contains eight essential amino acids. It binds and neutralizes various types of agents that are known to be carcinogenic to the colon. It is "nature's broom and deodorizer" which provides an excellent source of dietary fiber, chlorophyll, amino acids, and trace minerals. Overall, alfalfa is one of the most nutritious foods known.[20] It is also a good fiber laxative and a natural diuretic. Alfalfa has always been an important part of our health-building program. It is not a grass but a legume, important for those allergic to grass.

How to take. Start with two to three of the Alfalfa 500 mg tablets and increase to six to ten, then take that amount twice a day. The optimal dosage may be 20 or more tablets taken throughout the day, until your bowels are regular. Then cut back to as many as you need to keep you regular. The tablets may be taken at any time and are very inexpensive. Taking alfalfa is equivalent to eating a big green salad!

Bad breath and perspiration odor

People buy millions of dollars worth of breath fresheners and mouthwashes each year. Neither gargling nor sucking breath mints will keep breath from being offensive. Decayed teeth or food particles lodged in the teeth may be responsible for mouth odor. However, most often it is a result of the gas of putrefaction flooding from the bowels into the bloodstream, through which it enters the lungs, causing bad breath. Body odor results from the same problem when the food gases escape through the skin, one of the primary organs of elimination.

People who take acidophilus/bifidus and alfalfa for their bowels often find relief not only from constipation but also from bad breath and perspiration odors. Alfalfa, with its dark green color, is a very rich source of chlorophyll, which has for years been used as a natural deodorizer. You will notice your elimination will smell like "new hay" with no bad odor. Many believe it is the magnesium found in chlorophyll that gives it a deodorizing property.

Importance of fiber

The National Cancer Institute has recommended that we each consume at least 25 to 35 grams of fiber a day. Fiber is either water-soluble (oat bran, apple pectin, guar gum, psyllium husks, and glucomannan) or water-insoluble (cellulose as wheat bran). The water-soluble forms absorb water, carrying added moisture through your bowels, producing a softer stool. In the intestines, they will pass toxins and harmful forms of cholesterol as well. *Flaxseed Meal* is very effective. Grind one cupful of flaxseed (dry) in the blender or coffee grinder, and take a tablespoonful in a glass of water once or twice a day. This will help keep the bowels regular. The ground-up seeds should be kept in the freezer to avoid becoming rancid. Flaxseed meal is also another great source of fiber and essential fatty acids.

Natural herbal laxatives

These are good for emergencies or to take on a trip, and should only be used infrequently. *Cascara Sagrada* is one of the best herbs to use for chronic constipation. It is said to be non-habit forming and to help in painless evacuations. After extended use, the bowels will begin to function naturally and regularly from its tonic effect.[21] It can be used alone or in combination with other herbs. *Senna* leaves increase the intestinal peristaltic movements and have a strong laxative effect on the entire intestinal tract, especially the colon. Be careful to replenish your fluid levels since laxatives can cause a rapid loss of vital electrolytes, especially potassium.

The mineral magnesium

One of the benefits of too much magnesium is its laxative effect. Magnesium can have a relaxing and toning effect on all muscles including the colon. It can be purchased separately at your nutrition store.

Herbal teas

There are many herbal laxative teas available to help with elimination. Many of these are mild and effective for occasional use.

No mineral oil

Do NOT take mineral oil as a laxative. This undigested oil binds with the fat-soluble vitamins A, D, E, and K in the intestines where they are held captive and are later excreted in the feces, thereby creating deficiencies of these vitamins.

Help for Sleep Problems

I usually suggest my clients drink a small *Lindberg Protein Shake* before bed. If you eat your evening meal around 5 or 6 P.M. and go to bed near 10 or 11 P.M., then you need another small protein feeding before you retire. This keeps your blood sugar from dropping during the night. I personally enjoy the whey protein powder mixed with warm milk or warm water. It mixes quickly and easily, even with a spoon and tastes great.

A number of herbal products are available to help those who want to wean themselves from synthetic, addictive sleeping pills and tranquilizers. These herbals are non-habit forming. They are not as powerful as drugs; therefore most people wake up feeling refreshed after using them. Take these products an hour before bedtime.

Valerian root

Valerian root has been used a great deal in Europe as a sleep aid and to treat anxiety. It is reputed to be a relaxant for nervous tension and to act as a mild sedative or natural tranquilizer. For centuries, valerian has been the treatment of choice by herbalists for nervous tension and panic attacks.[22] It also has been used to relieve muscle cramps related to stress, menstrual cramps, PMS and it's non-addictive! Try the concentrated extract form.

Herbal combination or sleep formulas

These products often are combinations of different herbs such as *skullcap* which is said to help control nervous disorders and relax the mind. *Hops* has a sedative effect, helps restlessness, and calms the nerves for insomnia. *Passionflower* is quieting and soothing to the nervous system but does not bring on depression or disorientation. Look for sleep combination formulas at your nutrition store.

Herbal teas

There are many popular brands of tea which contain gentle herbal combinations that are naturally caffeine-free. A hot cup of these mild herbal blends may help a person relax. *Chamomile* tea is also helpful. Curl up with a good book and a cup of herb tea before bedtime and you will likely fall asleep easily and sleep more soundly! Traditional Medicinals make *Nighty Night Herb Tea*, which is a wonderful relaxing bedtime tea.

Homeopathic formulas

Several homeopathic formulas are available at nutrition stores to help with relaxation. They are a natural way to take the edge off restlessness and insomnia.

Melatonin

This is an exceptional sleep aid, which is particularly useful in overcoming jet lag. This hormone will help you sleep soundly and may produce vivid dreams. Some report that it may also improve one's mood.[23] If you are over 40, I know you will enjoy reading about melatonin's anti-aging benefits as well. Read more in chapter 8, *Anti-Aging Therapies*.

Minerals for sleep and bone building

Many recall their mothers giving them a glass of warm milk before bedtime. Milk is a natural source of the amino acid tryptophan, as well as a good source of calcium. A magnesium deficiency can cause overexcitement of the nervous system, which can lead to muscle spasms or cramps, even twitching of the muscles. Magnesium works as a nerve relaxer and is necessary for the sending of nerve impulses for normal brain functions, as well as for sleeping. Use a calcium and magnesium supplement with extra vitamin D, boron, manganese, zinc, copper and hydrochloric acid for assimilation. All of these minerals promote natural sleep in many people, but more importantly, they also build our bones!

A Review of the Keys to Your Good Health

A great response to our Lindberg Nutrition Program has always been: "I can live with this!" This is a program designed for excellent overall nutrition so that you can enjoy vibrant health the rest of your life.

If you try this program for a few months, you will be amazed at the change in the level of vitality and health you will experience. Many of our clients have reported a tremendous increase in their sense of well being, energy levels, and peace of mind, knowing they are practicing the best kind of preventative health care. Remember that you must take charge of your health, because nobody is going to do it for you. These health benefits will be valuable many years into the future. Decide which of the following you need to add to your lifestyle:

> **Eat breakfast.** Don't leave home without breakfast. If you

are in a hurry, a fortified protein shake is an excellent way to start your day. These protein shakes are a great breakfast.

- **Have a mid-afternoon feeding.** It is critical to your maintaining an even blood sugar level throughout the day. Try to space your feedings every three to four hours from the time you eat breakfast until you retire at night. This may mean a before bed feeding if you have an early dinner. Ice cream, cake and cookies are not what I am talking about. Remember some form of protein.

- **Take your vitamins every day.** I cannot stress enough their importance to your health. They make up for deficiencies in the diet and help protect you against the stresses of life. They are like a "health insurance policy" in many ways.

- **Be sure to take a mineral formula** that includes adequate amounts of calcium and magnesium in proper balance, to protect your body in many ways, including osteoporosis. Selenium is a valuable antioxidant and protects us against cancer. Chromium picolinate or polynicolinate stabilizes the blood sugar, especially important for diabetes. Zinc is for men's unique challenges and immunity. In other words all the minerals are essential. There is not enough space in a one or two capsule or table product. It takes several to get adequate potency, and I would suggest capsules for easier assimilation.

- **Eat your food in its natural form,** if possible. This means fresh, whole fruit eaten raw. Enjoy the abundance of the fresh fruits, organic if possible. Watermelon, cantaloupe, pears, grapes, cherries plus all the fresh dark berries are excellent. Of course, eat your apples, grapefruit and oranges, instead of fruit juice. Fresh pineapple and papayas are great for digestion. Eat five to six servings a day.

- **Enjoy all the fresh vegetables** in raw salads. Use organically grown vegetables if they are available. These natural vegetables are valuable complex carbohydrates. To cook your vegetables, steam them, or use a wok. Do not overcook or microwave your vegetables—both methods destroy enzymes. Frozen foods are second best, avoid canned if possible. Add large amounts of garlic and onions. The distinctive odor actually increases levels of enzymes that break down potential carcinogens and boosts the activity of cancer-fighting immune cells; they are a rich source of sulfur.

❧ **Avoid all refined carbohydrates.** This means anything made with white flour and white sugar, including candy, cakes, donuts, pies, cookies, sugared cereals, white flour, white pasta, and so forth. These foods trigger and elevate blood sugar levels, increase triglyceride levels, slow down our immune system and cause weight gain. Go back in this chapter and read about hypoglycemia.

❧ **Avoid as many chemicals added to foods as possible.** Artificial food colors and preservatives are synthetic additives. Read the labels carefully, if you cannot pronounce it, don't eat it. Avoid sodium nitrite and nitrate, which are potential carcinogenic substances (cancer-causing). Products that contain sodium nitrate and nitrite can cause the formation of nitrosamines inside the stomach. Nitrosamines are chemicals that may cause virtually any type of cancer. They are found in most cured and smoked meats, such as bacon, hot dogs, salami, corned beef, and deli-luncheon meats. The fat content of these foods also tends to be high.

Most nutrition stores sell frozen, chemical-free hot dogs and luncheon meats usually made from chicken or turkey meat. They also carry great veggie-burgers or hot dogs made with soy products, but they must be frozen. They are all good sources of protein. Give them a try!

❧ **Avoid artificial sweeteners**, especially Aspartame (Equal or NutraSweet) which can cause a long list of medical reactions. According to Dr. Whitaker, "It is broken down in the body into harmful components, including formalde-hyde (a known toxin and carcinogen), formic acid (the poison in ant stings), and methanol (a nervous system toxin also known as free methyl alcohol or wood alcohol). In addition, the two amino acids that comprise aspartame, phenylalanine and aspartic acid, can bypass the blood-brain barrier and enter the brain, upsetting the balance of neuro-transmitters and brain chemistry. High intake of aspartame has been linked with a number of adverse effects, including headache, vision loss, seizures, mood disorders, and other nervous system problems."[24]

Aspartame, Equal or Nutra Sweet is found in low fat and diet foods, soft drinks, pre-sweetened cereals, sugar free chewing gum, some toothpaste, drugs and some vitamin preparations–especially children's Tylenol, Liquid Motrin, etc. Be a wise consumer and read your labels. It is important we avoid feeding children this chemical sweetener.

- **Drink plenty of fresh pure water.** This usually means bottled water, not city tap water. Some water filters are good, but be sure to change the filters often. We do not recommend distilled water for daily consumption, as the trace minerals have been removed.

- **Include a variety of protein foods in your diet.** Eat fish (tuna, salmon, halibut, etc.) often. I personally have elimi-nated the scavenger shell fish like lobster, crab and shrimp. Add poultry—chicken, turkey, and other fowl. If possible, *avoid* meat and poultry products that have been fed synthetic hormones to speed growth. Look for hormone and antibiotic-free meat and poultry from organic producers. Red meat is an important source of heme iron (an easy-assimilated form of iron). Add soy protein foods to your diet. Try tofu, miso, tempeh, and textured soy protein.

- **Stop smoking.** It's time to rejuvenate your heart and lungs! Also, you will be sparing your family from the effects of "second hand smoke."

- **Reduce or eliminate your alcohol consumption.** Alcohol can be a destroyer of your liver and brain cells as well as lives and relationships.

- **Exercise daily.** A brisk walk before breakfast or after dinner is an excellent practice. The amount of daily exercise will depend to a great extent on your age and physical condition. Essentially your body has five fundamental requirements: air, water, food, rest, and movement. Every organ benefits from exercise—the heart and circulatory (cardiovascular), respiratory, skeletal, and digestive systems. Get started and get moving!

❧ **Get sufficient rest.** If you are older, small cat-naps are great. Those who have trouble sleeping should try a calcium/magnesium supplement, melatonin or an herbal or homeopathic product. Go back and read "Help for Sleep Problems" in this chapter. Avoid using drugs to help you sleep or relax. They can be highly addictive.

❧ **Have a positive mental attitude.** Decide that you are going to be in excellent health. Your mental attitude and emotional state go a long way toward making excellent health a reality. Your mind has a powerful influence on your body's well-being, on your immune system, and on your level of energy.

The Bible, the manufacturer's handbook, states that we each need to rid ourselves of all bitterness, anger, hate, resentment, strife, and unforgiveness, since these are negative emotions that may contribute to disease. Scientific studies are bearing out this truth! Adopt a spirit of love, joy, peace, patience, kindness, goodness, faithfulness, gentleness, forgiveness, and self-control (see Galatians 5:22–23). These attitudes can aid in building sound health! Develop your spiritual life, choosing to live spiritually the way our Lord designed you to live.

Start doing today what it is that you know to do, and stay with the program, believing for the very best health possible! The Bible states in the old testament, *"For I will restore health unto thee and will heal thee of thy wounds, saith the Lord"* (Jer. 30:17). One of my favorite scriptures is this lovely prayer: *"Beloved, I pray that you may prosper in all things and be in health, just as your soul prospers"* (3 Jn. 1:2, NKJV). These are my prayers for you and your family. You have the potential to create a vital, more vigorous and healthy life than ever before.

May you have God's abundant blessings throughout your journey!

Vitamin and Mineral Summary Chart

An Overview of All the Vitamins and Minerals and Their Importance to You!

This appendix provides you with a basic overview and description of all scientifically recognized vitamins and minerals. The following information is listed for each item.

UNDERSTANDING VITAMINS AND MINERALS

Name: the name of the vitamin or mineral, along with its number or letter designation.

Fat-soluble or water-soluble: Fat-soluble vitamins can be stored for longer periods of time in the body's fatty tissue and liver. Water-soluble vitamins must be taken into the body daily, as they are not stored over a long period of time.

Sources: the foods considered to be the richest natural sources for the vitamin or mineral.

What it does: the major function in the body of a particular vitamin or mineral.

Deficiency Symptoms: the common symptoms people suffer when deficient in a particular vitamin or mineral.

Optimal Daily Amount: a range is given, aimed not only at achieving general health but abundant health. This range is what we believe, after years of research and application, will help a person achieve optimal health and longevity. In some cases, the potency range suggested is quite wide. This is because our individual differences, genetic code, family history, body size, activity and stress level, pollutant-exposure factors, and general levels of health tend to vary widely. Keep in mind, too, that these optimal daily amounts are the best recommendations we have at the present time. New scientific information may yield new recommended amounts. Note especially that these are the recommended optimal amounts for adults, not children. The U.S. Government's RDAs (recommended dietary allowances) are also listed.

UNITS OF MEASURE

Units of vitamins and minerals are measured in the following ways:

- Fat-soluble vitamins are measured in International Units (IU)
- Water-soluble vitamins and minerals are measured by:
  1,000 micrograms (mcg) = 1 milligram (mg)
  1,000 milligrams (mg) = 1 gram (gm)

VITAMINS

VITAMIN A
(Retinol)

Fat-soluble

Sources: found only in animal sources—fish liver oils (as in cod liver oil), liver, milk, cream, cheese, butter, eggs.

What it does: is required for all situations that have to do with vision and the eyes, builds resistance to respiratory infections, increases immunity, protects against cancer, prevents birth defects, helps with skin conditions and acne. Is stored in the body.

Deficiency symptoms: night blindness or loss of adaptation to the dark, dry eye disease, sty in the eye, increased susceptibility to infection, sinus and bronchial infections, drying out of skin and mucous membranes, loss of taste and smell which leads to loss of appetite, loss of vigor, defective teeth and gums, slowed growth.

Optimal daily amount: 10,000 to 25,000 IU. RDA is 5,000 IU. Pregnant women should not take over the 10,000 IUs of vitamin A. The literature shows 500,000 IU of vitamin A can be absorbed and stored by an adult human liver. We recommend a mixture of both vitamin A and beta-carotene.

BETA-CAROTENE
(Provitamin A)

Fat-soluble

Sources: yellow fruit, dark green, yellow and leafy vegetables, such as carrots, yams, cantaloupe, yellow squash, spinach, apricots, spirulina, wheat grass, alfalfa and barley grass.

What it does: important free radical fighter for various forms of cancer, protects against ultraviolet damage, enhances immune system, many of the same functions as vitamin A. Beta-Carotene must be converted by the liver and the intestinal wall into usable vitamin A.[1]

Deficiency symptoms: intake of alcohol decreases beta-carotene in the liver; those with hypothyroidism and diabetes may have trouble converting beta-carotene into vitamin A.

Optimal daily amount: 20,000 to 50,000 IU. No RDA has been established. Nontoxic.

VITAMIN B$_1$
(Thiamin)

Water-soluble

Sources: brewer's or nutritional yeast, organ meats (especially liver), pork, dried beans, peas, soybeans, wheat germ, egg yolks, fish and seafood; dried yeast, brown rice, rice husks or rice bran, whole grain products, oatmeal, nuts, most vegetables, milk, raisins, prunes.

What it does: known as the "morale" vitamin, converts carbohydrates (sugar) into energy, promotes growth, aids digestion and is essential for nerve tissues, muscles and heart, helps repel insects and mosquitoes, used in the treatment of alcoholics and drug addicts.

Deficiency symptoms: loss of appetite, fatigue, weakness, neuritis, muscle atrophy, head pressures, poor sleep, feeling tense and irritable, aches and pains, subjectively poor memory, difficulty concentrating, constipation, impaired growth, pins and needles sensation in the toes and "burning" sensation in the feet; beriberi, which includes mental illness, paralysis of some eye muscles, foot drop and decreased sensation in the feet and legs. Alcohol consumption interferes with absorption of B$_1$.

Optimal daily amount: 25–100 mg. RDA is 1.4 mg with an additional 0.4 mg for pregnancy or lactation. Should be taken with the other vitamins.

VITAMIN B$_2$
(Riboflavin)

Water-soluble

Sources: milk, cheese and yogurt are rich sources, along with liver, kidney, meat, poultry, fish, eggs, bran, wheat germ, lentils, beans, peanuts, soy beans, green leafy vegetables, fruit.

What it does: helps convert protein, carbohydrates and fat into energy; protects against free radical damage; necessary for cellular respiration and good vision, skin, hair and nails; physical exercise increases need.

Deficiency symptoms: cracks and sores in the corners of the mouth, frayed or scaling lips, inflamed tongue with a purplish or magenta color, eczema or seborrhea, flaking skin around the nose, eyebrows, chin, cheeks, earlobes or hairline; oily appearance of nose, chin, and forehead with fatty deposits accumulating under the skin; bloodshot, watering, itching, burning, fatigued eyes with a keen sensitivity to light; increase in cataract formation; nervous symptoms such as "pins and needles" sensation, difficulty walking, muscular weakness, trembling and a lack of stamina or vigor; behavioral changes such as depression, moodiness, nervousness and irritability.

Optimal daily amount: 25–100 mg. RDA is 1.6 mg. Should be taken with the other B-vitamin complex vitamins.

VITAMIN B$_3$
(Niacin, Niacinamide, Nicotinic Acid, Nicotinamide)

Water-soluble

Sources: lean meats, organ meats, fish, brewer's yeast, whole grains, nuts, dried peas and beans, white meat of turkey or chicken, milk, milk products.

What it does: assists enzymes to break down proteins, fats, and carbohydrates into energy; helps lower cholesterol levels, lowers triglycerides and other cardiovascular disorders; for the nervous system, maintains healthy skin, tongue and digestive tissues; plays a role in the production of bile salts for synthesis of sex hormones; prevents or cures schizophrenia and some other mental disorders; alleviates arthritis.

Deficiency symptoms: pellagra (symptoms include dermatitis, diarrhea, and dementia [mental disorders]); bright red tongue; sore tongue and gums; inflamed mouth; throat and esophagus; canker sores; mental illness; perceptual changes in the five senses; schizophrenic symptoms; rheumatoid arthritis; muscle weakness; general fatigue; irritability; recurring headaches; indigestion; nausea; vomiting; bad breath; insomnia; small ulcers.

Optimal daily amount: 50–100 mg of niacinamide included in your daily B-complex supplement. To lower cholesterol, researchers use the niacin form, 250–1,200 mgs spread throughout the day. Various forms of "no flush" niacin are available. Inositol hexaniacinate exerts the benefits of niacin without flushing. RDA is 20 mg.

VITAMIN B₅
(Pantothenic Acid, Calcium Pantothenate, Panthenol)

Water-soluble

Sources: brewer's yeast, liver, kidney, wheat bran, crude molasses, whole grains, egg yolk, peanuts, peas, sunflower seeds, beef, chicken, turkey, milk, royal jelly.

What it does: vital for the adrenal glands and for production of cortisone; plays a role in creating energy from protein, carbohydrates and fats; helps synthesize cholesterol, steroids and fatty acids for a healthy digestive tract; essential to production of antibodies; helps with arthritis and is an anti-inflammatory.

Deficiency symptoms: burning sensation in the feet, enlarged beefy, furrowed tongue; skin disorders such as eczema; duodenal ulcers; inflammation of the intestines and stomach; decreased antibody formation; upper respiratory infections; vomiting; restlessness; muscle cramps; constipation; sensitivity to insulin; adrenal exhaustion; physical and mental depression; overwhelming fatigue; reduced production of hydrochloric acid in the stomach; allergies; arthritis; nerve degeneration; spinal curvature; disturbed pulse rate; gout; graying hair.

Optimal daily amount: 100–200 mg in a B-complex supplement or up to 1,000 mgs in divided doses. RDA is 10 mg.

VITAMIN B₆
(Pyridoxine, Pyridoxinal, Pyridoxamine)

Water-Soluble

Sources: brewer's yeast, sunflower seeds, wheat germ, liver and other organ meats, blackstrap molasses, bananas, walnuts, roasted peanuts, canned tuna, salmon.

What it does: metabolizes proteins, fats and carbohydrates; forms hormones for adrenaline and insulin; makes antibodies and red blood cells; helps in synthesis of RNA and DNA; regulates fluids in the body; needed for production of hydrochloric acid; relieves carpal tunnel syndrome; helps with PMS symptoms; helps asthmatics; helps prevent kidney stones in combination with magnesium.

Deficiency symptoms: greasy, scaly dermatitis between the eyebrows, and on the body parts that rub together; low blood sugar; numbness and tingling in the hands and feet; neuritis; arthritis; trembling hands in the aged; water retention and swelling during pregnancy; nausea; motion sickness; mental retardation; epilepsy; kidney stones; anemia; excessive fatigue; nervous breakdown; mental illness; acne; convulsions in babies; newborn infants may develop crusty yellow scabs on the scalp called "cradle cap."

Optimal daily amount: 25–100 mg combined with a B-complex supplement. RDA is 2 mg.

VITAMIN B₁₂
(Cobalamin or Cyanocobalamin)

Water-Soluble

Sources: organ meats, liver, beef, pork, eggs, whole milk, cheese, enriched whole wheat bread, fish.

What it does: metabolism of nerve tissue, protein, fat and carbohydrate metabolism; creates red blood cells; may stimulate appetite in children. An "intrinsic factor" must exist in the stomach for this vitamin to be absorbed.

Deficiency symptoms: pernicious anemia including weakness, a sore and inflamed tongue that appears smooth and shiny, numbness and tingling in extremities, pallor, weak pulse, stiffness, drowsiness, irritability, depression, mental deterioration, senile dementia, paranoid psychosis, chronic fatigue syndrome, diarrhea, poor appetite, growth failure in children.

Optimal daily amount: 500–2,000 mcg with a complete B-complex vitamin. Sublingual form is best absorbed with tablets placed under the tongue. RDA is 6 mcg.

BIOTIN

Water-Soluble

Sources: yeast, liver, organ meats, egg yolk, grains, nuts, fish.

What it does: needed for maintenance of hair and skin, for brittle fingernails, sweat glands, nerves, bone marrow, normal bone growth; may help with Sudden Infant Death Syndrome (SIDS) or crib death.

Deficiency symptoms: scaly dermatitis, inflamed sore tongue, loss of appetite, nausea, depression, muscle pain, sitophobia (morbid dread of food), pallor, anemia, abnormalities of heart function, burning or prickling sensations, sensitive skin, insomnia, extreme lassitude, increased cholesterol, depression of immune system.

Optimal daily amount: 50–200 mcg combined with B-complex. RDA is 3 mcg.

PABA
(Para-Amino-Benzoic Acid)

Water-Soluble

Sources: liver, brewer's yeast, wheat germ, molasses, eggs, organ meats, yogurt, green leafy vegetables.

What it does: stimulates intestinal bacteria which aids in production of pantothenic acid, coenzyme in making blood cells and metabolizing protein, important for skin health, hair pigmentation and health of intestines; may help with vitiligo; may restore gray hair to normal; used for many skin conditions.

Deficiency symptoms: similar to symptoms caused by a folic acid or pantothenic acid deficiency; also vitiligo, fatigue, irritability, depression, nervousness, headache, constipation, and other digestive disorders.

Optimal daily amount: 50–100 mg included in a B-complex vitamin. No RDA has been established.

FOLIC ACID
(Folacin, Folate)

Water-Soluble

Sources: deep, green leafy vegetables, liver, brewer's yeast, whole grains, bran, asparagus, lima beans, lentils, orange juice.

What it does: for synthesis of RNA and DNA, for red blood cell production, metabolism of protein, increases the appetite, for production of antibodies, prevents neural tube defects and birth defects in babies, reduces susceptibility to infection.

Deficiency symptoms: anemia, poor growth, weakness, an inflamed and sore tongue that may appear smooth and shiny, numbness or tingling in the hands and feet, indigestion, diarrhea, depression, irritability, pallor, drowsiness, a slow, weakened pulse; graying hair; mental illness; impaired wound healing; reduced resistance to infection; birth defects resulting in spina bifida and other neural tube defects, toxemia, insomnia, leg numbness and cramps in pregnant women, premature birth and after birth hemorrhaging, cervical cancer and dysplasia.

Optimal daily amount: 400–800 mcg combined with B-complex vitamin. RDA for men is 200 mcg; for women 180 mcg; RDA for pregnant women is 400 mcg, but should be 800 mcg.

CHOLINE

Water-Soluble

Sources: lecithin, brewer's yeast, fish, soybeans (tofu, tempeh, miso), peanuts, beef liver, egg yolk, wheat germ, cauliflower, cabbage.

What it does: for transport and metabolism of fats and cholesterol in the liver, prevents cardiovascular disease, detoxifies the liver, for a proper functioning nervous system, part of the nerve fluid for nerve impulses, prevents and treats memory loss and diseases of the nervous system, influences mood and depression (manic-depressives); strengthens capillary walls, accelerates blood flow, thereby lowering blood pressure; aids in the treatment of gallstones.

Deficiency symptoms: may cause high blood pressure, bleeding stomach ulcers, heart trouble, blocking of the tubes of the kidneys, hemorrhaging of the kidneys, hardening of the arteries, atherosclerosis, headaches, dizziness, ear noises, palpitations, constipation.

Optimal daily amount: 500–1,000 mg. No RDA has been established.

INOSITOL

Water-Soluble

Sources: lecithin, organ meats, wheat germ, whole grains, brewer's yeast, blackstrap molasses, peanuts, citrus fruit.

What it does: with choline helps to metabolize fats and cholesterol in the arteries and liver, helps promote the body's production of lecithin, for growth and cell survival in bone marrow, eye membranes and intestines; with vitamin E may help nerve damage in certain forms of muscular dystrophy; in certain cases may prevent thinning hair and baldness; helps with brain cell nutrition; with choline may help with menstrual problems.

Deficiency symptoms: none officially recognized; however, deficiency may cause constipation, eczema, abnormalities of the eyes, hair loss, high cholesterol.

Optimal daily amount: 500–1,000 mg. No RDA has been established.

VITAMIN C
(Ascorbic Acid)

Water-Soluble

Sources: rose hips, citrus fruit and juices, strawberries, blueberries, cantaloupe, raw vegetables such as red bell peppers.

What it does: a potent antioxidant to protect against cellular damage, formation and maintenance of collagen (the skin's "cement"), helps with wound healing and burns, especially those recovering from surgery; increases the absorption of iron and calcium; activates insulin; for a properly functioning nervous system; increases resistance to infections; raises HDL (good) cholesterol; helps protect from cardiovascular disease; prevents buildup of atherosclerotic plaque on the blood vessel wall; may help with cold and flu; may help with infertility; helps body produce interferon; for male fertility; protects us against industrial pollutants; for cataracts and other eye disorders; prevents bleeding gums; prevents many types of viral and bacterial infections; protects from many forms of cancer.

Deficiency symptoms: bruising easily, bleeding gums, tooth decay, nose bleeds, swollen or painful joints, anemia, poor wound healing, lowered resistance to infection, general weakening of connective tissue, scurvy, easily fractured bones, weakened arteries rupture or hemorrhage, extreme muscle weakness, painful joints, wounds and sores will not heal.

Optimal daily amount: 1,000–6,000 mg depending on your need. RDA is 60 mg (slightly higher for pregnancy and lactation).

BIOFLAVONOIDS
(Flavonoids, Rutin, Hesperidin, Vitamin P, Grape Seed Extract, Pycnogenol)

Water-Soluble

Sources: white part (including the center part) and pulp of oranges, lemon and grapefruit; apricots, rose hips, cherries, grapes, green peppers, tomatoes, papayas, broccoli, cantaloupe, and dark-pigmented fruit and vegetables.

What it does: decreases permeability and fragility of blood vessels and constricts the capillaries, protects vitamin C from oxidation, increases absorption of vitamin A, exhibits antiviral effects, free radical scavenger, natural antibiotic activity, may help ease pain of varicose veins, helps certain types of hemorrhoids, prevents bruising, may help relieve hot flashes, inhibits certain cataracts.

Deficiency symptoms: edema or accumulation of fluid in the tissue, bleeding into the tissue (noticeable as red spots and splotches when it occurs close under the skin) resulting from fragile, faulty capillaries.

Optimal daily amount: 500–2,000 mg, depending on your need. No RDA has been established.

VITAMIN D
(Ergocalciferol)

Fat-soluble

Sources: sunshine (manufactured through your skin); fish liver oils such as cod liver oil, liver, egg yolks.

What it does: enhances absorption of calcium and phosphorous, necessary for proper functioning of the thyroid and pituitary glands, improves psoriasis, maintenance of cell membrane fluidity.

Deficiency symptoms: osteomalacia (softening of the bones) in adults, rickets in children, irritability, restlessness, fitful sleeping, frequent crying, heavy perspiration behind the neck in babies, delayed eruption of teeth, soft and yielding skull, bowed legs, knock-knees, depressions in the chest, pigeon-chest deformity of the rib cage, swayback, overly prominent forehead causing the appearance of sunken eyes, delayed walking, may protect against colorectal and breast cancer.

Optimal daily amount: 400–800 IU from fish liver oil. RDA is 400 IU.

VITAMIN E
(Tocopherol)

Fat-Soluble

Sources: wheat germ oil, soybean oil, safflower oil, peanuts, whole grains (wheat, rice, oats), green, leafy vegetables, cabbage, spinach, asparagus, broccoli, eggs.

What it does: important for oxygen of the cells, preventing the oxidation of cells; may be useful in gangrene, coronary and cerebral thrombosis (clots), diabetes mellitus, congenital heart disease, arteriosclerosis, phlebitis, and other leg problems due to poor circulation; helps varicose veins; is a powerful antioxidant, protecting against air pollution, damage against radiation; protects polyunsaturated oils from breaking down; prevents clotting in blood vessels; melts fresh blood clots, frees blood platelets for normal clotting of wounds; prevents strokes; normalizes the activity of ovaries in women, improving periods, preventing excessive bleeding, and vaginal dryness; prevents miscarriages; helps proper functioning of the sex glands; improves male sperm cells; strengthens the immune system; applied externally it eliminates radiation burns and reduces scarring; may help with non-cancerous breast cysts; protects against nitrosamines in foods; alleviates pain in osteoarthritis; may help relieve menopausal symptoms; increased stamina in athletes; improves action of insulin.

Deficiency symptoms: may decrease survival time of red blood cells, faulty fat absorption, anemia in premature infants, degeneration of the brain and spinal cord, premature births and higher risk of miscarriage, decrease in sex hormones, higher risk of skin cancer.

Optimal daily amount: 400–1,200 IU. To obtain these potencies, you should use natural vitamin E supplements such as "d-alpha" tocopherol or the dry form, "d-alpha" tocopherol succinate. The synthetic is "dl-alpha" tocopherol, made from petrochemicals, and not as effective. RDA is 30 IU.

VITAMIN K
(Phylloquinone)

Fat-soluble

Sources: yogurt, kefir, acidophilus milk, alfalfa, spinach, cabbage, cauliflower, tomatoes, pork liver, lean meat, peas, carrots, soybeans, potatoes, egg yolks.

What it does: essential to blood clotting, for proper bone mineralization, has helped people with Crohn's disease and gastrointestinal disorders, for proper bone mineralization.

Deficiency symptoms: hypoprothrombinemia (condition in which the time it takes for the blood to clot is prolonged); hemorrhages, bloody urine and stools, nosebleeds, miscarriages, deficiency in newborn babies results in bloody stools or vomiting (fairly common since newborns have no intestinal bacteria).

Optimal daily amount: Most vitamin and mineral supplements do not contain vitamin K as it is easily available in the diet and synthesized in the body. RDA for women is 65 mcg, 80 mcg for men.

MINERALS

BORON

Sources: fresh fruit and vegetables.

What it does: helps retain calcium in bone and prevents against calcium and magnesium loss through the urine; helps bone mineralization; prevents osteoporosis; increases estrogen naturally in postmenopausal women.

Deficiency symptoms: none officially recognized.

Optimal daily amount: 3 mg daily combined with calcium, magnesium and all other minerals. No RDA has been established.

CALCIUM

Sources: milk, egg yolks, fish or sardines (eaten with bones), yogurt, soybeans, green leafy vegetables (such as turnip greens, mustard greens, broccoli, and kale), roots, tubers, seeds, soups and stews made from bones, blackstrap molasses, almonds, figs, beans.

What it does: maintains acid-alkaline balance in body, normalizes contraction and relaxation of the heart muscles, for strong bones and teeth; protects against osteoporosis, rickets and osteomalacia; helps lower high blood pressure; lowers cholesterol and helps prevent cardiovascular disease; helps relieve backaches, menstrual cramps and may help you sleep more soundly; natural tranquilizer; helps prevent cancer, especially colorectal-cancer.

Deficiency symptoms: nervous spasms, facial twitching, weak-feeling muscles, cramps, rickets, slow growth in children, osteoporosis (porous and brittle bones), osteomalacia (a bone-softening disease), heart palpitations and slow pulse rate, height reduction, colon cancer.

Optimal daily amount: 1,000–1,500 mg with half to equal parts of magnesium. Some researchers say menopausal women need 1,500 mg, with added boron and magnesium. RDA is 1,000 mg daily for adults; 1,200 mg for pregnancy and lactation; 1,200 mg for males and females from age 11 to 24.

CHLORIDE

Sources: most people obtain chloride from salt (sodium chloride) and salt substitute (potassium chloride); also found in large amounts in body.

What it does: stimulates production of hydrochloric acid for digestion; maintains fluid and electrolyte balance; helps the liver.

Deficiency symptoms: impaired digestion; loss of hair and teeth; rare as the body usually produces enough.

Optimal daily amount: The need nor the RDA has been established.

CHROMIUM

Sources: brewer's yeast, blackstrap molasses, black pepper, meat (especially liver), whole wheat bread and cereals, beets, mushrooms.

What it does: helps stabilize blood sugar levels, therefore is effective against diabetes and hypoglycemia; lowers cholesterol; increases level of high-density lipoproteins (HDLs) in humans (shown protective against cardiovascular disease); increases lean muscle tissue while decreasing body fat.

Deficiency symptoms: slowed growth, shortened life span, raised cholesterol levels, an array of symptoms related to low and high blood sugar such as diabetes and hypoglycemia.

Optimal daily amount: 200-600 mcg of GTF (glucose tolerance form) taken with other minerals. Chromium polynicotinate (bound to niacin) and chromium picolinate (bound to picolinic acid) are natural forms. RDA has not been established. The National Research Council tentatively recommends 50-200 mcg to be effective.

COPPER

Sources: nuts, organ meats, seafood, mushrooms, legumes.

What it does: with iron and protein it forms hemoglobin (red blood cells), forms melanin (pigment in skin and hair), helps form connective tissues such as collagen and elastin, helps lower cholesterol, helps prevent rancidity of fatty acids and maintains cellular structure, may help as anti-inflammatory against arthritis.

Deficiency symptoms: anemia, loss of hair, loss of taste, general weakness, impaired respiration such as emphysema, brittle bones, chronic or recurrent diarrhea, hair depigmentation, low white blood cell count which leads to reduced resistance to infection, retarded growth, water retention, nervous irritability, high cholesterol, abnormal ECG patterns, development of ischemic heart disease, birth defects, miscarriage and neural tube defects, antacid use creates copper deficiency.

Optimal daily amount: 2–3 mg taken with zinc at a 10:1 or 15:1 ratio (zinc:copper). RDA is 2 mg.

FLUORIDE

Sources: sometimes added to our drinking water which can be poisonous.

What it does: in toothpaste, helps prevent dental caries.

Deficiency symptoms: none.

Optimal daily amount: No RDA has been established. I do not recommend drinking fluoridated water.

IODINE
(Iodide)

Sources: seaweed (especially kelp), dulse, seafood, iodized sea salt, eggs, garlic, turnip greens, watercress.

What it does: stimulates the thyroid gland to produce thyroxin, protects against toxic effects from radioactive material, related to over 100 enzyme systems such as energy production, nerve function and hair and skin growth; stimulates conversion of body fat to energy; regulates basal metabolic rate; relieves pain and soreness associated with fibrocystic breast; loosens clogged mucous in breathing tubes.

Deficiency symptoms: goiter (characterized by enlarged thyroid gland which may thicken the neck, restrict breathing and cause bulging of the eyes); hypothyroidism (low thyroid); physical and mental sluggishness, poor circulation and low vitality; dry hair and skin, cold hands and feet, obesity; cretinism (characterized by physical and mental retardation in children born to deficient mothers); hearing loss.

Optimal daily amount: 150–300 mcg. RDA is 80–150 mcg. Liquid iodine for medicinal uses (as an antiseptic for wounds) should not be used orally.

IRON

Sources: liver, heart, kidney, lean meats, shellfish, dried beans, fruit, nuts, green, leafy vegetables, whole grains, blackstrap molasses.

What it does: helps form red-blood cells called hemoglobin and myoglobin (red pigment in muscles), cures and prevents iron-deficiency anemia, stimulates immunity, helps with muscular and athletic performance, prevents fatigue.

Deficiency symptoms: anemia (pallor, weakness, persistent fatigue, labored breathing on exertion, headaches, palpitation); young children suffer diminished coordination, balanced attention span, I.Q., and memory; older children have poor learning, reading and problem solving skills; depressed immune system with decreased ability to produce white blood cells to fight off infection; concave or spoon-like fingernails and toenails.

Optimal daily amount: RDA is 10 mg for men, 18 mg for women, and we feel this should be adequate. After menopause women should use 10 mg. As a supplement, do not use inorganic iron (ferrous sulfate) which destroys vitamin E. Use organic iron (ferrous fumarate, ferrous citrate or ferrous gluconate).

MAGNESIUM

Sources: chlorophyll from all plants, figs, lemons, grapefruit, green, leafy vegetables, alfalfa, yellow corn, soy flour, whole wheat, peas, beans, brown rice, almonds, oil-rich nuts and seeds, apples.

What it does: absolutely essential for life, a major mineral for the metabolism of glucose; production of cellular energy; to create protein; for nerve and muscle contraction; protective against cardiovascular disease; lowers high blood pressure; helps with PMS;

helps kidney stones; for nervous system; important for people taking diuretics and digitalis.

Deficiency symptoms: apathy, depression, apprehensiveness, confusion, disorientation, vertigo (a condition in which the room seems to spin around), muscular weakness and twitching, overexcitability of the nervous system which may lead to muscle spasms or cramps, insomnia, jumpiness, sensitivity to noise, irritability, poor memory, tremors or convulsions.

Optimal daily amount: 400–750 mg should be taken with twice as much calcium. RDA is 350 mg for men; 280 mg for women, plus 150 mg if pregnant or lactating. Large amounts of magnesium salts (3,000 to 5,000 mg daily) have a cathartic (laxative) effect.

MANGANESE

Sources: whole grains, wheat germ, bran, peas, nuts, green, leafy vegetables, beets, egg yolks, bananas, liver, organ meats, milk.

What it does: required for vital enzyme reactions, proper bone development and synthesis of mucopolysaccharides, for help with osteoarthritis, required for many enzyme reactions, for normal functioning of the pancreas and for carbohydrate metabolism, to manufacture collagen, important part in the formation of thyroxin, a hormone secreted by the thyroid gland; for thymus gland function; may improve memory and reduce nervous irritability.

Deficiency symptoms: weight loss, dermatitis, nausea, slow growth and color changes of hair, low cholesterol, disturbances in fat metabolism and glucose tolerance, deficiency suspected in diabetes; deficiency during pregnancy may be a factor in epilepsy in the offspring, myasthenia gravis (severe loss of muscle strength).

Optimal daily amount: 5–10 mg in combination with other minerals. No RDA has been established.

MOLYBDENUM

Sources: organ meats (liver, kidney), milk, dairy products, legumes, whole grains, leafy green vegetables.

What it does: required for the activity of several enzymes in the body, a vital part of the enzyme responsible for iron utilization; helps prevent anemia; a detoxifier of potentially hazardous substances we may come in contact with; may be an antioxidant;

protects teeth from cavities; aids in carbohydrate and fat metabolism.

Deficiency symptoms: possible esophageal cancer in those that have molybdenum deficient soil.

Optimal daily amount: Optimal intake is still uncertain; 50–200 mcg (not mg). No RDA has been established.

PHOSPHOROUS

Sources: high-protein foods such as meat, fish, poultry, eggs, milk, cheese, nuts, legumes, bone meal; many processed foods and soft drinks preserved with phosphates adversely affect the body's calcium-phosphorous balance.

What it does: essential for bone mineralization, for normal bone and tooth structure; involved in cellular activity; important for athletes and may help with muscular fatigue; important for heart regularity; needed for the transference of nerve impulses; aids in growth and body repair.

Deficiency symptoms: muscle weakness (to the point of respiratory arrest), anemia, increased susceptibility to infection. The typical diet usually makes a phosphorous deficiency rare in the United States; those with kidney failure or gastrointestinal diseases can have severe deficiencies; alcoholics and those taking antacids may be deficient.

Optimal daily amount: No supplementation needed as the diet should supply sufficient amounts. RDA is 800–1,200 mg for adults.

POTASSIUM

Sources: bananas, apricots, peaches, broccoli, potatoes, fresh fruit and fruit juices, sunflower seeds, unsalted peanuts, nuts, squash, wheat germ, brewer's yeast, desiccated liver, fish, bone meal, watercress, blackstrap molasses, unsulfured figs.

What it does: balances fluid with sodium inside the cells, for proper muscle and heart contraction, assists red blood cells in carrying oxygen, helps stimulate water waste through kidneys, for proper carbohydrate metabolism, for energy storage in the muscles and liver, helps reduce high blood pressure, helps colic in babies, prevents heart attacks, helps allergies, important for those using diuretics.

Deficiency symptoms: general weakness of muscles, mental confusion, muscle cramping, poor reflexes, nervous system disruption, soft, flabby muscles; constipation; acne in young people; dry skin in adults; severe deficiency leads to heart attack.

Optimal daily amount: 2,000–4,000 mg. Generally you get enough in foods. Athletes generally require more (3,000-6,000 mg) because of heavy perspiration. The maximum potency allowed by the government in supplement form is 99 mg. Discuss higher potencies with a physician. RDA is 2,000–2,500 mg.

SELENIUM

Sources: organ meats, tuna, seafood, brewer's yeast, fresh onions and garlic, mushrooms, wheat germ, some whole grains.

What it does: necessary for growth and protein synthesis, increases effectiveness of vitamin E (they are synergistic), an antioxidant for the cells to protect against oxygen exposure, protects against toxic pollutants, for sexual reproduction, reduces risk of cancer, helps against heart disease, reduces free radical damage that causes aging, alleviates hot flashes and some menopausal symptoms.

Deficiency symptoms: dandruff, enhanced damaging effects of ozone on the lungs, decreased growth, infant deaths associated with selenium and/or vitamin E deficiency, increased risk of cancer and heart disease.

Optimal daily amount: 100–200 mcg in high selenium areas; 200–400 mcg in low selenium areas. The Food and Nutrition board states that overt selenium toxicity may occur in humans ingesting 2,400–3,000 mcg. No RDA has been established.

SILICON
(Silica)

Sources: flaxseed, steel cut oats, almonds, peanuts, sunflower seeds, onions, alfalfa, fresh fruit, brewer's yeast, dietary fiber.

What it does: helps build connective tissue. Most people take silica as a form of silicon, to help with hair, skin and nails.

Deficiency symptoms: aging symptoms of skin (wrinkles), thinning or loss of hair, poor bone development, soft or brittle nails.

Optimal daily amount: We have no dietary recommendations. Adequate amounts are found in the diet. No RDA has been established.

SODIUM
(Sodium Chloride, Salt)

Sources: sea salt, most foods from animal sources, shellfish, meat, poultry, milk, cheese, kelp, powdered seaweed, most processed foods.

What it does: works with potassium to maintain proper fluid balance between cells, for nerve stimulation for muscle contraction, helps in keeping calcium and other minerals in the blood soluble, for weak muscles, stimulates the adrenal glands. High sodium usually accounts for high blood pressure. Aids in preventing heat prostration or sunstroke.

Deficiency symptoms: They are rare since most foods contain sodium. However, symptoms include headaches, excessive sweating, heat exhaustion, respiratory failure, muscular cramps, weakness, collapsed blood vessels, stomach and intestinal gas, chronic diarrhea, weight loss, kidney failure, tuberculosis of kidneys, streptococci infections.

Optimal daily amount: rarely needed, an ordinary diet provides enough sodium. A gram of sodium chloride has been suggested for each kilogram of water ingested. Sea salt (iodized) is the best form of sodium. RDA is 200–600 mg.

SULFUR

Sources: protein foods—especially eggs, lean beef, fish, onions, kale, soybeans, dried beans.

What it does: found in every cell of the body, helpful for musculoskeletal pain and inflammation, including rheumatoid arthritis, osteoarthritis, tendonitis and gout; helps nerves and muscles function properly, and normalizes glandular secretions; necessary for healthy hair, skin and nails; helps maintain oxygen balance necessary for brain function; the homeopathic supplement of sulfur helps with rashes and itching and other skin conditions.

Deficiency symptoms: rare but may be excessive sweating, chronic diarrhea, nausea, respiratory failure, heat exhaustion, muscular weakness, arthritis and mental apathy.

Optimal daily amount: a diet sufficient in protein should be sufficient in sulfur. No RDA has been established.

VANADIUM

Sources: fish, black pepper, and dill seed are richest source; middle range is whole grains, meats, dairy products.

What it does: in animal studies with diabetic rats, research showed it improved glucose tolerance and improved efficiency of insulin in the muscle cells. More research needs to be done.

Deficiency symptoms: little known at this time, but high blood pressure and hardening of the arteries have been suggested.

Optimal daily amount: More needs to be known before we can suggest an amount. No RDA has been established.

ZINC

Sources: fresh oysters, herring, wheat germ, pumpkin seeds, milk, steamed crab, lobster, chicken, pork chops, turkey, lean ground beef, liver, eggs.

What it does: promotes wound healing, helps with acne, affects impotence in men, and aids in increasing sperm count; helps infertility; may help with prostate problems; for increasing immunity; for colds and flu; prevents hair loss; may help with some forms of cancer; helps with macular degeneration.

Deficiency symptoms: fingernails with white spots or bands or an opaquely white appearance, loss of taste, smell and appetite; delayed sexual development in adolescence; underdeveloped penis and less full beard and underarm hair in boys; irregular menstrual cycle in girls; infertility and impaired sexual function in adults; poor wound healing; loss of hair; increased susceptibility to infection; reduced salivation; skin lesions; stretch marks; reduced absorption of nutrients; impaired development of bones; muscles and nervous system; deformed offspring; dwarfism.

Optimal daily amount: 30–50 mg (take with copper, a zinc:copper ratio of 10:1). RDA is 15 mg.

For further information regarding health issues or to obtain nutritional product information, request a nutritional products catalog, or order nutritional products, please visit:

www.JudyMcFarland.com

or

www.NutritionExpress.com

or call:

1 800-338-7979 (USA)

1 310-784-8500 (International)

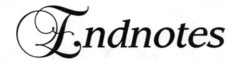

Endnotes

Chapter 1...Aging—Let's Slow It Down

1. Hayflick, Leonard. *Scientific American* 218 (1968).
2. Gelfant. Paper presented at the Miami Symposium on Theoretical Aspects of Aging, February 7, 1974.
3. Bosco, Dominick. *The People's Guide to Vitamins and Minerals*. Chicago: Contemporary Books, 1980, page 165.
4. Adams, Ruth. *The Big Family Guide to All the Vitamins*. New Canaan, CT: Keats Publishing, 1992, page 356.
5. "The Secret of the Human Cell." *Newsweek* (August 20, 1994) page 48.
6. Runestad, Todd. "Adverse Drug Reactions Kill More Than 100,000 Annually." *Industry News*.
7. Germano, Karl, R.D., CNS, LDN. *The Osteoporosis Solution—New Therapies for Prevention and Treatment*. New York: Kensington Publishing Corp., 1999.
8. Eisenberg, D. M., M.D., et al. "Trends in Alternative Medicine Use in the United States, 1990–1997: results of a follow-up national survey." *Journal of the American Medical Association* 280.18 (November 11, 1998): 1569–1575.
   Whitaker, J. *Health and Healing* 9.1 (Phillips Publishing, Inc., January 1999).
9. *Alternative Medicine Alert, A Clinician's Guide to Alternative Therapies* (Atlanta, GA: American Health Consultants).

Chapter 2...The Significance of Vitamins, Minerals, and Herbs

1. Szent-Gyorgi, Albert, M.D., Ph.D. "How New Understandings About the Biological Function of Ascorbic Acid May Profoundly Affect Our Lives!" *Executive Health* (May 1978).
2. *Journal of the American Medical Association* 253 (February 8, 1985): 6.
3. Rosenbaum, Michael E., M.D. and Dominick Bosco. *Super Supplements*. New York: New American Library, 1987, page 249.
4. Lindberg, Gladys and Judy McFarland. *Take Charge of Your Health*. San Francisco: Harper and Row, 1982, page 181.
   Prevention Magazine's *Complete Book of Vitamins and Minerals for Health*. New York: Wings Books, a division of Rodale Press Inc., 1988, pages 10–11.
5. U.S. Dept. of Agriculture Report of the Dietary Guidelines Advisory Committee on Dietary Guidelines for Americans, 2000.
6. Robbins, Michael. *The 1992 Top Ten Almanac*. Workman Publishing, 1992.
7. Gazella, Karolyn A. "Nutritional Supplements: Protecting the Core of American Health." *Health Counselor* 5.3: 27–31.
8. Harvey, Paul. "Vitamins are a 'health hazard'?" *Los Angeles Times Syndicate* (1992).
9. *Journal of the American Medical Association* 226 (1991): 2847–2851.
10. Whitaker, M.D., Julian. *Dr. Whitaker's Guide to Natural Healing*. Rocklin, CA: Prima Publishing, 1995, page 11.
11. Hoffer, Abram. *Journal of Orthomolecular Medicine* 7 (First quarter 1992): 1.
12. Adams, Ruth. *The Big Family Guide to All the Vitamins*. New Canaan, CT: Keats Publishing, 1992, page 144.

13.   Somer, Elizabeth. *The Essential Guide to Vitamins and Minerals.* New York: Harper-Perennial, a division of Harper Collins Publishers, 1992.
14.   Ashmead, Dwayne, Ph.D., et al. *Intestinal Absorption of Metal Ions and Chelates.* Springfield, IL: Charles Thomas Publisher, 1985, page 4.
        Murray, Frank. *The Big Family Guide to All the Minerals.* New Canaan, CT: Keats Publishing, Inc., 1995.
15.   *Herbal Gram* 12 (Austin, TX: Herb Research Foundation and the Journal of the American Botanical Council, Spring 1987).
16.   *Ibid.*
17.   *Ibid.*

Chapter 3...Promoting Longevity with Antioxidants

1.   Ames, Bruce N. "Understanding the Causes of Aging and Cancer." Paper presented at the Biological Oxidants and Antioxidants: New Developments in Research and Health Effects conference, Pasadena, CA, March 12–13, 1993.
        Ames, Bruce N. "Oxidants, Antioxidants, and the Degenerative Diseases of Aging." *Proceedings of the National Academy of Sciences* USA 90.17 (1993): 7915–7922.
2.   Braly, James and Laura Torbet. *Dr. Braly's Food Allergy and Nutrition Revolution.* New Canaan, CT: Keats Publishing, Inc., 1992, page 81.
        Ward, J. "Free radicals, antioxidants, and preventive geriatrics." *Australian Family Physician* 23 (July 1994): 1297–1301.
3.   Harman, D. "Free-Radical Theory of Aging: History." *Free-Radicals in Aging,* eds. I. Ement and B. Chance (Basel, Switzerland: Birkhauser Verlag, 1992).
        Harman, D. "The Aging Process: Major risk factor for disease and death." *Proceedings of the National Academy of Sciences* USA 88 (1991): 5360–5363.
        Harman, D. "Aging: Prospects for further increases in the functional life span." *Age* 17 (1994): 119–146.
4.   Hendler, Sheldon Saul, M.D., Ph.D. *The Doctors' Vitamin and Mineral Encyclopedia.* New York: Simon and Schuster, 1990, page 49.
5.   Ziegler, Regina. "Carotenoids, vegetables, fruits, and risk of cancer." Paper presented at the San Diego Conference, February 6–9, 1993.
        Patterson, G. H. "Fruits and Vegetables in the American Diet: Data from the NHANES II Survey." *American Journal of Public Health* 80 (1990): 1443–1449.
        Steinmetz, K. A. "Vegetables, Fruit, and Cancer—Part I: Epidemiology." *Cancer Causes and Control* 2 (1991): 325–327.
        Block, Gladys, Ph.D. "Fruit, vegetables, and cancer prevention: A review of the epidemiologic evidence." *Nutrition and Cancer* 18 (1992): 1–29.
6.   Prabhala, R. H. "Influence of beta-carotene on immune functions." *Annals of the New York Academy of Sciences* 691 (December 31, 1993): 262–263.
        Schroeder, D. J. "Cancer prevention and beta-carotene." *Annals of Pharmacotherapy* (April 28, 1994): 470–471.
7.   Henkel. *Antioxidant Update* (January/February, 1996). Used with permission.
8.   *Ibid.*
9.   Block, Gladys, Ph.D. "The data support for a role for antioxidants in reducing cancer risk." *Nutrition Review* 50 (1992): 207–213.
10.   Cohen, B. E. and I. K. Cohen. "Vitamin A: ajunvant and steroid antagonist in the immune response." *Journal of Immunology* 3 (1973): 1376–1380.
        Weiner, Michael A. *Maximum Immunity,* page 99.
        Nutrition and Cancer 11 (1988): 207–217.
11.   Hendler, Sheldon Saul, M.D., Ph.D. *The Doctors' Vitamin and Mineral Encyclopedia.* New York: Simon and Schuster, 1990, page 42.
12.   Block, Gladys, Ph.D. "Epidemiologic Evidence for Health Benefits of Antioxidants." Paper presented at the Biological Oxidants and Antioxidants: New Developments in Research and Health Effects conference, Pasadena, CA, March 12–13, 1993.
13.   Weiner, Michael A. *Maximum Immunity.* page 98.
14.   *Ibid.,* page 99.
        Beisel, W. R., R. Edelman, K. Nauss, and R. M. Suskin. *Journal of the American Medical Association* 245 (1981): 53–58.
15.   *Journal of the National Cancer Institute* 73 (December 1984): 1463–1468.

Hendler, Sheldon Saul, M.D., Ph.D. *The Doctors' Vitamin and Mineral Encyclopedia.* New York: Simon and Schuster, 1990, page 42.

Michsche, M., et al. "Stimulation of immune response in lung cancer patients by vitamin A therapy." *Oncology* 34 (1977): 234–238.

Shikelle, R. B., et al. "Dietary vitamin A and risk of cancer in the Western Electric study." *Lancet* 2 (1981): 1185.

16. Wald, N., M. Idle, and J. Boreham. *Lancet* (October 18, 1980): 813.

Hendler, Sheldon Saul, M.D., Ph.D. *The Doctors' Vitamin and Mineral Encyclopedia.* New York: Simon and Schuster, 1990, page 42.

17. *Ibid.*

18. *Journal of the National Cancer Institute* 73 (December 1984): 1463–1468.

19. Hendler, Sheldon Saul, M.D., Ph.D., *The Doctors' Vitamin and Mineral Encyclopedia.* New York: Simon and Schuster, 1990, page 42.

Michsche, M. et al. *Oncology* 34 (1977): 234–238.

Pastorino, A., et al. *Journal of Clinical Oncology* 11 (1993): 1216–1222.

20. Hendler, Sheldon Saul, M.D., Ph.D. *The Doctors' Vitamin and Mineral Encyclopedia.* New York: Simon and Schuster, 1990, page 42.

21. Bendich, A. and L. Langseth. "Safety of vitamin A." *American Journal of Clinical Nutrition* 49 (1989): 358–371.

22. "Committee on infectious diseases, American Academy of Pediatrics." *Pediatrics* 91 (May 1993): 1014–1015.

Challem, Jack. "Vitamin A and Pregnancy: How Many People Will the Panic Injure?" *The Nutrition Reporter* 6 (November 12, 1995).

23. Passwater, Richard A., Ph.D. *The New Supernutrition.* New York: Pocket Books, 1991, pages 288–289.

24. Bendich, A. and L. Langseth. "Safety of vitamin A." *American Journal of Clinical Nutrition* 49 (February 1989): 358–371.

25. *Ibid.*

26. Block, Gladys, Ph.D. *Nutrition Review* 50 (June 1992): 207–213.

27. Challem, Jack. "Vitamin A and Pregnancy: How Many People Will the Panic Injure?" *The Nutrition Reporter* 6 (November 12, 1995).

28. "Committee on infectious diseases, American Academy of Pediatrics." *Pediatrics* 91 (May 1993): 1014–1015.

Stone, Irwin. *The Healing Factor.* New York: Grosset & Dunlap, 1972, page 72.

Cameron, E. and L. Pauling. *Cancer and Vitamin C.* Warner Books, June 1981, page 114.

29. DiRenzo L, et al., The function of human NK cells is enhanced by beta-glucan, a ligand of CR3 (CD11b/CD18). *Eur J Immunol* 1997 Jul;21(7):1755–8.

30. Stone, Irwin. *The Healing Factor.* New York: Grosset & Dunlap, 1972, page 72.

Cameron, E. and L. Pauling. *Cancer and Vitamin C.* Warner Books, June 1981, page 114.

31. *Ibid.*

32. Stone, Irwin. *The Healing Factor.* New York: Grosset & Dunlap, 1972, page 72.

33. Szent-Gyorgi, Albert, M.D., Ph.D. "How New Understandings About the Biological Function of Ascorbic Acid May Profoundly Affect Our Lives!" *Executive Health* (May 1978).

34. *Ibid.*

35. Pauling, Linus. *Vitamin C & Cancer.* The Linus Pauling Institute of Science & Medicine Newsletter reprint, 1.2.

Block, Gladys, Ph.D. "Beyond deficiency: New views on the function and health effects of vitamins." *New York Academy of Sciences* (February 1992).

36. Cameron, E. and L. Pauling. *Cancer and Vitamin C.* Warner Books, June 1981.

37. Passwater, R. and C. Kandaswami. *Pycnogenol: The Super Protector Nutrient.* New Canaan, CT: Keats Publishing, Inc., 1994.

38. Schwitters, B. and J. Masquelier. "OPC in Practice: Bioflavonols and their application." Rome: *Alfa Omega* (1993).

49. Passwater, R. and C. Kandaswami. *Pycnogenol: The Super "Protector" Nutrient.* New Canaan, CT: Keats Publishing, Inc., 1994.

40. Murray, Michael T. "PCO Sources: Grape Seed vs Pine Bark—a review and comparison." Botanical Report in *Health Counselor* 7: 1.

Passwater, R. and C. Kandaswami. *Pycnogenol: The Super "Protector" Nutrient.* New Canaan, CT: Keats Publishing, Inc., 1994, pages 7–8.

41. Passwater, Richard and Chithan Kandaswami. *Pycnogenol: The Super "Protector" Nutrient.* New Canaan, CT: Keats Publishing, Inc., 1994, pages 7–8.
42. *Ibid.*
    Masquelier, Jacques. "Pycnogenols: Recent advances in the therapeutic activity of procyanidins." *Natural Products As Medicinal Agents,* J. L. Beal and E. Reinhard, eds. (Hippokrates Verlag Stuttart P., 1991): 343–356.
43. Martin, A. M. *The Truth about Pycnogenol.* Canada: R&T Press, 1996.
44. Murray, Michael T. "PCO Sources: Grape Seed vs Pine Bark—a review and comparison." Botanical Report in *Health Counselor* 7: 1.
45. Passwater, R. and C. Kandaswami. *Pycnogenol: The Super "Protector" Nutrient.* New Canaan, CT: Keats Publishing, Inc., 1994, pages 7–8.
46. Atkins, Robert C., M.D. *Dr. Robert Atkins' Vita-Nutrient Solution.* New York: Simon & Schuster, 1998.
47. Hendler, Sheldon Saul, M.D., Ph.D. *The Doctors' Vitamin and Mineral Encyclopedia.* New York: Simon and Schuster, 1990, page 102.
48. Clark, Linda. *Nutrition & Cancer.* 1984, 6: 13–21.
49. Meydani, Simin Bikbin, D.V.M., Ph.D. "Effect of Vitamin E Supplementation on Immune Responsiveness of Healthy Elderly Subjects." Paper read at a seminar conducted by the New York Academy of Sciences, November 2, 1988.
50. Wald, N., et al. *British Journal of Cancer* 49 (1989): 321–324.
51. Knekt, P., et al. *American Journal of Clinical Nutrition* 53 (1991): 283S–286S
52. *British Journal of Cancer* 49 (1984): 321–324.
    International Journal of Epidemiology 17 (1988): 281–286.
    Journal of the American College of Nutrition 4 (September–October 1985): 559–564.
53. Fredericks, Carlton. *Look Younger, Feel Healthier.* New York: Grosset & Dunlap, 1972, page 136.
54. Cooper, Kenneth H. *Antioxidant Revolution.* Nashville: Thomas Nelson, 1994, pages 138–139.
55. Cooper, Kenneth H. *Mutation Research* 346 (April 1995): 195–202. Found in *Antioxidant Revolution.*
56. "Selenium: A Quest for Better Understanding." *Alternative Therapies* 2.4 (July 1996): 59–67.
57. Passwater, Richard A., Ph.D. *Cancer Prevention & Nutritional Therapies.* New Canaan, CT: Keats Publishing, 1983, pages 59–67.
58. Passwater, Richard A., Ph.D. *The New Supernutrition.* New York: Pocket Books, 1991, pages 124–125.
59. Clark, L. C., et al. "Effects of Selenium Supplementation for Cancer Prevention in Patients with Carcinoma of the Skin." *Journal of the American Medical Association* 276.24 (December 25, 1996): 1957–1985.
60. Packer, Lester and Yuichiro Suzuki. "Alpha-Lipoic Acid and Inhibition of Gene Activating Transcription of HIV." Paper presented at Biological Oxidants and Antioxidants: New Developments in Research and Health Effects conference, Pasadena, CA, March 12–13, 1993.
61. Greenamyre, J. T., et al. *Neuroscience Letters* 171 (1994): 17–20.
    Passwater, Richard A. "Lipoic Acid, The Metabolic Antioxidant." *Good Health Guides* (New Canaan, CT: Keats Publishing, Inc., 1995): 1–47.
62. Packer, L., E. H. Witt, and H. J. Tritschler. "Lipoic acid as a biological antioxidant." *Free Radical Biology and Medicine* 19.2 (1995): 227–250.
63. Reschke, B., S. Zeuzem, C. Rosak, et al. "High-dose long-term treatment with thioctic acid in diabetic polyneuropathy." Borbe and Ulrich, eds. *Thioctsaure* (1989): 318–334.
64. Passwater, Richard A. "Lipoic Acid, The Metabolic Antioxidant." *Good Health Guides* (New Canaan, CT: Keats Publishing, Inc., 1995): 1–47.
65. Beach, Gershwin, Hurley. 1982: Rosenbaum 1984: in *Maximum Immunity,* page 116.
66. Folkers, Karl. *Clinical Investigator* (Supplement) 71 (1993): 51–54.
    Folkers, Karl, et al. *Biomedical and Clinical Aspects of Coenzyme Q.* 6 (Elsevier Publishing Co., New York, 1990).
    Bliznakof, Emile G., Ph.D. and Gerald Hunt. *The Miracle Nutrient: Coenzyme Q10.* New York: Bantam Books, 1987.
    Lockwood, K. and K. Folkers. *Biochemical and Biophysical Research Communications* 199 (1994): 1504–8. Found in *Lindberg Nutrition Newsletter* written by Danny Wells.

67. Folkers, K., R. Brown, W. V. Judy, and M. Morita. *Biochemical and Biophysical Research Communications* 192.1 (1993): 241–245.
68. Folkers, K., S. Moesgaard, and K. Lockwood. *Biochemical and Biophysical Research Communications* 199.3 (1994): 1504–1508.
69. Lockwood, Knud, M.D. *Biochemical and Biophysical Research and Communications* 212 (July 6, 1995): 172–177.
    Lockwood, Knud, M.D. *Biochemical and Biophysical Research and Communications* 199 (March 30, 1994): 1504–1508.
    Folkers, Karl, Ph.D. *Biochemical and Biophysical Research and Communications* 192 (April 15, 1993): 241–245.
70. Harman, D. "The Aging Process: Major risk factor for disease and death." *Proceedings of the National Academy of Sciences* USA 88 (1991): 5360–5363.
    Harman, D. "Aging: Prospects for further increases in the functional life span." *Age* 17 (1994): 119–146.
    Carper, Jean. *Stop Aging Now!* New York: HarperCollins, 1996.
71. Newsletter from the Linus Pauling Institute of Science and Medicine, Palo Alto, CA.
72. Julius, M. "Glutathione and Morbidity in a Community-based Sample of Elderly." *Journal of Clinical Epidemiology* 47.9 (1994): 1021–1026.
73. Carper, Jean. *Stop Aging Now!* New York: HarperCollins, 1996, page 124.
74. *Ibid.*
75. Braverman, E. R. and C. C. Pfeiffer. *The Healing Nutrients Within.* New Canaan, CT: Keats Publishing, Inc., 1987, page 99.
76. Jones, D. P. *Nutrition and Cancer* 17.1 (1992): 57–75.
77. Shabert, Judy, M.D., R.D. and Nancy Ehrlich. *The Ultimate Nutrient: Glutamine.* New York: Avery Publishing Group, 1994, page 51.
78. *Ibid.*
79. Welbourne, T. "Increased plasma bicarbonate and growth hormone after an oral glutamine load." *American Journal of Clinical Nutrition* 61.5 (1995): 1058–1061.
80. "The Soybean Solution to Aging." *International Journal of Anti-Aging Medicine* 1.2 (1998).
81. *Ibid.*
82. *Ibid.*

Chapter 4...Herbs and Other Nutrients to Building Immunity

1. *Cancer* 52 (1983): 70–73.
2. Weiss, Gaea and Shandor Weiss. *Growing and Using Healing Herbs.* Emmaus, PA: Rodale Press, 1986, 64–65.
   "Anti-Aging Herbs: The Proven Disease Fighters." *Longevity* (April 1991).
3. *Cancer* 52 (1983): 70–73.
4. Ritchason, Jack. *The Little Herb Encyclopedia,* 3rd ed. Pleasant Grove, UT: Woodland Health Books, 1994, page 14.
5. *Ibid.*
6. Hendler, Sheldon Saul, M.D., Ph.D. *The Doctors' Vitamin and Mineral Encyclopedia.* New York: Simon and Schuster, 1990, page 279.
7. Murray, Michael T., N.D. *Healing Power of Herbs.* Rocklin, CA: Prima Publishing, 1992, pages 86–88.
8. *Ibid.*
9. Mowrey, Daniel B. *Herbal Tonic Therapies.* New Canaan, CT: Keats Publishing Inc., 1993, pages 107–109.
10. Murray, Michael. *Healing Power of Herbs.* Rocklin, CA: Prima Publishing, 1992, pages 80–84.
11. Ritchason, Jack. *The Little Herb Encyclopedia,* 3rd ed. Pleasant Grove, UT: Woodland Health Books, 1994, page 14.
12. Ritchason, Jack. *The Little Herb Encyclopedia,* 3rd ed. Pleasant Grove, UT: Woodland Health Books, 1994, page 14.
13. Steinberg, Phillip N. "A Wondrous Herb from the Peruvian Rainforest." *Townsend Letter for Doctors* (An Informal Letter Magazine for Doctors Communicating with Doctors) 130: May 1994.
    "Plant Metabolites: New compounds and anti-inflammatory activity of Uncaria

tomentosa." *Journal of Natural Products* 54.2 (May/June 1991): 453–459.

"The alkaloids of uncaria tomentosa and their phagocytosis increasing effects." *Planta Medica* 51 (1985): 419–423.

14.   Davis, Brent W. "A New World Class Herb for AK Practice." (Summer 1992).

      "Phytochemical and biological research on uncaria tomentosa." *Bollettino—Societa Italiana Biologia Sperimentale* 65.6 (1989): 517–520.

15.   Lindberg, Gladys, and Judy McFarland. *Take Charge of Your Health.* San Francisco: Harper and Row, 1982, page 20.

      Airola, Paavo, M.D., Ph.D. *Every Woman's Book.* Phoenix: Health Plus, Publishers 1979, pages 440–442.

16.   Hendler, Sheldon, M.D., Ph.D. *The Doctors' Vitamin & Mineral Encyclopedia.* New York: Simon & Shuster, 1990, page 315.

      Vogel, G. "A Peculiarity among the flavonoids: silymarin, a compound active on the liver." *Munich Proceedings of the International Bioflavonoid Symposium* (1981): 461–480.

17.   Ritchason, Jack. *The Little Herb Encyclopedia,* 3rd ed. Pleasant Grove, UT: Woodland Health Books, 1994, page 146.

18.   Sonnenbichler, J., et al. *Biochemical Pharmacology* 35 (1986): 538–541.

19.   Feher, J. "Liver protective action of silymarin therapy in chronic alcoholic liver diseases." *Orvosi Hetilap* 130.51 (1989): 2723–7.

      Ferenci, R. "Randomized controlled trial of silymarin treatment inpatients with cirrhosis of the liver." *Journal of Hepatology* 9 (1989): 105–113.

20.   Carper, Jean. *Miracle Cures.* New York: HarperCollins Publishers, 1997.

21.   Salmi, H. A., et al. "Effect of silymarin on Chemical, Functional and Morphological Alteration of the Liver." *Scandinavian Journal of Gastroenterology* 17 (1982): 517–521.

22.   "Anti-Aging Physicians' Desk Reference." *International Journal of Anti-Aging Medicine* 1.2 (1998).

23.   Lieberman, Sheri, Ph.D. and Ken Babal, C.N. *Maitake: King of Mushrooms.* New Canaan, CT: Keats Good Health Guide, Keats Publishing, Inc., 1997.

24.   Nanba, H. "Maitake D-fraction, Healing and Preventing Potential for Cancer." *Townsend Letter for Doctors & Patients* (February/March 1996): 84–85.

25.   Nanba, H. et al. "The Chemical Structure of an Antitumor Polysaccharide in Fruit Bodies of Grifola Frondosa (Maitake)." *Chemical Pharmacology Bulletin* 35.3. (1987): 1162–1168.

      Lieberman, Sheri, Ph.D. and Ken Babal, C.N. *Maitake: King of Mushrooms.* New Canaan, CT: Keats Good Health Guide, Keats Publishing, Inc., 1997.

      Nanba, H., Maitake D-Fraction: Healing and Preventative Potential for Cancer. J. *Orthomol Med* 1997;12:43–49.

26.   Kaylor, Mark. "Maitake D-fraction: The Mushroom World's Gift for Today." Formulator for *Nature's Answer* 3.3. Mayell M., Maitake Extracts and Their Therapeutic Potential. *Altern. Medicine* Rev 2001;6:48–60.

      Jones, K., Maitake: A Potent Medicinal Food. *Alt Comp Ther* 1998;4:420–29

      Mayell M., Maitake Extracts and Their Therapeutic Potential. *Altern. Medicine* Rev 2001;6:48–60.

27.   Lieberman, Sheri, Ph.D. and Ken Babal, C.N. *Maitake King of Mushrooms.* New Canaan, CT: Keats Publishing, Inc., 1997.

28.   Zimmerman, Marcia, C.N. "Immune Enhancers." *Nutrition Science News* 4.2 (February 1999).

29.   Ritchason, Jack, N.D. *The Little Herb Encyclopedia Revised.* Pleasant Grove, UT: Woodland Health Books, 1994.

30.   F. Jordon, "An Immuno-Potentiating Super Hero-Beta-1,3/1,6-glucan Derived from Yeast Cell Wall," *Macrophage Technologies Publication* (1998): 1–4.

31.   Schultz et al., Association of Macrophage Activation with Anti-tumor Activity by Synthetic and Biologic Agents," *Cancer Res.* 37 (1997): 3338–3343.

32.   Life Extension, *Disease Prevention and Treatment,* 3rd Edition, 2000. Copyright 1997, 1998, 2000 Life Extension Media.

33.   *Alternative Medicine Review,* Volume 7, Number 2, 2002.

34.   Clark, Daniel, M.D., and Kaye Watt. *Colostrum: Life's First Food—The Ultimate Anti-aging Weight Loss and immune Supplement.* Salt Lake City: CRN Publications, 1998.

35.   Preston, R. "Bovine Colostrum; Human Consumption; Efficacy and Effects." *International Institute of Nutritional Research* (1987).

36. Reduction of Cell Proliferation and Enhancement of NK-Cell Activity, United States Patent # 5,082,833, Date of Patent: January 21, 1992, Inventor: Abulkalam M. Shamsuddin.
Shamsuddin AM. Metabolismans cellular functions of IP6: a review. Anticancer Res. 1999;19:3733–36
Jariwalla RJ. Inositol hexaphosphate (IP6) as an anti-neoplastic and lipid-lowering agent. Anticancer Res 1999;19:3699–702

Chapter 5...Mirror, Mirror on the Wall

1. Braverman, E. R. and C. C. Pfeiffer. *The Healing Nutrients Within*. New Canaan, CT: Keats Publishing, Inc., 1987, page 91.
2. Lindberg, Gladys and Judy McFarland. *Take Charge of Your Health*. San Francisco: Harper and Row, 1982, page 67.
3. Williams, Roger J., Ph.D. *Physicians Handbook of Nutritional Science*. Springfield, MO: C.C. Thomas, 1974, as found in *The Big Book of Vitamins* by Ruth Adams, New Canaan, CT: Keats Publishing, Inc., 1992, page 183.
4. *Ibid.*
5. Kuttan, R., et al. *Experientia* 37 (1981): 221–223.
6. *Prima Health*, 1998. A Division of Prima Publishing, U.S.A.
7. Murray, Frank. *The Big Family Guide to All the Minerals*. New Canaan, CT: Keats Publishing, Inc., 1995, pages 345–350.
Carlisle, E. M. "The Nutritional Essentiality of Silicon." *Nutrition Review* 40 (1982): 193–198.
8. Murray, Frank. *The Big Family Guide to All the Minerals*. New Canaan, CT: Keats Publishing, Inc., 1995, pages 345–350.
Ritchason, Jack. *The Little Herb Encyclopedia*, 3rd ed. Pleasant Grove, UT: Woodland Health Books, 1994, pages 121–122.
9. Erdmann, Robert, Ph.D. *The Amino Revolution*. New York: A Fireside Book by Simon & Schuster, Inc., 1987, page 194.
10. Braverman, E. R. and C. C. Pfeiffer. *The Healing Nutrients Within*. New Canaan, CT: Keats Publishing, Inc., 1987, page 91.
11. Pfeiffer, Carl C., Ph.D, M.D. *Mental and Elemental Nutrients*. New Canaan, CT: Keats Publishing, Inc., 1975, pages 84–85. (Note: in the body, cysteine will readily convert to cystine, and vice versa, so for the sake of convenience I will refer to either as cysteine.)
12. Ley, B. *The Forgotten Nutrient: MSM*. Viejo, CA: Health Learning Handbooks, BL Publications, 1998.
13. Vaughn, Sam and Janis Donnaud, eds. *The American Medical Association Encyclopedia of Medicine*. New York: Random House, 1989.
Ley, B. *The Forgotten Nutrient: MSM*. Viejo, CA: Health Learning Handbooks, BL Publications, 1998.
14. Newbold, H. L., M.D. *Mega Nutrients for Your Nerves*. New York: Peter H. Wyden, 1975, page 299.
15. Williams, Roger. *Nutrition Against Disease*. New York: Bantam Books, 1971.
Vaughn, Sam and Janis Donnaud, eds. *The American Medical Association Encyclopedia of Medicine*. New York: Random House, 1989.
16. Werbach, Melvyn R., M.D. *Nutritional Influences on Illness: A Sourcebook of Clinical Research*. Tarzana, CA: Third Line Press, 1993, pages 265–269.
Stewart, J. C. M., et al. "Treatment of severe and moderately severe atopic dermatitis with evening primrose oil (Epogram): a multi-center study." *Journal of Nutritional Medicine* 2 (1991): 9–15.
Allsion, J. R. "The relation of deficiency of hydrochloric acid and vitamin B-complex in certain skin diseases." *Southern Medical Journal* 38 (1945): 235–241.
17. Werbach, Melvyn R., M.D. *Nutritional Influences on Illness: A Sourcebook of Clinical Research*. Tarzana, CA: Third Line Press, 1993, pages 265–269.
18. *Ibid.*
19. Ellis, C. N., et al. *Journal of the American Academy of Dermatology* 29 (September 1992): 438–442.
Kurkcuoglu, N. and F. Alaybeyi. "Topical Capsaicin for Psoriasis." *British Journal of*

       Dermatology 123.4 (October 1990): 549–550.

20. Vaughn, Sam and Janis Donnaud, eds. *The American Medical Association Encyclopedia of Medicine.* New York: Random House, 1989.
21. Wright, Jonathan, M.D. *Dr. Wright's Guide to Healing with Nutrition.* Erasmus, PA: Rodale Press, 1984.
       Murray, Frank. "Acidophilus: The Friendly Bacteria." *Better Nutrition* (January 1987).
22. Lindberg, Gladys and Judy McFarland. *Take Charge of Your Health.* San Francisco: Harper and Row, 1982, page 233.
23. Davis, Adelle. *Let's Get Well.* New York: Signet, Published by the Penguin Group, 1972, pages 134–135.
24. Hendler, Sheldon Saul, M.D., Ph.D. *The Doctors' Vitamin and Mineral Encyclopedia.* New York: Simon and Schuster, 1990.
25. Smith, Lendon, M.D. *Feed Yourself Right.* New York: Dell Publishing Co., Inc., 1983, pages 363–367.
26. *U.S. Pharmacist* 15 (12): 27.
       Goldberg, Burton. *Alternative Medicine: The Definitive Guide.* Puyallup, WA: Future Medicine Pub., 1994. Contains information on all types of skin disorders.
27. Braverman, E. R. and C. C. Pfeiffer. *The Healing Nutrients Within.* New Canaan, CT: Keats Publishing, Inc., 1987, page 91.
       Buchanan, J. H. and M. S. Otterburn. "Some structural comparisons between cysteine-deficient and normal hair keratin." *IRCS Med Sci* 12 (1984): 691–692.
28. Information about all deficiency symptoms can be found in:
       Lindberg, Gladys and Judy McFarland. *Take Charge of Your Health.* San Francisco: Harper and Row, 1982, pages 184–241.
29. Lindberg, Gladys, and Judy McFarland. *Take Charge of Your Health.* San Francisco: Harper and Row, 1982.
30. Packer, Lester, Ph.D. and Carol Colman. *The Antioxidant Miracle.* New York: John Wiley & Sons, Inc., 1999.
31. *Ibid.*
32. Sepp, Dr. Dennis T. "Skin & The Aging Process." SkiKai Products.
33. Tenney, Louise. *Today's Herbal Health.* Provo, UT: Woodland Books, 1983, page 21.
34. Wesley-Hosford, Zia. *Fifty & Fabulous.* Rocklin, CA: Prima Publishing, 1995.
35. Wells, Danny. *Lindberg Newsletter* (December 1995).
       Brown, Royden. *Bee Hive Products Bible.* Garden City Park, NY: Avery Publishing Group Inc., 1993.
36. *Ibid.*
37. *Prevention* Magazine Health Books, eds. *Age Erasers for Women.* Rodale Press, Inc., 1994, page 487.
38. Belaiche, P. "Treatment of Vaginal Infections of Candida Albicans with the Essential Oil of Melaleuca Alternifolia." *Phylotherapie* 15 (1985).
       Pena, E. "Melaleuca Alternifolia Oil, Uses for Trichomonal Vaginitis and Other Vaginal Infections." *Obstetrics and Gynecology* (June 1962).
       Walker, M. "Clinical Investigation of Australian Melaleuca Alternifolia Oil for a Variety of Common Foot Problems." *Current Podiatry* (April 1972).

Chapter 6...Eyes—Our Windows to the World

1. Wertenbaker, Lael. *The Eye: Window to the World.* Washington, D.C.: U.S. News Books, division of *U.S. News & World Report,* Inc., page 7.
2. Vaughn, Sam and Janis Donnaud, eds. *The American Medical Association Encyclopedia of Medicine.* New York: Random House, 1989.
3. Pauling, L., M.D. *How to Live Longer and Feel Better.* New York: W.H. Freeman & Co., 1986, page 208.
4. Bouton, S. M., Jr. "Vitamin C and the Aging Eye." *Archives of Internal Medicine* 63 (1939): 930–945.
       Muhlmann, V., et al. "Vitamin C Therapy of Incipient Senile Cataract." *Archivos de Oftalmologia de Buenos Aires* 14 (1939): 552–575.
5. Adams, Ruth. *The Big Family Guide to All the Vitamins.* New Canaan, CT: Keats Publishing, 1992, page 241.
6. Bunce, G. E. "Nutrition and Eye Disease of the Elderly." *Journal of Nutritional*

Biochemistry 5 (February 1994): 66–76.

7. Adams, Ruth. *The Big Family Guide to All the Vitamins*. New Canaan, CT: Keats Publishing, 1992, pages 424–425.

8. Taylor, Allen. *Science News* vol. 135, from USDA Human Nutrition Research Center on Aging in Medford, MA.

9. Varma, S. D., D. Chand, Y. R. Sharma, J. F. Kuck, Jr. and R. D. Richards. "Oxidative Stress on Lens and Cataract Formation." *Current Eye Research* 3: 35–57.
Jacques, P. F., et al. "Antioxidant status in persons with and without senile cataract." *Archives of Ophthalmology* 106.3 (1988): 337–340.

10. *Archives of Ophthalmology* (February 1991).

11. Azar, Robert. *Prevention* (July 1983): 99–103. As found in Melvyn Werbach, *Healing Through Nutrition*. HarperCollins Publisher, 1993, page 71.

12. Cheraskin, E., M.D., W. M. Ringsdorf, Jr., and E. L. Sisley. *The Vitamin C Connection*. NY: Harper & Row, 1983.

13. Brietti, G. B., "Further Contributions on the Value of Osmotic Substances As Means to Reduce Intra–Ocular Pressure." *Ophthalmological Society of Australia* 26: 61–71.
Virno, M., et al. "Oral Treatment of Glaucoma with Vitamin C." *The Eye, Ear, Nose, and Throat Monthly* 46: 1502–1508.

14. Packer, Lester, Ph.D. and Carol Colman. *The Antioxidant Miracle*. New York: John Wiley & Sons, Inc., 1999.

15. Vaughn, Sam and Janis Donnaud, eds. *The American Medical Association Encyclopedia of Medicine*. New York: Random House, 1989, page 658.

16. Werbach, Melvyn. *Healing Through Nutrition*. New York: HarperCollins Publisher, 1993, page 114.

17. Levine, L. *Journal of Behavioral Optometry* 3 No. 5 (1992): 115–119.

18. *Physician's Desk Reference*, 46th ed. Montvale, NJ: Medical Economics Data, 1992.

19. Ritchason, Jack. *The Little Herb Encyclopedia*, 3rd ed. Pleasant Grove, UT: Woodland Health Books, 1994, pages 24–25.

20. *Ibid.*, pages 98–99.

21. Murray, Michael, N.D. and Joseph Pizzorno, N.D. *Encyclopedia of Natural Medicine*. Rocklin, CA: Prima Publishing, 1990, pages 408–409.

22. Seddon, Johanna M., M.D., et al. "Dietary Carotenoids, Vitamins A, C and E and Advanced Age-Related Macular Degeneration." *Journal of the American Medical Association* 272.18 (November 9, 1994): 1413–1420.

23. *Diet & Nutrition Letter* 12 (Tufts University, January 1995): 11.

24. "New Antioxidant defends against free radical damage." *Nutrition News* (1989).

25. Werbach, M. R., M.D. and M. Murray, N.D. *Botanical Influences on Illness: A Sourcebook of Clinical Research*. Tarzana, CA: Third Line Press (1994).

26. McBeth, Joyce, R.N., C.N., ed. "Antioxidants and Anti-Aging—The Fight Against Free-Radicals." *American Council on Collaborative Medicine* 1.8 (November 1995).

27. Gaby, A. R., M.D. and J. V. Wright. "Nutritional Factors in Degenerative Eye Disorders: Cataract and Macular Degeneration." *Journal of Advancement in Medicine* 6.1 (Spring 1993): 27–39.

28. Bunce, G. E., Ph.D. "Nutrition and Eye Disease of the Elderly." *Journal of Nutritional Biochemistry* 5 (February 1994): 66–77.
Schalch, Wolfgang. "Carotenoids in the Retina—A Review of Their Possible Role in Preventing or Limiting Damage Caused by Light and Oxygen." *Free-Radicals in Aging* (1992): 280–298.
Seddon, Johanna M., M.D., et al. "Dietary Carotenoids, Vitamins A, C and E and Advanced Age-Related Macular Degeneration." *Journal of the American Medical Association* 272.18 (November 9, 1994): 1413–1420.

29. Schalch, Wolfgang. "Carotenoids in the Retina—A Review of Their Possible Role in Preventing or Limiting Damage Caused by Light and Oxygen." *Free-Radicals in Aging* (1992): 280–298.

30. Lindberg, Gladys and Judy McFarland. *Take Charge of Your Health*. San Francisco: Harper and Row, 1982, pages 188–189.

31. Fredericks, Carlton, M.D. *The Prevention and Cure for Common Ailments & Diseases*. New York: A Fireside Book, Simon & Schuster, 1982, page 58.

32. Lindberg, Gladys and Judy McFarland. *Take Charge of Your Health*. San Francisco: Harper and Row, 1982, page 184.

33. Hendler, Sheldon Saul, M.D., Ph.D. *The Doctors' Vitamin and Mineral Encyclopedia.* New York: Simon and Schuster, 1990, page 199.
34. Lindberg, Gladys and Judy McFarland. *Take Charge of Your Health.* San Francisco: Harper and Row, 1982, page 65.
35. Hendler, Sheldon Saul, M.D., Ph.D., *The Doctors' Vitamin and Mineral Encyclopedia.* New York: Simon and Schuster, 1990, pages 224–225.
36. Bates, William H., M.D. *The Bates Method for Better Eyesight Without Glasses.* New York: Henry Holt & Co., 1981.

Chapter 7 ... Anti-Aging Nutrients for Our Brain

1.   Simon, Harvey B., M.D. *Staying Well.* Boston: Houghton Mifflin Co., 1992, pages 74–79.
2.   *Ibid.*
3.   *Ibid.*
4.   Crook, T. H., et al. "Recalling names after introduction: changes across the adult life span in two cultures." *Developmental Neuropsychology* 9 (1993): 103–13.
     Youngjohn, J. R., et al. "Test-retest reliability of computerized everyday memory measures and traditional memory tests." *Clinical Neuropsychologist* 6 (1992): 276–86.
     Ivnik, R. J., et al. "Traditional and computerized assessment procedures applied to the evaluation of memory change after temporal lobectomy." *Archives of Clinical Neuropsychology* 8 (1993): 69–81, as presented at the NNFA lecture in Nashville, TN, July 1996.
5.   Kreitsch, K., et al. "Prevalence, presenting symptoms, and psychological characteristics of individuals experiencing a diet-related mood disturbance." *Behavioral Therapy* 19 (1988): 593–604.
6.   Subar, A. F., et al. "Folate intake and food sources in the US population." *American Journal of Clinical Nutrition* 50 (1989): 508–516.
     Abou-Salen, M. T. and A. Coppen. "The biology of folate in depression: Implications for nutritional hypotheses of the psychoses." *Journal of Psychiatric Research* 20 (1986): 91–101.
     Godfrey, P. S. A., et al. "Enhancement of recovery from psychiatric illness by methylfolate," *Lancet* 336 (1990): 392–395.
     Botez, M. I., et al. "Neuropsychological correlates of folic acid deficiency: Facts and hypotheses." M. I. Botez, E. H. Reynolds, eds. *Folic Acid in Neurology, Psychiatry and Internal Medicine* (New York: Raven Press, 1979).
7.   Braverman, E. R. and C. C. Pfeiffer. *The Healing Nutrients Within.* New Canaan, CT: Keats Publishing, Inc., 1987, page 59.
8.   *Ibid.*
9.   Lemock, M. "The Mood Molecule." *Time* 74 (September 29, 1997).
     Babal, K. "The Fall and Rise of Tryptophan." *Nutrition Science News* 3.2 (February 1998).
10. Braverman, E. R. and C. C. Pfeiffer. *The Healing Nutrients Within.* New Canaan, CT: Keats Publishing, Inc., 1987, page 59.
     Hendler, Sheldon Saul, M.D. *The Doctors' Vitamin & Mineral Encyclopedia.* New York: Simon & Shuster, 1990, pages 228–234.
11. Pearson, D. and S. Shaw. *Life Extension: A Practical Scientific Approach.* New York: Warner Books, 1982.
12. Werbach, M. *Nutritional Influences on Mental Illness: A Sourcebook of Clinical Research.* Tarzana, CA: Third Line Press, 1991.
     Murray, Michael, N.D. *Ask the Doctor.* Vital Communications, Inc., 1998.
13. Hoebel, B. G. "Brain neurotransmitters in food and drug reward." *American Journal of Clinical Nutrition (Supplement)* 42.5 (1985): 1133–1150.
14. Sano, I. "L-5-hydroxytryptophan (L-5HTP) therapies." *Folia Psychiatrica et Neurologica Japonica* 26 (1972): 7–17.
15. Cangiano, C., et al. "Eating Behavior and Adherence to Dietary Prescriptions in Obese Subjects Treated with 5-Hydroxytryptophan." *American Journal of Clinical Nutrition* 56 (1992): 863–868.
16. Kahn, R. S., et al. "L-5 Hydroxytryptophan in the Treatment of Anxiety Disorders." *Journal of Affective Disorders* 8 (1985): 197–200.

17. Carper, Jean. *Miracle Cures*. New York: HarperCollins Publishers, 1997.
18. *Ibid.*
Woelk, H. "Benefits and risks of the hypericum extract LI 160: drug-monitoring study with 3250 patients." *Journal of Geriatric Psychiatry and Neurology (Supplement-1)* 7 (1994): S34–38.
Ernst, E. "St. John's wort, an antidepressant? A systematic, criteria-based review." *Phytomedicine* 2 (1995):67–71.
19. Carper, Jean. *Miracle Cures*. New York: HarperCollins Publishers, 1997.
Sommer, H. "Placebo-controlled double-blind study examining the effectiveness of an hypericum preparation in 105 mildly depressed patients." *Journal of Geriatric Psychiatry and Neurology (Supplement-1)* 7 (1994): S9–11.
20. Cowley, Geoffrey and Anne Underwood. "What Is SAMe?" *Newsweek* (July 5, 1999).
21. *Ibid.*
22. Jean Carper. *Your Miracle Brain*, Harper Collins Publishers, New N.Y.
23. *Dr. Murray's Total Body Tune-Up*, by Michael Murray, N.D., Bantam Books New York, 2000.
24. Fredericks, Carlton, Ph.D. *Program for Living Longer*. New York: Simon & Schuster, 1983.
Hendler, Sheldon Saul, M.D., Ph.D. *The Doctors' Vitamin and Mineral Encyclopedia*. New York: Simon and Schuster, 1990, pages 232–234.
25. Frank, O., et al. "Superiority of periodic intramuscular vitamin injections over daily oral vitamins in maintaining normal vitamin titers in a geriatric population." *American Journal of Clinical Nutrition* 30 (1977): 630.
26. Lindberg, Gladys and Judy McFarland. *Take Charge of Your Health*. San Francisco: Harper and Row, 1982.
27. Benton, D., et al. "The impact of long-term vitamin supplementation on cognitive function." *Psychopharmacology* 117: 298–305, 195
Meador, K. J., et al. "Evidence for a central cholinergic effect of high dose thiamine." *Annals of Neurology* 34 (1993): 724–26. This high dose may throw off the B vitamin balance, so be careful.
28. Hoffer, Abram, M.D., Ph.D. *Orthomolecular Medicine for Physicians*. New Canaan, CT: Keats Publishing, Inc., 1989, pages 149–152.
29. Adams, Ruth. *Big Family Guide to All the Vitamins*. New Canaan, CT: Keats Publishing, Inc., 1992, pages 127–128.
Hoffer, A. *Niacin Therapy in Schizophrenia*. Springfield, IL: Charles C. Thomas, 1962.
30. Hoffer, A. and H. Osmond. "Treatment of schizophrenia with nicotinic acid: a ten-year follow up." *Acta Psychiatrica Scandinavica* 40 (1964): 171–189.
31. Osmond, H. and A. Hoffer. "Massive niacin treatment in schizophrenia: review of a nine-year study." *Lancet* 1: 316–319.
32. Botez, M. I., et al. "Neuropsychological correlates of folic acid deficiency: Facts and hypotheses." M. I. Botez, E. H. Reynolds, eds. *Folic Acid in Neurology, Psychiatry and Internal Medicine* (New York: Raven Press, 1979).
Braverman, E. R. and C. C. Pfeiffer. *The Healing Nutrients Within*. New Canaan, CT: Keats Publishing, Inc., 1987, page 59.
33. Goodwin, James S., M.D. "On Nutrition & Memory." *Executive Health* (October 1984).
34. Pary, T. E. "Folate Responsive Neuropathy." *La Presse Medicale* 23.3 (Jan 29, 1994): 131–137.
35. Wright, Jonathan V., M.D. and Alan Gaby, M.D. *Nutrition & Healing* 2.3 (March 1995): 9.
36. Hendler, Sheldon Saul, M.D., Ph.D. *The Doctors' Vitamin and Mineral Encyclopedia*. New York: Simon and Schuster, 1990, page 69.
Beck, W. S. "Cobalamin and the nervous system (editorial)." *New England Journal of Medicine* 318 (1988): 1752–1754.
37. Garcia, C. A., M. J. Reding, and J. P. Blass. "Over diagnosis of dementia." *Journal of the American Geriatrics Society* 29 (1981): pages 407–410.
Dommisse, J. "Subtle vitamin B12 deficiency and psychiatry: A largely unnoticed but devastating relationship?" *Medical Hypotheses* 34 (1991): 131–140.
"Vitamin B12 deficiency often overlooked." *News* (University of Colorado Health Sciences Center, June 30, 1988).
38. Craig, G. M., C. Elliot, and K. R. Hughes. "Masked vitamin B12 and folate deficiency in the elderly." *British Journal of Nutrition* 54 (1985): pages 613–619.
39. Murray, Michael, N.D. and Joseph Pizzorno, N.D. *Encyclopedia of Natural Medicine*.

Rocklin, CA: Prima Publishing, 1990, page 133.

40. van Tiggelen, C. J. M., et al. "Assessment of vitamin B12 status in CFS." *American Journal of Psychiatry* 141 (1984): 136. As found in *Nutrition & Healing.* Wright, Jonathan V. and Alan R. Gaby. *Nutrition & Healing* 2.3 (March 1995).

41. Rogers, L. L. and R. B. Pelton. "Effect of Glutamine on I.Q. Scores of Mentally Deficient Children." *Texas Reports on Biology and Medicine* 15.1 (1957): 84–90.

42. Rogers, L. L., R. B. Pelton, and R. Williams. "Voluntary Alcohol Consumption by Rats Following Administration of Glutamine." *Journal of Biological Chemistry* 214.2 (1955): 503–506.

43. Werbach, Melvyn. *Healing Through Nutrition.* New York: HarperCollins Publisher, 1993, page 15.

44. Trunnell, J. B. and J. I. Wheeler. "Preliminary Report on Experiments with Orally Administered Glutamine in Treatment of Alcoholics." *Journal of the American Chemistry Society* (Houston, December 1955).

45. Young, L. S., et al. "Patients Receiving Glutamine Supplemented Intravenous Feedings Report an Improvement in Mood." *Journal of Parenteral and Enteral Nutrition* 17 (1993): 422–427.

46. Welbourne, T. "Increased Plasma Bicarbonate and Growth Hormone After an Oral Glutamine Load." *American Journal of Clinical Nutrition* 61 (1995): 1058–1061.

47. Pelton, Ross, R.Ph., Ph.D. and Taffy Clarke Pelton. *Mind Food & Smart Pills.* New York: Doubleday, 1989.

48. *Ibid.*

49. Gebner, A., et al. "Study of the Long-term Action of a Ginkgo Biloba Extract on Vigilance and Mental Performance as Determined by Means of Quantitative Pharmaco-EEG and Psychometric Measurements." *Arzeneimittel-Forschung* 35.9: 1459. Murray, Frank. *Ginkgo Biloba.* New Canaan, CT: Keats Publishing, 1993, pages 15–21.

50. Warburton, D. M. "Clinical Psychopharmacology of Ginkgo Biloba Extract." *La Presse Medicale* 15.31 (1986): 1595.

51. Schuitemaker, Dr. G. E. "Ginkgo Against Senility." Dutch and German magazine *Orthomolecular* (1988). A publication of the European Institute for Orthomolecular Science.
"Intermittent Claudication: Trental vs. Ginkgo biloba extract." *American Journal of Natural Medicine* 2.1 (January/February 1995): 10–13.

52. Hobbs, Christopher. *Ginkgo: Elixir of Youth.* Santa Cruz, CA: Botanica Press, 1995, page 57.

53. Wurtman, R. J. "The choline-deficient diet." *FASEB Journal* 5 (1991): 2612.

54. Lindberg, Gladys and Judy McFarland. *Take Charge of Your Health.* San Francisco: Harper and Row, 1982, pages 88–89.

55. Hendler, Sheldon Saul, M.D., Ph.D. *Purification Prescription.* New York: William Morrow and Co., Inc., 1991, pages 61–63.

56. *Nutrition Science News* 2.10 (October 1997).
Meck, W. H. "Choline and development of brain memory functions across the lifespan." Seventh International Congress of Phospholipids (Brussels, Belgium, September 1996).

57. *Nutrition Science News* 2.10 (October 1997).
Safford, F. and B. Baumel. "Testing the effects of dietary lecithin on memory in the elderly: An example of social work/medical research collaboration." *Research on Social Work Practice* 4 (1994): 349–358.

58. Passwater, Richard A., Ph.D. *The New Supernutrition.* New York: Pocket Books, 1991, pages 55–56.

59. Hendler, Sheldon Saul, M.D., Ph.D. *Purification Prescription.* New York: William Morrow and Co., Inc., 1991, pages 61–63.

60. Hendler, Sheldon Saul, M.D., Ph.D. *The Doctor's Vitamin and Mineral Encyclopedia.* New York: Simon & Schuster, 1990, page 263.

61. Kidd, Parris M., Ph.D. "Phosphatidyl serine and Aging." *Healthy & Natural Journal* 2.5.

62. Crook, T. H., et al. "Effects of phosphatidyl serine in age-associated memory impairment." *Neurology* 41 (1991): 644–649.

63. *Ibid.*

64. Cenacchi, B., et al. "Cognitive decline in the elderly: A double-blind placebo controlled multi-centered study on efficacy of phosphatidyl serine administration." *Aging—Clinical and Experimental Research* 5 (1993): 123–133.

65. *Ibid.*
66. Palmieri, G., et al. "Double-blind controlled trial of PS in subjects with senile mental deterioration." *Clinical Trials Journal* 24 (1987): 73–83.
67. Dean, Ward, M.D., John Morgenthaler, and Steven Fowkes. *Smart Drugs II: The Next Generation.* Menlo Park, CA: Smart Publications, 1993, pages 91–93.
68. Cipolli, C. and G. Chiari. "Effetti della L-acetilcarnitina sul deterioramento mentale dell'anziano: primi risultati (Effects of L-acetilcarnitine on mental deterioration in the aged: initial results) (6 Suppl)" *Clinica Terapeutica* 132 (March 1990): 479–510, 31. As found in *Smart Drugs II.*
69. Bella, R., R. Biondi, R. Raffaele, and G. Pennisi. "Effect of acetyl-L-carnitine on geriatric patients suffering from dysthymic disorders." *International Journal of Clinical Pharmacology Research* 10.6 (1990): 355–360.
70. Scrofani, A., R. Biondi, V. Sofia, F. D'Alpa, A. Grasso, and S. Filetti. "EEG patterns of patients with cerebrovascular damage. Effect of L-acetylcarnitine during sleep (Suppl. 1)." *Clinical Trials Journal* 25 (United Kingdom, 1988): 65–71.
71. Fulgente, T., M. Onofrj, M. L. Del Re, F. Ferrancci, S. Bazzano, M. F. Ghilardi, and G. Malatesta. "Laevo-acetylcarnitine (Nicetiel) treatment of senile depression." *Clinical Trials Journal* (United Kingdom) 27.3 (1990): 155–163.
    Garzya, G., D. Corallo, A. Fiore, G. Lecciso, G. Petrelli, and C. Zotti. "Evaluation of the effects of L-acetylcarnitine on senile patients suffering from depression." *Drugs Under Experimental and Clinical Research* 16.2 (Switzerland, 1990): 101–6.
    Villardita, C., P. Smirni, and I. Vecchio. "N-acetylcarnitine in depressed elderly patients (L'Acetil carnitina nei disturbi della sfera affettiva dell'anziano)." Italy: *European Review for Medical and Pharmacological Sciences* 6.2 (1984): 341–344.
    Tempesta, E., L. Casella, C. Pirrongelli, L. Janiri, M. Calvani, and L. Ancona. "L-acetyl-carnitine in depressed elderly subjects. A cross-over study vs. placebo." *Drugs Under Experimental and Clinical Research* 13.7 (1987): 417–423.
72. Sinforiani, E., M. Iannuccelli, M. Mauri, A. Costa, P. Merlo, G. Bono, and G. Nappi "Neuropsychological changes in demented patients treated with acetyl-L-carnitine." *International Journal of Clinical Pharmacology Research* 10.1–2 (1990): 69–74.
    Bonavita, E. "Study of the efficacy and tolerability of L-acetylcarnitine therapy in the senile brain." *Journal of Clinical Pharmacology, Therapy, and Toxicology* 24 (1986): 511–516.
    Bonavita, E., D. Bertuzzi, J. Bonavita, and A. Marani. "L-acetylcarnitine (L-Ac) (Branigen) in the long-term symptomatic treatment of senile dementia. Optimal treatment times and suspension periods." United Kingdom: *Clinical Trials Journal* 25.4 (1988): 227–237.
73. Passeri, M., D. Cucinotta, P. A. Bonati, M. Iannuccelli, L. Parnetti, and U. Senin. "Acetyl-L-carnitine in the treatment of mildly demented elderly patients." *International Journal of Clinical Pharmacology Research* 10.1–2 (1990): 75–79.
74. *Neuroscience Letters* 223 (1997): 3.
75. Bowman, B. A. B. "Acetyl-carnitine and Alzheimer's disease." *Nutrition Review* USA 50.5 (1992): 142–144.
    Rai, M. G., G. Wright, L. Scot, B. Beston, J. Rest, and A. N. Exton-Smith. "Double-blind, placebo controlled study of acetyl-L-carnitine in patients with Alzheimer's dementia." *Current Medical Research and Opinion* 11.10 (1990): 638–647.
    Sano, M., K. Bell, L. Cote, G. Dooneief, A. Lawton, L. Legler, K. Marder, A. Naini, Y. Stern, and R. Mayeux. "Double-blind parallel design pilot study of acetyl levocarnitine in patients with Alzheimer's disease." *Archives of Neurology* (United States) 49.11 (November 1992): 1137–1141.
76. Cabrero Lahuerta, M. C. and M. Crotes Blanco. "Current treatment of Alzheimer's disease (Aproximacion al estado actual del tratamiento de la demencia senil tipo Alzheimer)." *Ciencias Medica* (Spain) 9.3 (1992): 82–87.
    Cazzato, G., L. Bonfigli, M. Pasqua, and F. Iaiza. "Long-term treatment with acetyl-L-carnitine in patients suffering from dementia of the Alzheimer's type (Trattamento a lungo termine con L-acetilcarnitina in pazienti affetti da demenza di Alzheimer)." *Neurol Psichiatr Sci Um* (Italy) 10.2 (1990): 201–215.
77. Dean, Ward, M.D., John Morgenthaler, and Steven Fowkes. *Smart Drugs II: The Next Generation.* Menlo Park, CA: Smart Publications, 1993.
78. Regelson, William, M.D. and Carol Colman. *The Superhormone Promise.* New York: Simon & Schuster, 1996.

79. Flood, J. F., J. F. Morley, and E. Roberts. "Memory Enhancing Effects in Male Mice of Pregnenolone and Steroids Metabolically Derived From It." *Proceedings of the National Academy of Sciences* USA 89 (1992): 1567–1571.
80. *Prevention* Magazine's *Complete Book of Vitamins and Minerals for Health*. New York: Wings Books, a division of Rodale Press Inc., 1988, page 208.
81. Braly, James and Laura Torbet. *Dr. Braly's Food Allergy and Nutrition Revolution*. New Canaan, CT: Keats Publishing, 1992, page 153.
82. Pfeiffer, Carl C., et al. "Stimulant Effect of 2-Dimethyl-l-aminoethanol: Possible Precursor of Brain Acetylcholine." *Science* 126 (1957): 610–611.
83. Murphree, H. B., et al. "The Stimulant Effect of 2-Dimethylaminoethanol (Deanol) in Human Volunteer Subjects." *Clinical Pharmacology and Therapeutics* 1 (1960): 303–310.
84. Pelton, Ross, M.D., Ph.D. *Mind Food & Smart Pills*. 1st ed. New York: Doubleday, 1989, pages 76–79.
85. *DHA: Building Block of the Brain*. Columbia, MD: Mertek Biosciences.
86. Kraster, Caroline M. "Feed Your Head." *Whole Foods* (June, 1998).
87. Gormley, James J. "DHA and the Excitement of New Research." *Editor's Desk of Better Nutrition*.
88. Carlson, S. E., et al. "Synopsis: Dietary omega-3 fatty acids and the development of the brain and retina in human infants." NOAA technical memorandum, NMFS-SEFSC-367, NIH meeting on omega-3 fatty acid research, May 12, 1994.
    Information from Soft Gel Technologies found in *Whole Foods* (June 1998).
    Gormley, James J. "DHA and the Excitement of New Research." *Editor's Desk of Better Nutrition*.
89. Regelson, William, M.D. and Carol Colman. *The Superhormone Promise*. New York: Simon & Schuster, 1996, page 53.
90. "Problems with prescription drugs among elderly (editorial)." *American Family Physician* 28 (1986): 236.
91. Murray, Michael, N.D. and Joseph Pizzorno, N.D. *Encyclopedia of Natural Medicine*. Rocklin, CA: Prima Publishing, 1990, page 128.
92. *Ibid*.
93. Wells, C., F. A. Davis, R. D. Terry, and R. Katzman. "Senile dementia of the Alzheimer type." *Annals of Neurology* 14 (1983): 497–506.
    King, R. G. "Do raised brain aluminum levels in Alzheimer's Dementia contribute to cholinergic neuronal deficits?" *Medical Hypotheses* 14 (1984): 301–306.
    Hershey, C. O., L. A. Hershey, A. Varnes, et al. "Cerebrospinal fluid trace element content in dementia: clinical, radiologic, and pathologic correlations." *Neurology* 33 (1983): 1, 350–353.
    Candy, J. M., J. Klinowski, R. H. Perry, et al. "Aluminosilicates and senile plaque formation in Alzheimer's disease." *Lancet* 1 (1986): 354–357.
94. Klatzo, I., et al. *Journal of Neuropathology and Experimental Neurology* 24 (1965): 187–199.
95. Lester Packer, Ph.D., *The Antioxidant Miracle*, John Wiley & Sons, Inc., New York.
96. Regelson, William, M.D. and Carol Colman. *The Superhormone Promise*. New York: Simon & Schuster, 1996, pages 54–55.
97. David Perlmutter, M.D., *BrainRecovery.com*, The Perlmutter Health Center, Naples, Florida, 2000.

Chapter 8...Protecting Your Heart and Keeping It Healthy

1. Rath, Matthias, M.D. "Eradicating Heart Disease." *Health Now* (San Francisco, CA, 1993).
2. Barnes, Broda, M.D. and Lawrence Galton. *Hypothyroidism: The Unsuspected Illness*. New York: Thomas Y. Crowell Co., 1976, pages 168–169.
3. Pinckney, Cathey and Edward R. Pinckney. *The Patient's Guide to Medical Tests*. New York: Facts on File Publishers, 1986, pages 83–85.
   Passwater, Richard A., Ph.D. *The New Supernutrition*. New York: Pocket Books, 1991.
   Langer, Stephen, Ph.D. and James F. Scheer. *Solved: The Riddle of Illness*. New Canaan, CT: Keats Publishing, 1995, page 99.
4. Atkins, Robert C., M.D. *Dr. Atkins' Nutrition Breakthrough*. New York: Morrow, 1981, pages 213–214.
   Passwater, Richard, Ph.D. *Supernutrition for Healthy Hearts*, pages 37–38, 318–319.

Bland, Jeffrey. *Your Health Under Seige: Using Nutrition to Fight Back*. Brattleboro, VT: The Stephen Greene Press, 1981, pages 62–63.

Pauling, Linus. "Vitamin C and Heart Disease." *Executive Health* (January 1978).

5. Lommis, H. "Preferential Utilization of Free Cholesterol from High-Density Lipoproteins for Biliary Cholesterol Secretion in Man." *Science* (April 7, 1978): 62-64.

6. Pinckney, Cathey and Edward R. Pinckney. *The Patient's Guide to Medical Tests*. New York: Facts on File Publishers, 1986, 83–85.

7. *American Journal of Clinical Nutrition* 53 (January 1991): 326S–334S.

8. Passwater, Richard A., Ph.D. *The New Supernutrition*. New York: Pocket Books, 1991, page 139.

9. *Ibid.*
    Langer, Stephen, Ph.D. and James F. Scheer. *Solved: The Riddle of Illness*. New Canaan, CT: Keats Publishing, 1995, page 99.

10. Pauling, L., M.D. *How to Live Longer and Feel Better*. New York: W.H. Freeman & Co., 1986, page 195.

11. Fredericks, Carlton, Ph.D. "Hotline to Health." *Prevention* (January 1975): 97.

12. Passwater, Richard A., Ph.D. *The New Supernutrition*. New York: Pocket Books, 1991, page 139.

13. Yudkin, J. *Lancet* 2 (1957): 155.
    Cohen, A. M. *American Heart Journal* 65 (1962): 291.
    Antar, M. A., et al. *American Journal of Clinical Nutrition* 14 (1964): 169.

14. Yudkin, John. *Sweet and Dangerous*. New York: Peter H. Wyden, 1972, page 91.

15. Tzagournis, Manuel. "Triglycerides in Clinical Medicine." *American Journal of Clinical Nutrition* (August 1978).

16. *Ibid.*

17. Rath, Matthias, M.D. *Eradicating Heart Disease*. San Francisco: Health Now Publishers, 1993, page 101.

18. *Annals of Nutrition and Metabolism* (May–June 1984): 186–191.

19. Shute, E. V. *Heart & Vitamin E*. London, Canada: The Shute Foundation for Medical Research, 1969.
    Shute, Wilfrid E. and Harold T. Shute. *Vitamin E for Ailing and Healthy Hearts*. New York: Pyramid House, 1969.
    Shute, W. E. *Vitamin E Book*. New Canaan, CT: Keats Publishing, 1978.
    Adams, Ruth. *The Big Book on Vitamins*. New Canaan, CT: Keats Publishing.

20. *Cardiovascular Research* 25.2 (February 1991): 89–92.

21. Passwater, Richard A., Ph.D. *The New Supernutrition*. New York: Pocket Books, 1991.

22. Shute, E. V. *Heart & Vitamin E*. London, Canada: The Shute Foundation for Medical Research, 1969.
    Shute, W. E. and H. J. Taub. *Vitamin E for Ailing and Healthy Hearts*. New York: Pyramid House, 1969.
    Shute, W. E. *Vitamin E Book*. New Canaan, CT: Keats Publishing, 1978.
    Adams, Ruth. *The Big Book on Vitamins*. New Canaan, CT: Keats Publishing.

23. Hodis, Howard N., et al. *Journal of the American Medical Association* 273 (June 21, 1995): 1849–1854.
    "Vitamin E Seems to Benefit Heart, Two Studies Show." *New York Times* (November 19, 1992).

24. Gey, E. Fred, et al. "Inverse Correlation Between Plasma Vitamin E and Mortality from Ischemic Heart Disease in Cross Cultural Epidemiology." *American Journal of Clinical Nutrition* 53 (January 1991): 326–334.

25. Jialal, I. "The effect of dietary supplementation with alpha-tocopherol on the oxidative modification of low density lipoprotein." *Journal of Lipid Research* 6 (1992): 899–906.

26. Jialal, I. "The effect of a-tocopherol supplementation on LDL oxidation and vitamin E: a dose response study." *Arteriosclerosis, Thrombosis, and Vascular Biology* 15.2 (1995): 190–198.

27. *Arteriosclerosis, Thrombosis, and Vascular Biology* 15 (1995): 325–333.

28. *Journal of the American College of Nutrition* 11 (1992): 130–137.

29. Jialal, I. "The effect of a-tocopherol supplementation on LDL oxidation and vitamin E: a dose response study." *Arteriosclerosis, Thrombosis, and Vascular Biology* 15.2 (1995): 190–198.

30. *Research* 49 (1988): 393–404.

31. *Lancet* 347 (1996): 781–786.
32. Hennekens, Charles. Presentation to the New York Academy of Sciences, February 1992.
33. *Ibid.*
34. *Lancet* 346 (July 1995): 57–81.
35. Rath, Matthias, M.D. "Eradicating Heart Disease." *Health Now* (San Francisco, CA, 1993): 42–46.
36. *Proceedings of the National Academy of Sciences* USA (August 1990).
    Rath & Pauling. "Solution to the puzzle of human cardiovascular disease: Its primary cause is ascorbate deficiency, leading to the deposition of lipoprotein(a) and fibrinogen/fibrin in vascular wall." *Journal of Orthomolecular Medicine* 6 (1991): 125–134.
37. The Linus Pauling Institute of Science and Medicine Newsletter, March 1992.
    Rath, M., M.D. "Lipoprotein(a)—a reduction by ascorbate." *Journal of Orthomolecular Medicine* 7: 73–80.
38. *Ibid.*
39. Pauling, Linus, Ph.D. *How to Live Longer and Feel Better.* New York: W. H. Freeman and Co., 1986, page 152.
40. The Linus Pauling Institute of Science and Medicine Newsletter, March 1992.
    Rath, M. and Pauling, L. "A Unified Theory of Human Cardiovascular Disease Leading the Way to the Abolition of This Disease As a Cause for Human Mortality." *Journal of Orthomolecular Medicine* (1992).
41. Ginter, Emil, M.D. "The Effects of Ascorbic Acid on Humans in a Long-Term Experiment." *International Journal for Vitamin and Nutrition Research* 47.2.
    Ginter, E. "Vitamin C in the Control of Hypercholesteremia in Man." *Vitamin C: New Clinical Applications in Immunology, Lipid Metabolism, and Cancer,* A. Hanck, Hans Huber, ed. (Bern, 1982): 137–152.
42. Norden, R. *International Journal of Microbiology* 3 (1984): 425.
43. Bordia, A. and S. K. Verma. *Clinical Cardiology* 8.10 (October 1985): 552–554.
44. Folkers, Karl, et al. *Biomedical and Clinical Aspects of Coenzyme Q* 6 (New York: Elsevier Publishing Co., 1990).
    Bliznakof, Emile G., Ph.D. and Gerald Hunt. *The Miracle Nutrient: Coenzyme Q10.* New York: Bantam Books, 1987.
    Folkers, Karl. Co-chairman's Opening Remarks, Fifth International Symposium on Biomedical and Clinical Aspects of Coenzyme Q, 1987.
    Folkers, K., P. Langsjoen, Y. Nara, K. Muratsu, J. Komorowski, P. C. Richardson, and T. H. Smith. *Biochemical and Biophysical Research Communications* 153 (1988): 888–896.
    Mortensen, S. A., and S. Vadhanavikit, K. Nuratsu, and K. Folders. "Coenzyme Q10: clinical benefits with biochemical correlates suggest a scientific breakthrough in the management of chronic heart failure." *International Journal of Tissue Reactions* 22.3: 155–162.
    Folkers, Karl. "Contemporary Therapy with Vitamin B_6, Vitamin B12 and Coenzyme CoQ10." *Chemical & Engineering News* 64.16 (April 21, 1986): 27–30, 55–56.
45. Folkers, Karl. (Priestly Medal Address) "Contemporary Therapy with Vitamin B_6, Vitamin B12, and Coenzyme Q10." *Chemical & Engineering News* 64.16 (April 21, 1986): 27–30, 55–56.
46. Folkers, Karl, et al. *Biomedical and Clinical Aspects of Coenzyme Q* 6 (New York: Elsevier Publishing Co., 1990).
47. Bliznakof, Emile G., Ph.D. and Gerald Hunt. *The Miracle Nutrient: Coenzyme Q10.* New York: Bantam Books, 1987.
48. The Linus Pauling Institute of Science and Medicine Newsletter.
    Folkers, Karl, et al. *Biomedical and Clinical Aspects of Coenzyme Q* 6 (New York: Elsevier Publishing Co., 1990).
49. Mortensen, S. A., S. Vadhanavikit, K. Nuratsu, and K. Folkers. "Coenzyme Q10: Clinical Benefits with Biochemical Correlates suggesting a scientific breakthrough in the management of chronic heart failure." *International Journal of Tissue Reactions* 22.3 (1990): 155–162.
50. *Ibid.*
51. Leviton, Richard. "High Blood Pressure, Lower it Naturally." *Alternative Medicine Digest* 16: 44.
    Sinatra, Stephen. *Heartbreak & Heart Disease.* New Canaan, CT: Keats Publishing, 1996.

52. Mortensen, S. A., S. Vadhanavikit, K. Nuratsu, and K. Folkers. "Coenzyme Q10: Clinical Benefits with Biochemical Correlates suggesting a scientific breakthrough in the management of chronic heart failure." *International Journal of Tissue Reactions* 22.3 (1990): 155–162.

53. Linnane, Antony W. *Center for Molecular Biology and Medicine,* Clayton, Australia: Monash University.

54. *International Clinical Nutrition Review* 2.3 (1982): 14.

55. Ghidino, O., M. Azzurro, A. Vita, and G. Sartori. "Evaluation of the therapeutic efficacy of L-carnitine in congestive heart failure." *International Journal of Clinical Pharmacology, Therapy and Toxicology* 26 (1988): 217–220.

56. Walker, Morton. *The Chelation Way.* Garden City Park, NY: Avery Publishing Group, Inc., 1990, page 211.

57. Cherchi, A., C. Lai, F. Angelino, et al. "Effects of L-carnitine on exercise tolerance in chronic stable angina: a multicenter, double-blind, randomized, placebo controlled crossover study." *International Journal of Clinical Pharmacology, Therapy and Toxicology* 23 (1985): 569–572.
Orlando, G. and C. Rusconi. "Oral L-carnitine in the treatment of chronic cardiac ischaemia in elderly patients." *Clinical Trials Journal* 23 (1986): 338–344.
Kamikawa, T., Y. Suzuki, A. Kohayashi, et al. "Effects of L-carnitine on exercise tolerance in patients with stable angina pectoris." *Japanese Heart Journal* 25 (1984): 587–597.
Kosolcharoen, P., J. Nappi, P. Peruzzi, et al. "Improved exercise tolerance after administration of carnitine." *Current Therapeutic Research* 30 (1981): pages 753–764.
Pola, P., L. Savi, M. Serricchio, et al. "Use of physiological substance, acetyl-carnitine, in the treatment of angiospastic syndromes." *Drugs Under Experimental and Clinical Research* X (1984): 213–217.

58. *Ibid.*
Ghidino, O., M. Azzurro, A. Vita, and G. Sartori. "Evaluation of the therapeutic efficacy of L-carnitine in congestive heart failure." *International Journal of Clinical Pharmacology, Therapy and Toxicology* 26 (1988): 217–220.

59. Cherchi, A., et al. "Effects of L-carnitine on exercise tolerance in chronic stable angina: A multicenter, double-blind, randomized, placebo-controlled, crossover study." *International Journal of Clinical Pharmacology, Therapy and Toxicology* 23 (1985): 569–572.
Orlando, G. and C. Rlusconi. "Oral L-carnitine in the treatment of chronic cardiac ischaemia in elderly patients." *Clinical Trials Journal* 23 (1986): 338–344.
Kamikawa, T., et al. "Effects of L-carnitine on exercise tolerance in patients with stable angina pectoris." *Japanese Heart Journal* 25 (1984): 587–597.
Pola, P., et al. "Use of physiological substance, acetylcarnitine, in the treatment of angiospastic syndromes." *Drugs Under Experimental and Clinical Research* X (1984): 213–217.
Folkers, K. and Y. Yamamura, eds. *Biomedical and Clinical Aspects of Coenzyme Q10* 1–4 (Amsterdam: Elsevier Science Publishers, 1977, 1980, 1982, 1984).
Littarru, G. P., L. Ho, and K. Folkers. "Deficiency of coenzyme Q10 in human heart disease: Part II." *International Journal for Vitamin and Nutrition Research* 42 (1972): 413.
Kamikawa, T., A. Kobayashi, T. Yamashita, et al. "Effects of coenzyme Q10 on exercise tolerance in chronic stable angina pectoris." *American Journal of Cardiology* 56 (1985): 247.

60. Whitaker, M.D., Julian. *Dr. Whitaker's Guide to Natural Healing.* Rocklin, CA: Prima Publishing, 1995, page 157.

61. Hendler, Sheldon Saul, M.D., Ph.D., *The Doctors' Vitamin and Mineral Encyclopedia.* New York: Simon and Schuster, 1990, page 157.

62. Iseri, L. T. "Magnesium and Cardiac Arrhythmias." *Magnesium* 5: 111–126.
Iseri, L. T. and J. H. French. "Magnesium: Nature's Physiologic Calcium Blocker." *American Heart Journal* 109: 188–193.

63. Dudley, A. and R. Solomon. "Magnesium, myocardial ischaemia and arrhythmias: the role of magnesium in myocardial infarction." *Drugs* 37 (1989): 1–7.
Hendler, Sheldon Saul, M.D., Ph.D., *The Doctors' Vitamin and Mineral Encyclopedia.* New York: Simon and Schuster, 1990, page 159.

64. Rasmussen, H. S., et al. "Intravenous Magnesium in Acute Myocardial Infarction." *Lancet* 1 (1986): 234–235.

65. Passwater, Richard A., Ph.D. *The New Supernutrition.* New York: Pocket Books, 1991, pages 144–146.

66. *Ibid.*
67. Folkers, Karl. "Contemporary Therapy with Vitamin B_6, Vitamin B_{12} and Coenzyme Q_{10}." *Chemical & Engineering News* 64.16 (April 21, 1986): 27–30, 55–56.
68. McCully, K., Homocysteine, folate, vitamin B_6, and cardiovascular disease (editorial) *JAMA*. 1998; 279:392–393.
69. *Ibid.*
70. Stampfer M, Malinow M, Can lowering homocysteine levels reduce cardiovascular risk? *New England Journal of Medicine,* 1995; 332:328–329.
71. Stampfer M, Malinow M, Willeff W, et al. A prospective study of plasma homocyst(e)ine and risk of myocardial infarction in US physicians. *JAMA*. 1992; 268:877–881.
72. Murray, Michael, N.D., *The Encyclopedia of Nutritional Supplements.* Rocklin, CA: Prima Publishing, 1996; p.93.
     Welsh, A. L. and M. Ede. "Inositol hexanicotinate for improved nicotinic acid therapy." *Int Record Med* 174 (1961): 9–15.
     El-Enein, A. M. A., et al. "The role of nicotinic acid and inositol hexaniacinate as anti-cholesterolemic and antilipemic agents." *Nutr Rep Intl.* 28 (1983): 899–911.
     Sunderland, G. T., J. J. F. Belch, R. D. Sturrock, et al. "A double blind randomized placebo controlled trial of hexopal in primary Raynaud's disease." *Clinical Rheumatology* 7 (1988): 46–49.
     O'Hara, J. P. N. Jolly, and C. G. Nichol. "The therapeutic effect of inositol nicotinate (Hexopal) on intermittent claudication: A controlled trial." *British Journal of Clinical Practice 42* (1988): 377–383.
73. *Ibid.*
74. *Dr. Whitaker 's Guide to Natural Healing* by Julian Whitaker, M.D., Prima Publishing Rocklin, CA. 1995.
75. Passwater, Richard A., Ph.D. *The New Supernutrition.* New York: Pocket Books, 1991, page 179.
76. Horlick, L., Circulation 10, 30, 1956, Duff, G. L. et al., *Am. Jour. Med.* 11, 92, 1951, Adlersberg, D., et. al., *Jour. Nut.* 25, 255, 1943.
77. Lindberg, Gladys and Judy McFarland. *Take Charge of Your Health.* San Francisco: Harper and Row, 1982, pages 88–90.
78. Passwater, Richard A., Ph.D. *The New Supernutrition.* New York: Pocket Books, 1991, page 105–106.
     Yates, John. "Lecithin Works Wonders." *Prevention* (February 1980): 55–59.
     Morrison, Lester M. "Serum Cholesterol Reduction with Lecithin." *Geriatrics* (January 1958): 12–19.
79. Davis, Adelle, *Let's Get Well,* A Signet Book, New York. 1972.
     Hirsch. E. F., et. al., *Physiol, Rev,* 23, 185, 1943.
80. Davis, Adelle, *Let's Get Well,* A Signet Book, New York. 1972.
81. Kesten, H. D., et al., Proc. Soc, *Exp. Biol. Med.* 49, 71, 1942.
82. Davis, Adelle, *Let's Get Well,* A Signet Book, New York. 1972.
     Wagner, A.L.,et al., *J. Lab. Clin. Med.* 40, 324, 1952, Gross, K.L, et al, *N.Y. State J Med* 30, 2683, 1950, Sinclair, H. M., *Lancet* 2, 271, 281, 1956.
83. *Family Practice News.* Kalevi Pyorala, June 1979, *The Complete Book of Minerals for Health* by Sharon Faelten, Rodale Press Emmaus, PA 1981.
84. Clin. Chem., 24(4), 1978, p.541, *The People's Guide to Vitamins and Minerals From A to Zinc,* Dominick Bosco, Contemporary Books, Inc. Chicago, Ill, 1980.
85. Castano G, et al. 1999. a double blind, placebo-controlled study of the effects of policosanol in patients with intermittent claudication. *Angiology* 50:123–30. Mas R, et al. 1999 Pharmacoepidemiologic study of policosanol. *Curr Ther Res* 60:456–67. Mas R. 2000. Policosanol. *Drugs of the Future* 25:569–86.
86. *Ibid.*
87. Burnham TH, Sjweain SL, Short RM (eds.) Monascus. In: *The Review of Natural Products.* St. Louis, MO: Facts and Comparisons, 1997.
88. *Ibid.*
89. Wang J, Lu Z, Chi J, et al. Multicenter clinical trial of the serum lipid lowering effects of a *Monascus purpureus* (red yeast) rice preparation from traditional Chinese medicine. *Curr Ther Res* 1997;58:964–77.
90. Heber D, Yip I, Ashley JM, et al. Cholesterol lowering effects of a proprietary Chinese red-yeast-rice dietary supplement. *Am J Clin Nutr* 1999;69:231–6

91. Wang J, Lu Z, Chi J, et al. Multicenter clinical trial of the serum lipid lowering effects of a *Monascus purpureus* (red yeast) rice preparation from traditional Chinese medicine. *Curr Ther Res* 1997;58:964–77.

92. Tenny, Louise. *Todays Herbal Health, Provo,* UT: Woodland Books, 1992

93. Murray, Michael, N.D., *Encyclopedia of Natural Medicine,* Rocklin, CA, Prima Publishing 1990, p. 146

94. Davis, Adelle, *Let's Get Well,* A Signet Book, New York. 1972, Wagner, A.L.,et al., *J. Lab. Clin. Med.* 40, 324, 1952, Gross, K.L, et al, *N.Y. State J Med* 30, 2683, 1950, Sinclair, H. M., *Lancet* 2, 271, 281, 1956
Lancet II 800 (1969): 962.
Journal of Traditional Chinese Medicine 6 (1986): 117.
Journal of the American Chemistry Society 106 (1984: 82–95.

95. *Ibid.*

96. Syckner, T. and P. O. Wester. *British Medical Journal* 286 (1983): 1847.

97. Carper, Jean. *Stop Aging Now,* Harper Collins, New York, NY 1995.

98. Whitaker, Julian. *Health & Healing* 6.2 (February 1996).
Sanders, T. A. B. "Cod Liver Oil, Platelet Fatty Acids, and Bleeding Time." *Lancet* 1 (1980): 1189.

99. Kang, J. X. "Antiarrhythmic effects of polyunsaturated fatty acids. Recent Studies." *Circulation* 94 (1996): 1774–1780.

100. Leaf, A. "Omega-3 fatty acids and prevention of ventricular fibrillation." *Prostaglandins, Leukotrienes and Essential Fatty Acids* 52 (1995): 197–198.

101. Carper, Jean. *Miracle Cures.* New York: HarperCollins Publishers, 1997.

102. Sugano, M., et al. *Annals of Nutritional Medicine* 30 (1986): 289–299.

103. Daviglus, M. L., J. Stamler, A. L. Orencia, et al. *New England Journal of Medicine* 336.15 (April 10, 1997): 1046–1053.

104. *Family Practice News.* Kalevi Pyorala, June 1979, *The Complete Book of Minerals for Health* by Sharon Faelten, Rodale Press Emmaus, PA 1981

105. Lecture at the National Nutritional Foods Association convention in Las Vegas, Nevada, 1995.

106. Nelson, M. E., et al. *American Journal of Clinical Nutrition* 43 (1986): 910–916.

Chapter 9 ... If the Pressure Is Up, Let's Turn It Down!

1. Alderman, M. H. "Which antihypertensive drugs first—and why." *Journal of the American Medical Association* 267 (1992): 2786–2787.

2. Raeburn, Paul, Associated Press. "Doctors: Popular drug isn't working." *The Daily Breeze* (November 20, 1995): A1–A7.
Whitaker, M.D., Julian. *Dr. Whitaker's Guide to Natural Healing.* Rocklin, CA: Prima Publishing, 1995, page 11.

3. Leviton, Richard. "High Blood Pressure: Lower it Naturally." *Alternative Medicine Digest* 16: 44.

4. Carlson, Wade. "A Nutritional Approach to Lowering Blood Pressure." *Better Nutrition* (February 1987).

5. Ackley, S., E. Barrett-Conner, and L. Suarez. "Dairy Products, calcium and blood pressure." *American Journal of Clinical Nutrition* 38 (1983): 457.
Norman, Kaplan, M.D. "Non-drug treatment of hypertension." *Annals of Internal Medicine* 102 (March 1985): 359–373.

6. Vaughn, Sam and Janis Donnaud, eds. *The American Medical Association Encyclopedia of Medicine.* New York: Random House, 1989, page 188.

7. Langer, Stephen, M.D. "Don't Gamble with Hypertension." *Better Nutrition for Today's Living* (November 1995): 48–52.

8. Vaughn, Sam and Janis Donnaud, eds. *The American Medical Association Encyclopedia of Medicine.* New York: Random House, 1989, page 948.

9. *Ibid.*

10. Hendler, Sheldon Saul, M.D., Ph.D., *The Doctors' Vitamin and Mineral Encyclopedia.* New York: Simon and Schuster, 1990, page 176.
Horowitz, Nathan. "Dietary Potassium Is Said to Protect Against Stroke." *Medical Tribune* (August 17, 1989): 6.

11. *Ibid.*

12. Khaw, Kay-Tee, M.D. and Elizabeth Barrett-Connor, M.D. "The Association Between Blood Pressure, Age and Dietary Sodium and Potassium: A Population Study." *Circulation* 77 (1988): 53–61.
13. Khaw, Kay-Tee, M.D. and Elizabeth Barrett-Connor, M.D. "Dietary Potassium and stroke-associated mortality: A 12–year prospective population study." *New England Journal of Medicine* 316 (1987): 235–240.
     Khaw, Kay-Tee, M.D. and S. Thom. "Randomized double-blind cross-over trial of potassium on blood pressure in normal subjects." *Lancet* 2 (1982): 1127–1129.
14. McLaughlin, Lloyd. "USDA Finds Salt and Potassium Intake Askew in Adult Diets." *USDA News* (December 19, 1984).
15. Hendler, Sheldon Saul, M.D., Ph.D. *The Doctors' Vitamin and Mineral Encyclopedia.* New York: Simon and Schuster, 1990, page 182.
     Kirschmann, Gayla J. and John D. Kirschmann. *Nutrition Almanac.* McGraw-Hill, 1996.
16. John JH et al. Effects of fruit and vegetable consumption on plasma antioxidant concentrations and blood pressure. *Lancet* 2002; 359:1969–74.
17. Cappuccio, F. P., et al. "Epidemiological Association Between Dietary Calcium Intake and Blood Pressure: A Meta-Analysis of Published Data." *American Journal of Epidemiology* 142.9 (1995): 935–845.
18. *Science* 224 (June 29, 1984): 12–17.
19. Lieberman, Shari and Nancy Burning. *The Real Vitamin and Mineral Book.* Garden City Park, NY: Avery Publishing Group Inc., 1990. As excerpted in *American Journal of Clinical Nutrition* 42 (July 1985): 12–17.
     Ackely, S., E. Barrett-Conner, and L. Suarez. "Dairy products, Calcium and Blood Pressure." *American Journal of Clinical Nutrition* 38 (1983): 457.
20. Dyckner, T. and P. O. Wester. *British Medical Journal* 286 (1983): 1847.
     American Journal of Clinical Nutrition 42 (July 1985): 12–17.
21. Ruddell, H., et al. "Effect of magnesium supplementation in patients with labile hypertension." *Journal of the American College of Nutrition* 6 (1987): 445.
22. *Ibid.*
     Resnick, L. M., R. K. Gupta, and J. H. Laragh. "Intracellular free magnesium in erythrocytes of essential hypertension: Relation of blood pressure and serum divalent cations." *Proceedings of the National Academy of Sciences* USA 81 (1984): 6511.
23. *International Journal for Vitamin and Nutrition Research* 54 (1984): 343–347.
24. *American Journal of Clinical Nutrition* 48 (November 1988): 1226–1232.
25. McCarron, D. A., C. D. Morris, H. U. Henry, and J. L. Stanton. "Blood Pressure and Nutrient Intake in the United States." *Science* 224 (1984): 1392–1398. As seen in *Eradicating Heart Disease,* by Matthias Rath.
26. *Nutrition Research* 3 (1983): 653–661.
27. Murray, Michael, N.D. and Joseph Pizzorno, N.D. *Encyclopedia of Natural Medicine.* Rocklin, CA: Prima Publishing, 1990, page 382.
28. Folkers, K., T. Watanabe, and M. Kaji. "Critique of coenzyme Q10 in biochemical and biochemical research and in ten years of clinical research on cardiovascular disease." *Journal of Molecular Medicine* 2 (1977): 431–460.
     Folkers, Karl, et al. *Biomedical and Clinical Aspects of Coenzyme Q 6* (Amsterdam: Elsevier Publishing Co., 1984).
29. Langsjoen, P., et al. "Treatment of Essential Hypertension With Coenzyme Q10." *Life Extension Magazine* 2.2 (February 1996): 49.
30. Leviton, Richard. "High Blood Pressure: Lower it Naturally." *Alternative Medicine Digest* 16 (1999): page 44.
     Sinatra, Stephen. *Heartbreak & Heart Disease.* New Canaan, CT: Keats Publishing, 1996.
31. Berger, Stuart, M.D. *How to Be Your Own Nutritionist.* New York: Avon Books, 1987, page 92.
32. *Atherosclerosis* 49 (1983). *Circulation* (March 1983).
33. *Lancet* II (1969): 962, 800.
     Journal of Traditional Chinese Medicine 6 (1986): 117.
34. Gottlieb, Bill, ed. *New Choices in Natural Healing.* Emmaus, PA: Rodale Press, 1995, page 361.
35. Langer, Stephen, M.D., contributing writer. "Don't Gamble with Hypertension." *Better Nutrition for Today's Living* (November 1995).
36. Murray, Michael, N.D. and Joseph Pizzorno, N.D. *Encyclopedia of Natural Medicine.*

Rocklin, CA: Prima Publishing, 1990, page 383.

37. Leviton, Richard. "High Blood Pressure: Lower it Naturally." *Alternative Medicine Digest* 16 (1999): 44.

38. Langer, Stephen. "Don't gamble with hypertension." *Better Nutrition for Today's Living* (November 1995): 48–52.

39. Gottlieb, Bill. *New Choices in Natural Healing.* Emmaus, PA: Rodale Press, 1995, page 363.

40. Rothenberg, Mikel A., M.D. and Charles F. Chapman. *Dictionary of Medical Terms for the Nonmedical Person.* New York: Barron's Educational Series, Inc., 1994.

41. Ackley, S., E. Barrett-Conner, and L. Suarez. "Dairy Products, calcium and blood pressure." *American Journal of Clinical Nutrition* 38 (1983): 457.
Norman, Kaplan, M.D. "Non-drug treatment of hypertension." *Annals of Internal Medicine* 102 (March 1985): 359–373.

42. Davis, Adelle. *Let's Get Well.* New York: Signet, Published by the Penguin Group, 1972, pages 278–279.

43. Wright, Jonathan V., M.D. with Alan R. Gaby M.D. *Nutrition & Healing* 3.5 (May 1996): 12.

44. Salaman, Maureen Kennedy. *All You Health Questions Answered Naturally.* MKS, Inc., 1998.
Healton, Edward B., et al. "Neurologic Aspects of Cobalamin Deficiency," *Medicine.* 70.4 (1991): 229–244.

Chapter 10...Importance of a Properly Functioning Thyroid

1. Ratcliff, J. D. "I Am Joe's Thyroid." *Reader's Digest* (Pleasantville, NY, March 1973).

2. Barnes, Broda. *Hypothyroidism: The Unsuspected Illness.* New York: Thomas Y. Crowell Company, 1976.
Langer, Stephen, Ph.D. and James F. Scheer. *Solved: The Riddle of Illness.* New Canaan, CT: Keats Publishing, 1995, page 15.
Shefrin, David, N.D. Seminar for Broda Barnes research Foundation, Fall Physician Teaching Seminar (Scottsdale, AZ, September 22–24, 1995).

3. Jackson, A.S. "Hypothyroidism." *Journal of the American Medical Association* (1957): 121–165.

4. Israel, Murray, M.D. *The Thyroid-Vitamin Approach to Cholesterol, Atheromatosis and Chronic Disease: A Ten Year Study.* New York: The George Press, Inc., 1960.

5. *Ibid.*

6. *Ibid.*

7. *Ibid.*

8. *Ibid.*

9. *Ibid.*

10. Barnes, Broda O. and Lawrence Galton. *Hypothyroidism: The Unsuspected Illness.* New York: Thomas Y. Crowell Co., page 43.

11. *Ibid.*

12. *Ibid.*
Braverman, E. R. and C. C. Pfeiffer. *The Healing Nutrients Within.* New Canaan, CT: Keats Publishing, Inc., 1987, page 51.

13. Barnes, Broda. *Hypothyroidism: The Unsuspected Illness.* New York: Thomas Y. Crowell Company, 1976.

14. Whitaker, Julian. *Health & Healing* (May 1994).
Harby, K. "New proactive guidelines urge thyroid screening." *Medical Tribune* (January 19, 1995).

15. *Ibid.*

16. Braverman, E. R. and C. C. Pfeiffer. *The Healing Nutrients Within.* New Canaan, CT: Keats Publishing, Inc., 1987, page 51.

17. Israel, Murray, M.D. *The Thyroid-Vitamin Approach to Cholesterol, Atheromatosis and Chronic Disease: A Ten Year Study.* New York: The George Press, Inc., 1960.

18. Gaby, Alan, M.D. *Preventing and Reversing Osteoporosis.* Rocklin, CA: Prima Publishing, 1994, page 143.

19. Haddow, J. E., et al. "Maternal Thyroid Deficiency During Pregnancy and Subsequent Neuropsychological Development of the Child." *New England Journal of Medicine* 341.8 (1999): 549–555.

20. Peat, Ray, Ph.D. "Thyroid: Misconceptions." *Townsend Letter for Doctors* 124

(November 1993): 1120–1122.

Balch, James F., M.D. and Phyllis A. Balch, C.N.C. *Prescription for Nutritional Healing.* Garden City, NY: Avery Publishing Group, Inc., 1990, pages 213–214.

Goodhart, Robert S., M.D. and Maurice E. Shils, M.D. *Modern Nutrition in Health and Disease,* 6th ed. Philadelphia: Lea & Febiger, 1978, pages 406, 473.

21. Barnes, Broda O. and Lawrence Galton. *Hypothyroidism: The Unsuspected Illness.* New York: Thomas Y. Crowell Co., 1976, page 176.

Israel, Murray. *The Thyroid-Vitamin Approach to Cholesterol Atheromatosis and Chronic Disease: A Ten Year Study.* New York: The George Press, 1960.

Israel, Murray, M.D. "An Effective Therapeutic Approach to the Control of Atherosclerosis Illustrating Harmlessness of Prolonged Use of Thyroid Hormone in Coronary Disease." *American Journal of Digestive Diseases* 22 (1955): 161–168.

22. Israel, Murray, M.D. *The Thyroid-Vitamin Approach to Cholesterol, Atheromatosis and Chronic Disease: A Ten Year Study.* New York: The George Press, Inc., 1960, page 9.

23. Lindberg, Gladys, and Judy McFarland. *Take Charge of Your Health.* San Francisco: Harper and Row, 1982, page 223.

24. Murray, Michael, N.D. *Encyclopedia of Nutritional Supplements.* Rocklin, CA: Prima Publishing, 1996.

Chapter 11...Nutritional Help for All Forms of Arthritis

1. Schiedermayer, David, M.D., FACP. *Alternative Medical Alert, A Clinician's Guide to Alternative Therapies* 1.11 (November 1998): 121–132.

2. Lewis, R. *FDA Consumer* 25 (July/August 1991): 18–26.

3. Whitaker, Julian. *Health & Healing* 7.8 (August 1997).

Bloom, M. S. "Direct medical cost of disease and gastrointestinal side effects during treatment for arthritis." *American Journal of Medicine* 84 (1988): 23.

McKenzie, L. S., Horsburgh, B.A., Ghosh, P., and Taylor, T.K.F. "Osteoarthrosis: Uncertain Rationale for Anti-inflammatory Drug Therapy." *Lancet* 1 (1976): 908–909.

4. Whitaker, Julian. *Health & Healing* 7.8 (August 1997).

5. Roger, J. Williams. *Nutrition Against Disease.* New York: Pitman Publishing Corp., 1971, pages 122–123.

6. *Arthritis Information: Rheumatoid Arthritis.* Atlanta, GA: The Arthritis Foundation, Brochure No. 4020, May 1995.

7. Balch, J., P. Balch. *Prescription for Nutritional Healing.* Garden City Park, NY: Avery Publishing Group, 1997.

8. Lindberg, Gladys and Judy McFarland. *Take Charge of Your Health.* San Francisco: Harper and Row, 1982, page 24.

9. Pfeiffer, Carl. *Mental and Elemental Nutrients.* New Canaan, CT: Keats Publishing, Inc., 1975, page 452.

10. Follis, Richard, Jr. *Deficiency Disease.* Springfield, IL.: Charles C. Thomas Publishers, 1958.

11. Fredericks, Carlton. *Arthritis: Don't Learn to Live With It.* pages 97–98.

12. Pauling, Linus. *How to Live Longer and Feel Better.* New York: W. H. Freeman and Co., 1986, page 25.

13. *Ibid.*

14. *Ibid.*

15. Pfeiffer, Carl. *Mental and Elemental Nutrients.* New Canaan, CT: Keats Publishing, Inc., 1975, pages 454–455.

16. *Ibid.*

17. , Robert. "The Conquest of Arthritis by Nutritional therapy." *Arthritis News Today* (July 1980).

Bingham, R. *Fight Back Against Arthritis.* Desert Hot Springs, CA: Desert Arthritis Medical Clinic, 1984.

Bingham, R. "New and Effective Approaches in the Prevention and Treatment of Arthritis." *Journal of Nutrition* 28 (1976): 38–47.

Bingham, R. "Arthritis News Today." *Arthritis and Health News* 1–5.1–65 (1978–1983). Yorba Linda, CA: Arthritis Patients Association.

18. Kaufman, W. "The Use of Vitamin Therapy to Reverse Certain Concomitants of Aging." *Journal of the American Geriatrics Society* 3.11 (November 1955): 927–936.

Kalliomaki, J. L., et al. "Urinary excretion of thiamin, riboflavin, nicotinic acid, and pantothenic acid in patients with rheumatoid arthritis." *Acta Medica Scandinavica* 166 (1960): 275.

Pauling, Linus. *How to Live Longer and Feel Better.* New York: W. H. Freeman and Co., 1986, page 204.

Kaufman, W. "Niacinamide, A Most Neglected Vitamin." *International Academy of Preventive Medicine* 8 (1983): 5–25.

Kaufman, W. "Niacinamide therapy for joint mobility: Therapeutic reversal of a common clinical manifestation of the 'normal' aging process." *Conn St Med J* 17 (1953): 584.

D'Agostino, L. "The vascular or erthremic effect of nicotinic acid upon various portions of the body of men in health and various diseases." *Acta Vitaminologica et Enzymologica* 1 (1947): 130.

19.   Hoffer, A. "Treatment of arthritis by nicotinic acid and nicotinamide." *Canadian Medical Association Journal* 81 (1959): 235.

20.   *Ibid.*

Ellis, J. M. and J. Presley. *Vitamin B_6, the Doctor's Report.* New York: Harper and Row, 1973.

21.   Aaseth, J., et al. Research paper presented at the Second International Symposium on Selenium in Biology and Medicine, May 1980.

22.   *Scandinavian Journal of Rheumatology* 14 (April–June 1985): 97–101.

23.   *Biological Trace Element Research* 7 (May–June 1985): 195–198.

24.   Passwater, Richard A., Ph.D. *The New Supernutrition.* New York: Pocket Books, 1991, pages 253–254.

25.   Schiedermayer, David, M.D., FACP. "Glucosamine Sulfate for the Treatment of Osteoarthritis." *Alternative Medicine Alert* 1.11 (November 1998).

26.   Pujalte, J. M., et al. "Double-blind clinical evaluation of oral glucosamine sulphate in the basic treatment of osteoarthrosis." *Current Medical Research and Opinion* 7 (1980): 110–114.

Drovanti, A., et al. "Therapeutic activity of oral glucosamine sulfate in osteoarthrosis: A placebo-controlled double-blind investigation." *Clinical Therapeutics* 3 (1980): 260–272.

27.   O'Ambrosia, E. et al. "Glucosamine sulfate: a controlled clinical investigation in arthritis." *Pharmatherapeutica* 2 (1991): 504–8.

28.   Rovati, et al. *International Journal of Tissue Reactions* 14 (1992): 243–245.

Vaz, A. L. "Double blind-clinical evaluation of the relative efficacy of ibuprofen and glucosamine sulfate in the management of osteoarthrosis of the knee in out-patients." *Current Medical Research and Opinion* 8 (1982): 145–149.

Qiu, et al. *Arzneimittel-Forschung* 48.5 (1998): 469.

29.   Werbach, Melvyn. *Healing Through Nutrition.* New York: HarperCollins Publisher, 1993, page 284.

Vaz, A. L. "Double blind-clinical evaluation of the relative efficacy of ibuprofen and glucosamine sulfate in the management of osteoarthrosis of the knee in out-patients." *Current Medical Research and Opinion* 8 (1982): 145–149.

30.   Murray, Michael T., N.D. "Natural Relief for Osteoarthritis." *Health Counselor.* Impakt Communications, Inc. (1997).

31.   Schiedermayer, David, M.D., FACP. "Glucosamine Sulfate for the Treatment of Osteoarthritis." *Alternative Medicine Alert* 1.11 (November 1998).

32.   Murray, Michael, N.D. *Encyclopedia of Nutritional Supplements.* Rocklin, CA: Prima Publishing, 1996, page 342.

33.   Murray, Michael T., N.D. "Glucosamine Sulfate: Nature's Arthritis Cure." *Ask the Doctor.* Impakt Communications Inc. (1998).

34.   Schiedermayer, David, M.D., FACP. "Glucosamine Sulfate for the Treatment of Osteoarthritis." *Alternative Medicine Alert* 1.11 (November 1998).

35.   Crolle G. and E. d'Este. "Glucosamine sulfate for the management of arthrosis: a controlled clinical investigation." *Current Medical Research and Opinion* 7 (1980): 104–114.

Tapadinhas, M. J., I. C. Rivera, and A. A. Ginamini. "Oral glucosamine sulfate in the management of arthrosis: report on a multi-center open investigation in Portugal." *Pharmatherapeutica* 3 (1982): 157–168.

D'Ambrosia, E. D., B. Casa, R. Bompani, G. Scali, and M. Scali. "Glucosamine sulfate, a controlled clinical investigation in arthrosis." *Pharmatherapeutica* 2 (1982): 504–508.

Murray, Michael, N.D. *Encyclopedia of Nutritional Supplements.* Rocklin, CA: Prima

            Publishing, 1996, page 342.
36.   Theodosakis, Jason, M.D., M.S., M.P.H., et al. *The Arthritis Cure*. New York: St. Martin's
        Press, 1997.
37.   Ley, Beth M. *MSM: Our Way Back to Health With Sulfur*. Aliso Viejo, CA: Health
        Learning Handbooks, BL Publications, 1998.
38.   *Federation Proceedings* 44.3 (1985): 692.
        Journal of Laboratory and Clinical Medicine 110 (1987): 1.
        Annals of the NY Academy of Sciences 411 (1983).
39.   Privitera, James, M.D., D.C. "James Coburn: Cinema's Tough Guy Takes On Arthritis."
        Journal of Longevity 5:3 (1999).
40.   Erdmann, Robert, Ph.D. *The Amino Revolution, A Fireside Book*. New York: Simon &
        Schuster Inc., 1987.
        Ley, Beth M. *MSM: Our Way Back to Health With Sulfur*. Aliso Viejo, CA: Health
        Learning Handbooks, BL Publications, 1998.
        Challem, Jack. "MSM: The Newest Arthritis Cure." *Let's Live* magazine (no date).
        Jacobs, Stanley W. and Robet Herschler. *MSM: DMSO2 After 20 Years*. Portland, OR:
        Department of Surgery, Oregon Health Science University. As reported in the *Journal
        of the New York Academy of Sciences*.
        Jacobs, Stanley W., M.D., Ronald M. Lawrence, M.D., Ph.D., and Martin Zucker. *The
        Miracle of MSM: The Natural solution of Pain*. New York: G.P. Putman's Sons Publishers,
        1999.
41.   Ley, Beth M. *MSM: Our Way Back to Health With Sulfur*. Aliso Viejo, CA: Health
        Learning Handbooks, BL Publications, 1998.
42.   Challem, Jack. "MSM: The Newest Arthritis Cure." *Let's Live* magazine (no date).
        Jacobs, Stanley W., M.D., Ronald M. Lawrence, M.D., Ph.D., and Martin Zucker. *The
        Miracle of MSM: The Natural solution of Pain*. New York: G.P. Putman's Sons Publishers,
        1999.
43.   Jacobs, S. W. and R. Herschler. *Annals of the New York Academy of Sciences* 411.xiii (1983).
44.   Christy, Martha M. *MSM, The Super-Supplement of the Decade!* Scottsdale: Wishland
        Publishing, Inc., 1997.
        Jacobs, Stanley W., M.D., Ronald M. Lawrence, M.D., Ph.D., and Martin Zucker. *The
        Miracle of MSM: The Natural solution of Pain*. New York: G.P. Putman's Sons Publishers,
        1999.
45.   Jacobs, Stanley W., M.D., Ronald M. Lawrence, M.D., Ph.D., and Martin Zucker. *The
        Miracle of MSM: The Natural solution of Pain*. New York: G.P Putman's Sons Publishers,
        1999.
46.   Ammon HP, et al., Mechanism of anti-inflammatory actions of curcumine and boswellic
        acids. Biochem Pharmacol 1989 Oct 15; 38(20):3527–34.
47.   Ruby AJ, et al., Anti-tumor and antioxidant activity of natural curcuminoids. Cancer
        Lett 1995 Jul 20; 94(1):79–83.
48.   Bliddal H, et al., A randomized, placebo-controlled, cross-over study of ginger extracts
        and ibuprofen in osteoarthritis. Osteoarthritis Cartilage 2000 Jan; 8(1):9–12.
49.   Goldberg, Burton. *Alternative Medicine: The Definitive Guide*. Puyallup, WA: Future
        Medicine Pub., 1994, page 535.
50.   Murray, Michael, N.D. and Joseph Pizzorno, N.D. *Encyclopedia of Natural Medicine*.
        Rocklin, CA: Prima Publishing, 1990, page 337.
51.   Gabor, M. "Pharmacologic effects of flavonoids on blood vessels." *Angiologia* 9 (1972):
        355–374.
        Kuhnau, J. "The flavonoids. A class of semi-essential food components: their role in
        human nutrition." *World Review of Nutrition and Dietetics* 24 (1976): 117–191.
        Havsteen, B. "Flavonoids, a class of natural products of high pharmacological
        potency." *Biochemical Pharmacology* 32 (1983): 1141–1148.
52.   Gabor, M. "Pharmacologic effects of flavonoids on blood vessels." *Angiologia* 9 (1972):
        355–374.
        Kuhnau, J. "The flavonoids. A class of semi-essential food components: their role in
        human nutrition." *World Review of Nutrition and Dietetics* 24 (1976): 117–191.
        Kuhnau, J. "The flavonoids. A class of semi-essential food components: their role in
        human nutrition." *World Review of Nutrition and Dietetics* 24 (1976): 1141–1148.
        Middleton, E. "The flavonoids." *Trends in Pharmacological Sciences*.
53.   Vaughn, Sam and Janis Donnaud, eds. *The American Medical Association Encyclopedia of*

Medicine. New York: Random House, 1989, page 653.

54. Murray, Michael, N.D. and Joseph Pizzorno, N.D. *Encyclopedia of Natural Medicine*. Rocklin, CA: Prima Publishing, 1990, page 339.

55. *Ibid.*, page 469.

56. Regelson, William, M.D. and Carol Colman. *The Superhormone Promise*. New York: Simon & Schuster, 1996, pages 94–98.
van Vollenhoven, Ronald T., et al. "An open study of dehydroepiandrosterone in systemic lupus erythematosus." *Arthritis & Rheumatism* 37 (1994): 1305–1310.

57. Greenwood, J., Jr. "Optimum Vitamin C Intake as a Factor in the Preservation of Disc Integrity." *Medical Annals of the District of Columbia* 33 (1964): 274.
Greenwood, J., Jr. "Intervertebral Disc Lesions: Adjuncts to Conservative, Operative and Postoperative Management." Proceedings of the Third International Congress of Neurological Surgery. Copenhagen, *Exerpta Medica*, abstract 1965, page 807.
Greenwood, J., Jr. "On Osteoarthritis, the 'Wear and Tear' Disease ... Can Vitamin C Help?" *Executive Health* 16.7 (April 1980).
Houssay, A. B., et al. "Ascorbic acid concentrations in different periods of experimental arthritis in rats." *Acta Physiologica et Pharmacologica Latinoamericana* 16 (1966): 43.
Ballabio B. C. and G. Sala. "Research on arthritis treatment." *Lancet* 258 (1950): 644.
Gallini, R. and B. Grego. "Chorionic gonadtropin and ascorbic acid in experimental arthritis of the rat." *Sperimentale* 101 (1951): 169.
Williams R. J., and G. Deason. "Individuality in vitamin C needs." *Proceedings of the National Academy of Sciences* USA 57 (1967): 1638.
Pauling, Linus. *How to Live Longer and Feel Better*. New York: W.H. Freeman and Co., 1986.

58. Ellis, J. M., et al. "The Effect of Pyridoxine Therapy in the Management of Carpal Tunnel Syndrome." *Proceedings of the National Academy of Sciences* USA 79 (1982): 7494–7498.

59. *Proceedings of the National Academy of Sciences* USA 81 (November 1984).
Ellis, J. M. "Treatment of carpal tunnel syndrome with vitamin B_6." *Southern Medical Journal* 80 (1987): 882–884.
Ellis, John M. *The Doctor Who Looked at Hands*. New York: Vantage Press, 1966.
Amadio, P. C. "Pyridoxine as an adjunct in the treatment of carpal tunnel syndrome." *Journal of Hand Surgery* 10 (1985): 237–241.
Kasdan, M. L. and C. J. James. "Carpal tunnel syndrome and vitamin B_6." *Plastic and Reconstructive Surgery* 80 (1987): 882–884.
Ellis, J. M., et al. "Response of Vitamin B_6 Deficiency and the Carpal Tunnel Syndrome to Pyridoxine." *Proceedings of the National Academy of Sciences* USA 79 (1982): 7479–7498.

60. Lee, T. H., et al. "The Effect of Dietary Enrichment with Eicosapentaenoic and Docosahexaenoic Acids on In Vitro Neutrophil and Monocyte Leukotriene Generation and Neutrophil Function." *New England Journal of Medicine* 312.19 (May 9, 1985): 1216–1224.

61. Kremer, J., et al. *Clinical Research* 33 (1985): A778.

62. Kremer, J., A. V. Michaelek, L. Lininger, et al. "Effects of manipulation of dietary fatty acids on clinical manifestations of rheumatoid arthritis." *Lancet* (January 26, 1985): 184–187.
McCormick, J. N., et al. *Lancet* 2 (1977): 508.

63. Kremer, J., A. V. Michaelek, L. Lininger, et al. "Effects of manipulation of dietary fatty acids on clinical manifestations of rheumatoid arthritis." *Lancet* (January 26, 1985): 184–187.
McCormick, J. N., et al. *Lancet* 2 (1977): 508.
Cleland, L., et al. *Journal of Rheumatology* 15 (October 1988): 1471–1475.
Lancet (January 26, 1985): 184–187.
Annals of Internal Medicine 106 (April 1987): 497.
Journal of Immunology 134.3 (March 1985).

64. McCormick, J. N., et al., *Lancet* 2 (1977): 508.

65. Belch, J., et al. *Annals of the Rheumatic Diseases* 47 (October 1988): 94–104.
Bingham, R. *Fight Back Against Arthritis*. Desert Hot Springs, CA: Desert Arthritis Medical Clinic, 1984.
Lancet (January 25, 1985): 184–187.

66. Rosen, J., W. T. Sherman, J. F. Prudden, and G. J. Thorbecke. "Immuno-regulatory Effects of Catrix." *Journal of Biological Response Modifiers* 7 (1988): 498–512.
Heinerman, J. *Science of Herbal Medicine*. Orem, UT: BiWorld Publishers, 1984, page 97.

67.   Bingham, Robert. "Yucca Extract." *Journal of the Academy of Rheumatoid Disease* 2.1
       (1990): 20.
       Bingham, R. "Yucca Plant Saponin in the Management of Arthritis." *Journal of Applied
       Nutrition* 17 (1985): 45–51.
       Bingham, R. "Yucca in the Treatment of Hypertension and Hypercholesterolemia."
       Journal of the American Academy of Applied Nutrition 30 (1978): 3–4.
68.   Murray, Michael, N.D., Joseph Pizzorno, N.D. *Encyclopedia of Natural Medicine.*
       Rocklin, CA: Prima Publishing, 1990, page 339.
69.   Ritchason, Jack. *The Little Herb Encyclopedia,* 3rd ed. Pleasant Grove, UT: Woodland
       Health Books, 1994, pages 73–74.
70.   *Ibid.,* page 250.
71.   Bingham, R. "The Conquest of Arthritis by Nutritional Therapy," Arthritis News
       Today, July 1980.
       Bingham, R. *Fight Back Against Arthritis.* Desert Hot Springs, CA: Desert Arthritis
       Medical Clinic, 1984.
       Bingham, R. "New and Effective Approaches in the Prevention and Treatment of
       Arthritis." *Journal of Nutrition* 28 (1976): 38–47.
       Bingham, R. "Arthritis News Today." *Arthritis and Health News* 1–5.1–65 (Yorba Linda,
       CA: Arthritis Patients Association, 1978–1983).
72.   Childers, Norman. "A Relationship of Arthritis to the Solanacaea (Nightshades)."
       Journal of the International Academy of Preventive Medicine (November 1982): 31–37.

Chapter 12 . . . Anti-Aging Therapies

 1.   Hodes, Richard. "The National Institute on Aging and Their Position on Growth
       Hormone Replacement Therapy in Adults." *Journal of American Geriatrics Society* 42
       (1994): 1208–1211.
 2.   *Ibid.*
 3.   Regelson, William, M.D. and Carol Colman. *The Superhormone Promise.* New York:
       Simon & Schuster, 1996, page 41.
 4.   Ley, Beth M. *DHEA—Unlocking the Secrets to the Fountain of Youth.* Newport Beach, CA:
       BL Publications, 1996, pages 28–29.
 5.   Kalimi, M., and W. Regelson. *The Biological Role of Dehydroepiandrosterone.* New York:
       de Gruyter, 1990.
       Regelson, W., R. Loria, and M. Kalimi. "Dehydroepiandrosterone (DHEA) The 'Mother
       Steroid' I: Immunologic Action." *Annals of the New York Academy of Sciences* 719
       (1994): 553–563.
 6.   Schwartz, A. G., L. Pashko, and J. M. Whitcomb. "Inhibition of tumor development
       by dehydroepiandrosterone and related steroids." *Toxicological Pathology* 14 (1986):
       357–362.
       Loria, R. M., et al. "Protection against acute lethal viral infections with the native steroid
       dehydroepiandrosterone (DHEA)." *Journal of Medical Virology* 26 (1988): 301–314.
       Schwartz, A., et al. "Dehydroepiandrosterone: An anti-obesity and anti-carcinogenic
       agent." *Nutrition and Cancer* 3.1 (1981): 46–53.
       Nestler, J. E., et al. "Dehydroepiandrosterone reduces serum low density lipoprotein
       levels and body fat but does not alter insulin sensitivity in normal men." *Journal of
       Clinical Endocrinology and Metabolism* 66 (1988): 57–61.
       Sunderland, T., et al. "Reduced plasma dehydroepiandrosterone concentrations in
       Alzheimer's disease (Letter)." *Lancet* 2 (1989): 570.
       Flood, J. F. and E. Roberts. "Dehydroepiandrosterone sulfate improves memory in
       aging mice." *Brain Research* 448 (1988): 178–181.
 7.   Reiter, Russel J., et al. "A review of the evidence supporting melatonin's role as an
       anti-oxidant." *Journal of Pineal Research* 18 (1995): 1–11.
       "DHEA Replacement Therapy." *Life Extension Magazine* 13.9 (September 1993).
 8.   Reff, M. E. and E. L. Schneider. "Biological markers in aging." (Bethesda HIH Pub.,
       1980): 82 ff.
 9.   Kalimi, M. and W. Regelson. *The Biological Role of Dehydroepiandrosterone.* New York:
       Walter de Gruyter, 1990.
10.   Regelson, W., M. Kalimi, and R. Loria. "Dehydroepiandrosterone (DHEA): the
       precursor steroid: introductory remarks." In: *The Biologic Role of Dehydroepiandrosterone*

(DHEA). Kalimi, M., Regelson, W., eds., New York: Walter de Gruyter, 1990, pages 1–6.

11. *Science News* 19.3 (1981): 39.

12. Gaby, Alan, M.D., *Preventing and Reversing Osteoporosis,* Prima Publishing, Rocklin, CA, 1994, pages 157–172.

13. Orentriech, N., et al. "Age changes and sex differences in serum dehydroepiandrosterone sulfate concentrations throughout adulthood." *Journal of Clinical Endocrinology and Metabolism* 59 (1984): 551–555.

    Yen, S. S., A. J. Morales, and J. C. Nolan Nelson. "Effects of replacement dose of dehydroepiandrosterone in men and women of advancing age." *Journal of Clinical Endocrinology and Metabolism* 78.6 (June 1994): 1360–1367.

    Regelson, William, M.D. and Carol Colman. *The Superhormone Promise.* New York: Simon & Schuster, 1996, pages 47–48.

14. Coleman, D. L., R. W. Schwizer, and E. H. Leiter. "Effect of genetic background on the therapeutic effects of dehydroepiandrosterone (DHEA) in diabetes-obesity mutants and in aged normal mice." *Diabetes* 33 (1984): 26–32.

    Gordon, G. B., D. E. Bush, and H. F. Weisman. "Reduction of atherosclerosis by administration of dehydroepiandrosterone." *Journal of Clinical Investigation* 82 (1988): 712–720.

    Regelson, W., R. Loria, and M. Kalimi. "Hormonal intervention, buffer hormones or state dependency: The role of dehydro-epiandrosterone (DHEA), thyroid hormone, estrogen and hypophysectomy in aging." *Annals of the New York Academy of Sciences* 521 (1988): 260–273.

15. Sunderland, T., et al. "Reduced plasma dehydroepiandrosterone concentrations in Alzheimer's disease (Letter)." *Lancet* 2 (1989): 570.

    Roberts, E. et al. "Effects of Dehydroepiandrosterone and Its Sulfate on Brain Tissue in Culture and on Memory in Mice." *Brain Research* 406 (1987): 357–362.

16. Merril, C. R., M. G. Harrington, and T. Sunderland. "Reduced plasma dehydroepiandrosterone concentrations in HIV infection and Alzheimer's disease." In *The Biological Role of Dehydroepiandrosterone,* Kalimi, M., Regelson, W., eds., New York: Walter de Gruyter, 1990, pages 101–105.

    Gaby, Alan, M.D. *Preventing and Reversing Osteoporosis.* Rocklin, CA: Prima Publishing, 1994, page 158.

    Nordin, B.E.C., et al. "The relation between calcium absorption, serum dehydroepiandrosterone, and vertebral mineral density in postmenopausal women." *Journal of Clinical Endocrinology and Metabolism* 60 (1985): 651–657.

17. Regelson, William, M.D. and Carol Colman. *The Superhormone Promise.* New York: Simon & Schuster, 1996, pages 50–51.

    Baulieu, E. F. and P. Robel. "Neurosteroids: A new brain function?" *Journal of Steroid Biochemistry and Molecular Biology* 37 (1990): 305–430.

    Majewska, M. "Neuronal Actions of DHEA. Possible Role in Brain Development, Aging and Memory." *Annals of the New York Academy of Sciences* 774 (1995): 111–120.

18. Loria, R. M., et al. "Protection against acute lethal viral infections with the native steroid dehydroepiandrosterone (DHEA)." *Journal of Medical Virology* 26 (1988): 301–314.

19. Klatz, R. and R. Goldman. *Stopping the Clock.* New Canaan, CT: Keats Publishing Inc., 1996, page 62.

    Khorram, O., A. L. Vu and S.S.C. Yen. "Activation of Immune Function by Dehydroepiandrosterone (DHEA) in Age Advanced Men." *Journal of Gerontology* (1996).

20. Feo, F and R. Pastale. "Glucose–6–phosphate dehydrogenase and the relation of dehydroepiandrosterone to carcinogenesis." In *The Biologic Role of Dehydroepiandrosterone (DHEA).* Kalimi, M., Regelson, W., eds., New York: Walter de Gruyter, 1990, pages 331–360.

21. Bulbrook, R. D., J. L. Hayward, and C. C. Spicer. "Relation between urinary androgen and corticoid excretion and subsequent breast cancer." *Lancet* 2 (1971): 395–398.

    Adams, J. and J. B. Brown. "Increase in urinary excretion of estrogen on administration of dehydroepiandrosterone sulphate to an adrenalectomized, oephorectomized patient with breast cancer." *Steroidologia* 2 (1971):1–6.

    Schwartz, A. G., L. Pashko, and J. M. Whitcomb. "Inhibition of tumor development by dehydroepiandrosterone and related steroids." *Toxicological Pathology* 14 (1986): 357–362.

22. Schwartz, A. G. and L. L. Pashko. "Cancer chemoprevention with the adrenocortical steroid dehydroepiandrosterone and structural analogs (Supplement)." *Journal of Cellular Biochemistry* 17G (1993): 73–9.

Schwartz, A. G. "Inhibitions of spontaneous breast cancer formation in female C3H (Avy'a) mice by long-term treatment with dehydroepiandrosterone." *Cancer Research* 39 (1979): 1129–1132.

23. Schwartz, A. G., J. M. Whitcomb, J. W. Nyce, M. L. Lewbart, and K. K. Pashko. "Dehydroepiandrosterone and structural analogs: a new class of cancer chemopreventive agents." *Advances in Cancer Research* 51 (1988): 391–424.

24. Regelson, William, M.D. and Carol Colman. *The Superhormone Promise.* New York: Simon & Schuster, 1996, page 73.

Boone, C. W., G. H. Kelloff, and W. E. Malone. "Identification of candidate cancer chemopreventive agents and their evaluation in animal models and human clinical trials: a review." *Cancer Research* 1 (1990 Jan): 50(1)2–9.

Gordon, G. B., L. M. Shantz, and P. Talalay. "Modulation of growth, differentiation, and carcinogenesis by dehydroepiandrosterone." *Advances in Enzyme Regulation* 26 (1987): 355–382.

Hastings, L. A., L. L. Pashko, M. L. Lewbart, and A. G. Schwartz. "Dehydroepiandrosterone and two structural analogs inhibit 12–0–tetradecanoylphorba–13–acetate stimulation of prostaglandin G2 content in mouse skin." *Carcinogenesis* 9 (1988): 1099–1102.

25. Schwartz, A., et al. "Dehydroepiandrosterone: An anti-obesity and anti-carcinogenic agent." *Nutrition and Cancer* 3.1 (1981): 46–53.

Jakubowicz, D. J., N. A. Beer, and J. Nestler. "Disparate Effects of Weight Reduction by Diet on Serum DHEAS Levels in Obese Men and Women." *Journal of Clinical Endocrinology and Metabolism* 80 (1995): 3373–3376.

26. Cleary, M. P. "The antiobesity effect of dehydroepiandrosterone in rats." *Proceedings of the Society for Experimental Biology and Medicine* 196.1 (January 1991): 8–16.

Cleary, M. P., P. Shepherd, and B. Jenits. "Effect of dehydroepiandrosterone on growth in lean and obese Zucker rats." *Journal of Nutrition* 114 (1984): 1242–1251.

Cleary, M. P. "The role of DHEA in obesity." *The Biologic Role of Dehydroepiandrosterone (DHEA).* Kalimi, M., Regelson, W., eds., New York: Walter de Gruyter, 1990, pages 281–298.

27. Schwartz, A., et al. "Dehydroepiandrosterone: An anti-obesity and anti-carcinogenic agent." *Nutrition and Cancer* 3.1 (1981): 46–53.

28. Gaby, Alan, M.D. *Preventing and Reversing Osteoporosis.* Rocklin, CA: Prima Publishing, 1994, pages 157–172.

Mortola, J. F. and S.S.C. Yen. "The effects of oral dehydroepiandrosterone on endocrine-metabolic parameters in postmenopausal women." *Journal of Clinical Endocrinology and Metabolism* 71 (1990): 696–704.

29. Gaby, Alan, M.D. *Preventing and Reversing Osteoporosis.* Rocklin, CA: Prima Publishing, 1994, pages 163–171.

30. *Ibid.*

31. Sambrook, P. N., et al. "Sex Hormone Status and Osteoporosis in Postmenopausal Women with Rheumatoid Arthritis." *Arthritis & Rheumatism* 31 (1988): 973–978.

Gaby, Alan, M.D. *Preventing and Reversing Osteoporosis.* Rocklin, CA: Prima Publishing, 1994, page 166.

32. *Ibid.*

33. Crilly, R. G., D. H. Marshall, and B.E.C. Nordin. "Metabolic effects of corticosteroid therapy in post-menopausal women." *Journal of Steroid Biochemistry and Molecular Biology* 11 (1979): 429–433.

34. E. Barrett-Connor, et al. "A prospective study of dehydroepiandrosterone sulfate, mortality, and cardiovascular disease." *New England Journal of Medicine* 315 (1986): 1519–1524.

35. Mitchelle, L.E., et al. "Evidence for an association between dehydroepiandrosterone sulfate and non-fatal, premature myocardial infraction in males." *Circulation* 89: 89–93.

Hendler, Sheldon Saul, M.D., Ph.D., *The Doctors' Vitamin and Mineral Encyclopedia.* New York: Simon and Schuster, 1990, page 371.

36. Regelson, William, M.D. and Carol Colman. *The Superhormone Promise.* New York: Simon & Schuster, 1996, page 80.

37. *Ibid.*, page 49.

Gordon, G. B., D. E. Bush, and H. F. Weisman, "Reduction of atherosclerosis by

administration of DHEA." *Journal of Clinical Investigation* 82 (1988): 712–720.
38. Interview with Dr. Ray Sahelian on DHEA, *Nutritional News* 10.4 (July 1996).
39. Regelson, William, M.D. and Carol Colman. *The Superhormone Promise*. New York: Simon & Schuster, 1996, pages 88–89.
   Mortola, J. and S.S.C. Yen. " The effects of oral dehydroepiadrosterone on endrocrine-metabolic parameters in postmenopausal women." *Journal of Clinical Endocrinology and Metabolism* 71 (1990): 696–704.
   Casson, P. R., et al. "Oral dehydroeplandrosterone in physiologic doses modulates immune function in postmenopausal women." *American Journal of Obstetrics and Gynecology* 169 (1993): 1536.
40. Regelson, William, M.D. and Carol Colman. *The Superhormone Promise*. New York: Simon & Schuster, 1996, page 89.
41. Gaby, Alan, M.D. *Preventing and Reversing Osteoporosis*. Rocklin, CA: Prima Publishing, 1994, page 164.
42. *Ibid.*, pages 168–169.
43. Whitaker, M.D., Julian. *Dr. Whitaker's Guide to Natural Healing*. Rocklin, CA: Prima Publishing, 1995.
   Morales, Arlene J. "Effects of Replacement Dose of Dehydroepiandrosterone in Men and Women of Advancing Age." *Journal of Clinical Endocrinology and Metabolism* 78.6 (1994).
44. Kent, Saul, editor/publisher. *Life Extension Magazine* 13.9 (September 1993): 70.
45. Chaitow, Leon, N.D., D.O., M.B.N.O.A. *Amino Acids in Therapy*. New York: Thorsons Publishers Inc., 1985.
46. McBeth, Joyce. "Melatonin Madness." *American Council on Collaborative Medicine* 1.6 (September 1995).
   Kent, Saul. "How Melatonin Combats Aging." *Life Extension Magazine* (December 1995): pages 10–27.
47. Reiter, Russel J., et al. "A Review of the Evidence Supporting Melatonin's Role As an Anti-oxidant." *Journal of Pineal Research* 18 (1995): 1–11.
   Reiter, Russel J., et al. *Melatonin*. New York: Bantam Books, December 1995.
48. Pierpaoli, Walter, and William Regelson. *Melatonin Miracle*. New York: Simon & Schuster, 1995, pages 57–58.
49. *Ibid.*
50. *Ibid.*
   Reiter, Russel J. "The Pineal Gland and Melatonin in Relation to Aging: A Summary of the Theories and of the Data." *Experimental Gerontology* 30.3,4 (1995): 199–212.
51. *Ibid.*
   Reiter, Russel J. "The Pineal Gland and Melatonin in Relation to Aging: A Summary of the Theories and of the Data." *Experimental Gerontology* 30.3,4 (1995): 199–212.
52. *Ibid.*
   Reiter, Russel J. "The Pineal Gland and Melatonin in Relation to Aging: A Summary of the Theories and of the Data." *Experimental Gerontology* 30.3,4 (1995): 199–212.
53. McBeth, Joyce. "Melatonin Madness." *American Council on Collaborative Medicine* 1.6 (September 1995).
   Lissoni, P., S. Megegalli, S. Barni, and F. Frigerino. "A Randomized Study of Immuno-therapy with Low–Dose Subcutaneous Interleukin–2 Plus Melatonin vs. Chemotherapy with Cisplatin and Etoposide as First-Line Therapy for Advanced Non-Smal Cell Lung Cancer." *Tumori* 80 (1994): 464–467.
54. Chein, Edmund Y. M. *Total Hormone Replacement Therapy*. United States Patent #5,855,920, January 5, 1999.
55. Massion, A. O., et al. *Medical Hypotheses* 44.1 (1995): 39–46.
   Chen, L. D., et al. *Cancer Letters* 91.2 (1995): 153–159.
56. Reiter, J. J. *Reviews on Environmental Health* 10.3,4 (July–December 1994): 171–186.
57. Lissoni, P., S. Barni, S. Meregalli, et al. "Modulation of Cancer Endocrine Therapy by Melatonin: A Phase II Study of Tamoxifen Plus Melatonin in Metastatic Breast Cancer Patients Progressing under Tamoxiden Alone." *British Journal of Cancer* 71 (1995): 854–856.
58. Praast, G., et al. *Experientia* 51.4 (1995): 349–355.
   Pierpaoli, Walter, and William Regelson. *Melatonin Miracle*. New York: Simon & Schuster, 1995.

59. Chein, Edmund Y. M. *Total Hormone Replacement Therapy*, United States Patent #5,855,920, January 5, 1999.
60. Brock, Steven J. and Michael Boyette. *Stay Young the Melatonin Way*. New York: Dutton—Penguin Group, 1995.
    Sahelian, Ray, M.D. "Melatonin: The Natural Sleep Medicine." *Total Health* 17.4 (August 1995): 30.
    Zhdanova, I. V., R. J. Wurtman, and D. L. Schomer. "Sleep-inducing Effects of Low Doses of Melatonin Ingested in the Evening." *Clinical Pharmacology and Therapeutics* 57 (1995): 552–558.
61. Pierpaoli, Walter, and William Regelson. *Melatonin Miracle*. New York: Simon & Schuster, 1995, page 161.
62. *Ibid.*, page 162.
63. Chein, Edmund Y. M. *Total Hormone Replacement Therapy*, United States Patent #5,855,920, January 5, 1999.
64. Chein, Edmund, M.D., J.D. *Control the Aging Process Through Age Reversal*. Palm Springs, CA: Palm Springs Life Extension Institute, 1997.
65. Walker, Morton. *The Chelation Way*. Garden Park, NY: Avery Publishing Group, Inc., 1990, page 93.
    Null, Gary. "Chelation Therapy: One of Medicine's Best Kept Secrets." *OmniMedicine* 16.2 (November 1993).
    Atkins, Robert C. *Dr. Atkins Health Revolution*. Boston: Houghton Mifflin Co., 1988, page 219.
66. *Ibid.*
67. Personal Conversation with Dr. Casdorph in Long Beach, CA.
68. Null, Gary. "Chelation Therapy: One of Medicine's Best Kept Secrets." *OmniMedicine* 16.2 (November 1993).
69. Atkins, Robert C. *Dr. Atkins Health Revolution*. Boston: Houghton Mifflin Co., 1988, page 219.
    Chein, E.Y., M.D., Palm Springs Life Extension Institute pamphlet, Palm Springs, CA.
70. Schmid, K., and J. Stein, eds. *Cell Research and Cell Therapy* (Thoune, Switzerland: Ott Publishers, 1967): 19.
71. *Ibid.*
72. *Ibid.*
73. Cazzola, P., P. Mazzanti, and G. Bossi. "In vivo modulating effect of a calf thymus and lysate on human T lymphocyte subsets and CD4+/CD8+ ratio in the course of different diseases." *Curr Ther Res* 42 (1987): 1011–1017.
    Genova, R., and A. Guerra. "Thymomodulin in management of food allergy in children." *International Journal of Tissue Reactions* 8 (1986): 239–242.
    Valesini, G., V. Barnaba, M. Levrero, et al. "Clinical improvement and partial correction of the T-cell defects of acquired immunodeficiency syndrome (AIDS) and lymphadenopathy syndrome (LAS) by a calf thymus lysate." *European Journal of Clinical Oncology* 22 (1986): 531–532.
    Fiocchi, A., E. Borcella, E. Riva, et al. "A double-blind clinical trial for the evaluation of the therapeutic effectiveness of a calf thymus derivative (Thymomodulin) in children with recurrent respiratory infections." *Thymus* 8 (1986): 831–839.

Chapter 13...Men's Unique Challenges

1. Davis, Adelle. *Let's Get Well*. New York: Signet, Published by the Penguin Group, 1972, pages 338–339.
2. Pfeiffer, Carl, Ph.D., M.D. *Zinc and Other Mental and Elemental Nutrients*. New Canaan, CT: Keats Publishing, 1975.
3. Pfeiffer, Carl, Ph.D., M.D. *Zinc and Other Miro-Nutrients*. New Canaan, CT: Keats Publishing, 1978. Found in Lindberg, Gladys, and Judy McFarland. *Take Charge of Your Health*. San Francisco: Harper and Row, 1982, page 239.
4. Vaughn, Sam, and Janis Donnaud, eds. *The American Medical Association Encyclopedia of Medicine*. New York: Random House, 1989.
5. Rothenberg, Mikel A., M.D., Charles F. Chapman. *Dictionary of Medical Terms for the Nonmedical Person*. New York: Barron's Educational Series, Inc., 1994.
    Ibid.

6. Newbold, H. L. *Mega-Nutrients for Your Nerves.* New York: Peter H. Wyden Publishers, 1975.
7. *Ibid.*
8. *Stopping the Clock,* Klatz, Ronald, Goldman, Robert, Keats Publishing Inc. New Canaan, Con. 1996
9. Regelson, William, M.D. and Carol Colman. *The Superhormone Promise.* New York: Simon & Schuster, 1996, page 123.
10. Phillips, Dr. Gerald, Department of Medicine at Columbia University. *Atherosclerosis and Thrombosis* 14.15 (May 1994).
    Chein, Edmund, M.D., J.D. "Testosterone—Male Menopause (Andropause)." Article in a book from the Life Extension Institute, 2825 Tahquitz Canyon Way, Suite A, Palm Springs, CA 92262.
11. White, J.R., et al. "Enhanced sexual behavior in exercising men." *Archives of Sexual Behavior* 19 (1990): 193–209.
12. Chein, Edmund, M.D., J.D. "Testosterone—Male Menopause (Andropause)." Article in a book from the Life Extension Institute, 2825 Tahquitz Canyon Way, Suite A, Palm Springs, CA 92262.
    Phillips, Dr. Gerald, Department of Medicine at Columbia University. *Atherosclerosis and Thrombosis* 14.15 (May 1994).
13. Klatz, Ronald, and Robert Goldman. *Stopping the Clock.* New Canaan, CT: Keats Publishing, Inc., 1996
14. Ref: United States Patent #5,855,920, January 5, 1999, Dr. Edmund Y. M. Chein.
15. Regelson, William, M.D. and Carol Colman. *The Superhormone Promise.* New York: Simon & Schuster, 1996, page 123.
16. Singh A, et al., Magnesium, Zinc and Copper Status of U.S. Navy SEAL Trainees, *Am J Clin Nutr* (1989) 49:695–700.
    Singh A, et al., Biochemical Indices of Selected Trace Minerals in Men: Effect of Stress, *Am J Clin Nutr* (1991) 53:126–131
    Haralambie G, Serum Zinc in Athletes in Training, *Inter J Sports Med* (1981) 2:135–138
    Lefavi R, et al., Reduced Serum Mineral Levels in Basketball Players After Season, *Med Sci Sports Exercise* (1995) 27:5.
    Van Loan M, et al., The Effects of Zinc Depletion on Peak Force and Total Work of Knee and Shoulder Extensor and Flexor Muscles, *Int J Sport Nutr* (1999) 2:125–135
    Brilla L, et al., A Novel Zinc and Magnesium Formulation (ZMA) Increases Anabolic Hormones and Strength in Athletes, *Sports Med Train Rehab J,* (in press).
    Brilla L, et al., Effects of Zinc-Magnesium (ZMA) Supplementation on Muscle Attributes of Football Players, *Med Sci Sports Exer* (1999), 31(5):483
17. "30 Years to Immortality." *Anti-Aging & Longevity Newsletter.* Found in the *International Journal of Anti-Aging Medicine* (Summer 1998).
18. Rudman, Daniel, M.D. "Effects of Human Growth Hormone in Men Over 60 Years Old." *New England Journal of Medicine* 32.1 (July 5, 1990): 1–6.
    Rudman, Daniel M.D. "Growth hormone, body composition, and aging." *Journal of the American Geriatrics Society* (1995).
    Rudman, D., M. H. Kutner, C. M. Rogers, et al. "Impaired growth hormone secretion in the adult population: relation to age and adiposity." *Journal of Clinical Investigation* 67 (1981): 1361–1369.
19. Katz, Dr. Ronald. *Grow Young with HGH.* New York: Harper Collins, 1997, page 5.
20. Regelson, William, M.D. and Carol Colman. *The Superhormone Promise.* New York: Simon & Schuster, 1996, page 203.
21. *Ibid.*
    Schwartz, A. G., K. K. Fairinan, and L. L. Pashko. "The Biologic Significance of Dehydrolprandrosterone." *The Biologic Role of Dehydrolprandrosterone (DHEA).* Kalimi, M., Regelson, W., eds., New York: Walter D. Gruyter, 1990, pages 7–12.
22. Klatz, Ronald, and Robert Goldman. *Stopping the Clock.* New Canaan, CT: Keats Publishing, Inc., 1996, page 19.
23. Klatz, Ronald, and Robert Goldman. *Stopping the Clock.* New Canaan, CT: Keats Publishing, Inc., 1996, page 19.
24. Welbourne, T. "Increased plasma bicarbonate and growth hormone after an oral glutamine load." *American Journal of Clinical Nutrition* 61 (1995): 1058–1061.
25. Castell, L., et al. "Does glutamine have a role in reducing infection in athletes?" *European Journal of Applied Physiology* 73 (1996): 488–490

26. Murray, Michael T., N.D. *Health Counselor* (September/October 1991).
27. Regelson, William, M.D. and Carol Colman. *The Superhormone Promise.* New York: Simon & Schuster, 1996, page 49.
28. *Ibid.,* pages 118–119.
     McLure, R. D., R. Oses, and M. L. Ernst. "Hypogonadal Impotence Treated by Transdermal Testosterone." *Urology* 37 (1991): 224–228.
29. Erdmann, Robert, Ph.D. and Meirion Jones. *The Amino Revolution.* New York: A Fireside Book—Simon & Schuster Inc., 1989, pages 164–165.
30. *Ibid.*
31. *Ibid.*
32. Passwater, Richard A., Ph.D. *The New Supernutrition.* New York: Pocket Books, 1991, page 82.
33. Hendler, Sheldon Saul, M.D., Ph.D., *The Doctors' Vitamin and Mineral Encyclopedia.* New York: Simon and Schuster, 1990, pages 214–215.
     Schachter, A., et al. "Treatment of oligospermia with the amino acid arginine." *Journal of Urology* 110 (1973): 311–313.
     Adams, Ruth. *The Big Family Guide to All the Vitamins.* New Canaan, CT: Keats Publishing, 1992, page 299.
34. *Let's Have Healthy Children,* Adelle Davis, Harcourt Brace, Jovanovicy, New York, N.Y. 1972
35. Reid, K., et al. "Double-blind trial of Yohimbine in Treatment of Psychogenic Impotence." *Lancet* II.8556 (August 22, 1987): 421–423.
     Kronhausen, Eberhard, and Phyllis Kronhausen. *Formula for Life—Science Rediscovers a Natural Aphrodisiac.* New York: William Morrow and Co., 1989, pages 551–557.
36. *Today's Herbal Health,* Louise Tenney, M.H., 5th Edition New and Revised Woodland Publishing, Pleasant Grove, Utah 2000 p132–133
     Michael T. Murray, *Sexual Vitality for Men and Women Let's Live,* May 1994
37. Reid, K., et al. "Double-blind trial of Yohimbine in Treatment of Psychogenic Impotence." *Lancet* II.8556 (August 22, 1987): 421–423.
     Ritchason, Jack. *The Little Herb Encyclopedia,* 3rd ed. Pleasant Grove, UT: Woodland Health Books, 1994, page 263.
38. Geller, J. "Overview of benign hypertrophy (Supplement)." *Urology* 34 (1989): 57–68.
     Sikora, R., M. Sohn, F. J. Deutz, D. Rohrmann, and W. Schafer. "Ginkgo biloba extract in the therapy of erectile dysfunction." *Journal of Urology* 141 (1989): 188A.
39. Brown, Donald J., N.D. *Herbal Prescriptions for Better Health.* Rocklin, CA: Prima Publishing, 1996, pages 253–257.
     Wright, Jonathan V., M.D. *Nutrition & Healing* 1.2 (September 1994): 3, 8.
40. Shibata, S., et al. "Chemistry and Pharmacology of Panax." *Econ Med Plant Res* 1 (1985): 217–284.
41. Brown, Donald J., N.D. *Herbal Prescriptions for Better Health.* Rocklin, CA: Prima Publishing, 1996, pages 253–257.
42. Hendler, Sheldon Saul, M.D., Ph.D., *The Doctors' Vitamin and Mineral Encyclopedia.* New York: Simon and Schuster, 1990, pages 291–292.
     Ritchason, Jack. *The Little Herb Encyclopedia,* 3rd ed. Pleasant Grove, UT: Woodland Health Books, 1994, page 70.
43. Hendler, Sheldon Saul, M.D., Ph.D., *The Doctors' Vitamin and Mineral Encyclopedia.* New York: Simon and Schuster, 1990, page 198.
44. Bush, I. M. "Zinc and the Prostate." Paper read at the annual meeting of the American Medical Association, Chicago, 1974.
45. Fahim, M., et al. "Zinc Treatment for the Reduction of Hyperplasia of the Prostate." *Federation Proceedings* 35 (1976): 361.
46. Passwater, Richard A., Ph.D. *The New Supernutrition.* New York: Pocket Books, 1991, page 79.
47. Champlault, G., J. C. Patel, and A. M. Bonnard. "A double-blind trial of an extract of the plant Serenoa repens in benign prostatic hyperplasia." *British Journal of Clinical Pharmacology* 18 (1984): pages 461–462.
     Tasca, A., M. Barulli, A. Cavazzana, et al. "Treatment of obstructive symptomatology caused by prostatic adenoma with an extract of Serenoa repens. Double-blind clinical study vs. placebo." *Minerva Urologica E Nefrologica* 37 (1985): pages 87–91.
     Boccafoschi, C., and S. Annoscia. "Comparison of Serenoa repens extract with

placebo by controlled clinical trial in patients with prostatic adenomatosis." *Urologia Internationalis* 50 (1983): pages 1257–1259.
Braeckman, J. *Current Therapeutic Research* 55 (1994): 776–785.

48. Whitaker, M.D., Julian. *Dr. Whitaker's Guide to Natural Healing.* Rocklin, CA: Prima Publishing, 1995, page 22.
49. *Ibid.*
50. Vanderhaege, Lorna R. and Patrick J. D. Bouic, PhD. *The Immune System Cure.* New York: Kensington Books, 1999.
51. Weil, Andrew, M.D. *Spontaneous Healing.* New York: Fawcett Columbine, 1995, page 260.
    Murray, Michael T. *The Healing Power of Herbs.* Rocklin, CA: Prima Publishing, pages 150–151.
    Murray, Michael T. *Natural Alternatives to Over-the-Counter and Prescription Drugs.* New York: William Morrow and Co., Inc., page 215.
52. Lange, J. and M. Bardeaux. "Clinical Experimentation with V1326 in Prostatic Disorders." *Bordeaux Medical* 3.11 (November 1970): 2807–2808. In French.
53. Ritchason, Jack. *The Little Herb Encyclopedia,* 3rd ed. Pleasant Grove, UT: Woodland Health Books, 1994, pages 190–191.
54. Ingwall, J. "Creatine and the muscle-specific protein synthesis in cardiac and skeletal muscle." *Circulation Research* 38 (1976): 115–122.
    Earnest, C., et al. "The Effect of creatine monohydrate ingestion on anaerobic powder indices, muscular strength and body composition." *Acta Physiologica Scandinavia* 153 (1995): 2207–2209.
    Volek, J. et al. "Creatine supplementation enhances muscular performance during high-intensity resistance exercise." *Journal of the American Dietetic Association*; 97: 765–770, 1997.
    Harris, R. et al. "The effect of oral creatine supplementation on running performance during maximal short-term exercise in man." *Journal of Physiology*; 467: 74P, 1993.
    Harris, R.C., et al. "Elevation of creatine in resting and exercised muscle of normal subjects by creatine supplementation." *Clinical Science*; 83; 367–374, 1992.
55. Sahelian, R., and D. Tuttle. *Creatine: Nature's Muscle Builder.* Garden City, NY: Avery Publishing Group, 1998, pages 34, 88.
56. Earnest, C., et al. "The Effect of creatine monohydrate ingestion on anaerobic powder indices, muscular strength and body composition." *Acta Physiologica Scandinavia* 153 (1995): 2207–2209.
57. Earnest, C. et al. ob cit.
58. Birch, R. et al. "The influence of dietary creatine supplementation on performance during repeated bouts of maximal isokinetic cycling in man." *European Journal of Applied Physiology*; 69: 268–270, 1994.

Chapter 14...Young Women's Special Needs

1. Northrup, Christiane, M.D. *Women's Bodies, Women's Wisdom.* New York: Bantam Books, 1998.
2. Fredericks, Carlton, Ph.D. *Nutrition Guide for the Prevention & Cure of Common Ailments & Diseases.* New York: Simon and Schuster, 1982.
3. *Ibid.*
   Rossignol, A. M. "Caffeine-Containing Beverages and Premenstrual Syndrome in Young Women." *American Journal of Public Health* 75.11 (1985): 1335–1337.
4. Northrup, Christiane, M.D. *Women's Bodies, Women's Wisdom.* New York: Bantam Books, 1998, page 136.
5. Stephen Berger, M.D. *What Your Doctor Didn't Learn in Medical School.* New York: William Morrow and Co., 1988.
6. Stephen Berger, M.D. *What Your Doctor Didn't Learn in Medical School.* New York: William Morrow and Co., 1988.
7. Gaby, Alan, M.D. B_6: *The Natural Healer.* New Canaan, CT: Keats Publishing, Inc., 1987, pages 28–29.
8. Gaby, Alan, M.D. B_6: *The Natural Healer.* New Canaan, CT: Keats Publishing, Inc., 1987.
9. Hendler, Sheldon Saul, M.D., Ph.D. *The Doctor's Vitamin and Mineral Encyclopedia.* New York: Simon and Schuster, 1990.
10. Passwater, Richard, Ph.D. *The New Supernutrition.* Pocket Books, New York, 1991, p.275.
    Bush, M., et al. *British Journal of Clinical Pathology* 42 (1988):448–45.

11.   Abraham, G. E., Hargrove, J. T. "Effect of Vitamin B on Premenstrual Tension Syndrome: A Double Blind Crossover Study." *Infertility* 3 (1980): 155.
12.   *The Practitioner* 228 (April 1984): 425–427.
13.   Passwater, Richard, Ph.D. *The New Supernutrition*. New York: Pocket Books, 1991.
14.   Piesse, J. W. *International Clinical Nutrition Review* 4 (1984): 54–81.
15.   Hendler, Sheldon Saul, M.D., Ph.D. *The Doctor's Vitamin and Mineral Encyclopedia*. New York: Simon and Schuster, 1990, page 64.
       Abraham, G. E., and J. Hargrove. *Infertility* 3 (1980):155–165.
16.   Hendler, Sheldon Saul, M.D., Ph.D. *The Doctor's Vitamin and Mineral Encyclopedia*. New York: Simon and Schuster, 1990, page 66.
17.   Ellis, John M., M.D. *The Doctor Who Looked at Hands* New York: Vantage Press, 1966.
18.   Horrobin, D. F, ed. *Clinical Uses of Essential Fatty Acids*. Montreal: Eden Press, 1982, pages 155–161.
       Horrobin, D. F. "The Role of Essential Fatty Acids and Prostaglandins in the PMS Syndrome." *Journal of Reproductive Medicine* 28 (1983): 465–481.
19.   Passwater, Richard, Ph.D. *Evening Primrose Oil*. New Canaan, CT: Keats Publishing, page 12.
20.   *Journal of Reproductive Medicine* 39 (1985): 149–153.
21.   Facchinetti, F., et. al. "Oral Magnesium Successfully Relieves Premenstrual Mood Changes." *Obstetrics and Gynecology* 78.2 (August 1991): 177–181.
22.   Hendler, Sheldon Saul, M.D., Ph.D. *The Doctor's Vitamin and Mineral Encyclopedia*. New York: Simon and Schuster, 1990, page 160.
       Lubran, M., and G. Abraham. "Serum and Red Cell Magnesium Levels in Patients with Premenstrual Tension." *American Journal of Clinical Nutrition* 34 (1982): 2364.
23.   *American Journal of Clinical Nutrition* 34 (November 1981): 2364–2366.
24.   *Medical World News* (Sept.ember 13, 1975) page 32.
       Journal of Reproductive Medicine 28 (1983): p 446.
25.   *Journal of the American College of Nutrition* 3 (1984): 351–356.
26.   Shute, Evan, F.R.C.S. *Your Heart and Vitamin E*. New Canaan: Keats Publishing, Inc., 1977, page 120–122.
27.   *Journal of the American College of Nutrition* 4 (September/October 1985): 559–564.
28.   *The Vitamin E Fact Book*. La Grange, IL: Henkel Corporation.
       Journal of Reproductive Medicine 32 (1987): 400.
29.   *Journal of the American College of Nutrition* 2 (1983): 115–123.
30.   Lee, John, M.D. *What Your Doctor May Not Tell You About Menopause*. New York: Warner Books, 1996.
31.   Martin, Raquel. *The Estrogen Alternative*. Rochester, VT: Healing Arts Press, 1997.
       Dalton, Katharina. "Premenstrual Syndrome and Postnatal Depression." *Health and Hygiene* 11 (1990): 199–201.
32.   Lee, John, M.D. *What Your Doctor May Not Tell You About Menopause*. New York: Warner Books, 1996, page 229.
33.   Williams, Dr. David G. *Alternatives For The Health Conscious Individual* 4.6 (Mountain Home Publishing, December, 1991).
34.   Norris, R. "Progesterone for Premenstrual Tension." *Journal of Reproductive Medicine* 28.8 (August 1983): 509–515.
35.   *International Journal of Clinical Nutrition* 84.4: 54–81.
       Journal of Reproductive Medicine 83.28: 446–464.
36.   Lauerson, Niels, M.D. *PMS: Premenstrual Syndrome and You*. New York: Simon & Schuster, 1983, page 170.
37.   Hargrove, Dr. Joel. *American Journal of Obstetrics & Gynecology* 161.4 (October 1989): 948–951.
       Lee, John, M.D. *What Your Doctor May Not Tell You About Menopause*. New York: Warner Books, 1996.
38.   Dalton, K., M.D., and R. Greene. "The Premenstrual Syndrome." First published in the *British Medical Journal* 1 (1953): 1007.
       Dalton, Dr. K., M.D., and R. Greene. *The Premenstrual Syndrome and Progesterone Therapy*. Chicago: Year Book Medical Publishers, Inc., 1977.
39.   Lauersen, Niels H. *Premenstrual Syndrome and You; Next Month Can Be Different*. New York: Simon & Schuster, 1983, page 170.
40.   *Physician's Desk Reference*, 49th edition, 1995.

41. Lauersen, Niels H. *Premenstrual Syndrome and You; Next Month Can Be Different.* New York: Simon & Schuster, 1983.
42. Lee, John, M.D. *What Your Doctor May Not Tell You About Menopause.* New York: Warner Books, 1996.
43. Martin, Raquel. *The Estrogen Alternative.* Rochester, VT: Healing Arts Press, 1997.
    Lee, John, M.D. *What Your Doctor May Not Tell You About Menopause.* New York: Warner Books, 1996.
44. Northrup, Christiane, M.D. *Women's Bodies, Women's Wisdom.* New York: Bantam Books, 1998.
    Lee, John, M.D. *What Your Doctor May Not Tell You About Menopause.* New York: Warner Books, 1996.
45. Northrup, Christiane, M.D. *Women's Bodies, Women's Wisdom.* New York: Bantam Books, 1998, page 138.
    Arafat, E. S., J. T. Hargrove, W.S. Maxon, et al. *American Journal of Obstetrics and Gynecology* 159 (1988): 1203.
46. Braverman, E. R. and C. C. Pfeiffer. *The Healing Nutrients Within.* New Canaan, CT: Keats Publishing, Inc., 1987, pages 50–53.
47. Gelenberg, A. L., et al. *American Journal of Psychiatry* 137 (1980): 622–623.
    Goldberg, I. K. *Lancet* 2 (1980): 364.
48. *American Journal of Public Health* 75.11 (1985).
49. London, R. S., et al. *Nutrition Research* 2 (1982): 243–247.
    Passwater, Richard, Ph.D. *The New Supernutrition.* New York: Pocket Books, 1991, page 280.
50. Werbach, Melvyn R., M.D. *Nutritional Influences of Illness: A Sourcebook of Clinical Research.* New Canaan: Keats Publishing, Inc., 1988.
51. Passwater, Richard, Ph.D. *The New Supernutrition.* New York: Pocket Books, 1991.
52. Fredericks, Carlton, Ph.D. *Breast Cancer: A Nutritional Approach.*
53. Davis, Adelle. *Let's Get Well. New York:* Signet, Penguin Group, 1972.
54. Northrup, Christiane, M.D. *Women's Bodies, Women's Wisdom.* New York: Bantam Books, 1998, page 157.
    Lithgow, D. M. and W. M. Polizer. *South African Medical Journal* 51 (1977): 191.
    Fumii, T. *Journal of Vitaminology* 18 (1972): 125–30.
55. Cohen, J. D. and H. W. Rubin, H. W. "Functional Menorrhagia: Treatment with Bioflavonoids and Vitamin C." *Current Therapeutic Research* 2 (1960): 539.
56. Davis, Adelle. *Let's Get Well.* New York: Harcourt, Brace & World, Inc., 1965, page 305.
57. *Journal of the American Medical Association* 219 (1972): 216–217.
    California Medicine 111 (1969): 87–91.
58. Perry, Susan and Katherine O'Hanlan, M.D. *Natural Menopause.* New York: Addison-Wesley Publishing Company, Inc., 1992.
59. Jovanovic, Lois, M.D., and Genell J. Subak-Sharpe. *Hormones: The Woman's Answer Book.* New York: Fawcett Columbine,1987, pages 102–103.
    Lachtigall, Lila, M.D. *Estrogen: The Facts Can Change Your Life.* 1988, pages 28–36.

Chapter 15 . . . Natural Approaches to Menopause

1. Lee, John, M.D. *What Your Doctor May Not Tell You about Menopause.* New York: Warner Books, 1996, page 117.
2. Gittleman, Ann Louise. *Super Nutrition for Menopause.* New York: Simon & Schuster, Inc., 1993.
3. *Ibid.*
4. Shute, Wilfrid E. *Complete Updated Vitamin E Book.* New Canaan, CT: Keats Publishing, 1975.
    Finkler, R. S. "The Effect of Vitamin E in Menopause." *Journal of Endocrinological Metabolism* 9 (1949): 89–94.
5. *Agents and Actions* 12 (1982): 298–302.
6. Barnes. "Soybeans inhibit mammary tumor growth in models of breast cancer." *Mutagens and Carcinogens in the Diet.* (New York: Wiley-Lis, 1990).
7. Kalimi, M. and W. Regelson. *The Biological Role of Dehydroepiandrosterone (DHEA).* New York: Walter de Gruyter, 1990.
8. Northrup, Christiane, M.D. *Women's Bodies, Women's Wisdom.* New York: Bantam

Books, 1998.

9. Balch, James F., M.D., Balch, Phyllis A., C.N.C., *Prescription for Nutritional Healing*, Avery Publishing, Garden City, New York, 1997, p 336.

10. Balch, James F., M.D., Balch, Phyllis A., C.N.C., *Prescription for Nutritional Healing*, Avery Publishing, Garden City, New York, 1997, p 336.

11. Sheehy, Gail. *The Silent Passage*. New York: Pocket Books, 1993, page 19.

12. *Ibid.*
    Celso-Ramon, Garcia and Winnifred Cuttler. "Preservation of the Ovary: A Re-evaluation." *Fertility and Sterility* 42.4 (October 1984): 510–514.
    Ob/Gyn News (November 15–30, 1984).

13. *Ibid.*, page 174.

14. Goldberg, Burton. *Alternative Medicine: The Definitive Guide*. Puyallup, WA: Future Medicine Pub., 1994, page 668.
    Charles, Allan. "Estrogen Replacement after Menopause. When Is It Warranted?" *Postgraduate Medicine* 85 (1989): 101.

15. Premarin (Conjugated estrogen tablets) insert, Pl 4060–1, issued June 6, 1990, and text from the Physicians insert, Cl 4079, May 23, 1991. Wyeth-Ayerst Laboratories, Philadelphia, PA 19101.

16. "Primary Care & Cancer" June 1991, reprinted with permission from *The Cancer Bulletin* Volume 42, Number 6 (1990). The publication of M.D. Anderson Cancer Center.

17. Rodriguez Calle, E. E., R. J. Contes, H. L. Manacle-McMahill, M. J. Wun, and C. W. Heath, Jr. "Estrogen Replacement Therapy and Fatal Ovarian Cancer." *American Journal of Epidemiology* 141 (1995): 828–835.

18. American Cancer Society, *Cancer Facts and Figures,* 1991.

19. Love, Susan, M.D. Public Broadcasting System (PBS), October 1993.

20. Fredericks, Carlton, Ph.D. *Breast Cancer: A Nutritional Approach*. New York; Grosset & Dunlap, 1977.

21. Premarin (Conjugated estrogen tablets) insert, Pl 4060-1, issued June 6, 1990, and text from the Physicians insert, Cl 4079, May 23, 1991. Wyeth-Ayerst Laboratories, Philadelphia, PA 19101.

22. *Ibid.*

23. *Medical Tribune* (November 26, 1992).

24. 30. 31. Bliznakov, E. G. and G. L. Hunt. *The Miracle Nutrient Coenzyme Q10*. New York: Bantam Books, 1987.

25. *Ibid.*

26. *Newsweek*, July 22, 2002, p 38.

27. Bergkvist, Leif, et al. "The risk of breast cancer after estrogen and estrogen-progestin replacement." *New England Journal of Medicine* (August 3, 1989):293–297.
    Marx, Jean L. "Estrogen Use Linked to Breast Cancer" *Science* 245, August 11, 1989, p 593.

28. *Ibid.*
    Estrogen Drugs: Do They Increase the Risk of Cancer? *Science* 191, Feb 27, 1976, p 838.

29. Laux, Marcus, N.D., Conrad, Christine *Natural Woman, Natural Menopause*, Harper Perennial, New York, NY 1997.

30. Begley, Sharon. "A Clear Signal on Estrogen." *Newsweek* (June 30, 1997).

31. Follingstad, A. H. "Estriol, the forgotten estrogen." *Journal of the American Medical Association* 239 (1978): 29–30.
    Gaby, Alan, M.D. *Preventing and Reversing Osteoporosis*. Rocklin, CA: Prima Publishing, 1994, pages 131–133.

32. Murray, Michael, N.D., *Total Body Tune-Up*, Bantam Books, New York, NY 2000, p 349.

33. Fredericks, Carlton. *Breast Cancer: A Nutritional Approach*. New York: Grosset & Dunlap, A Filmways Co. Publishers, 1977.

34. *Ibid.*

35. *British Journal of Cancer* 49 (1984): 321–324.

36. Murray, M. *The Healing Power of Herbs*. Rocklin, CA: Prima Publishing, 1995, page 375.

37. Lieberman, Shari, Ph.D., *Get Off the Menopause Roller Coaster*, Avery Publishing, New York, 2000, pp 34–35.

38. "Isoflavones Have Emerged as the Most Interesting Phytoestrogen." *Phytoestrogen Update* (Novogen, Inc., Stamford, CT, 1998).

39. Murray, Michael T., N.D. *Ask the Doctor*. Vital Communication, Inc., 1997.

Stoll, W. "Phytopharmacon influences on atrophic vaginal epithelium. Double-blind study—Cimicifuga vs. estrogen substances." *Therapeuticum* 1 (1987): 23–31.

Duker, E. M., et al. "Effects of extracts from Cimicifuga racemosa on gonadotropin release in menopausal women and ovariectomized rats." *Planta Medica* 57 (1991): 420–424.

40. Murray, Michael T., N.D. *Ask the Doctor.* Vital Communication, Inc., 1997.

Neselhut, T., S. Borth, and W. Kuhn. "Influence of Cimicifuga racemosa extracts with estrogen-like activity on the in vitro proliferation of mamma carcinoma cells." *Institute of Tumor Immunology* (Duderstact, Germany, 1994).

Korn, W. D. "Six month oral toxicity study with Remifemin-granulate in rats followed by an 8-week recovery period." *International Bioresearch* (Hannover, Germany, 1991).

41. Murray, Michael T., N.D. *The Healing Power of Herbs.* Rocklin, CA: Prima Publishing, 1995.

42. Ritchason, Jack, N.D., *The Little Herb Encyclopedia,* Woodland Health Books, 1995.

43. Mindell, Earl, Ph.D., *Earl Minedell's Herb Bible,* A Fireside Book, Simon Schuster, 1992.

44. Hobbs, Christopher. *Vitex, The Women's Herb.* Capitola, CA: Botanica Press, 1990.

45. Murray, M. *The Healing Power of Herbs.* Rocklin, CA: Prima Publishing, 1995, page 159.

Kumagai, A., K. Nishino, A. Shimomura, T. Kin, and Y. Yamamura. "Effect of glycyrrhizin on estrogen action." *Endocrinologia Japonica* 14 (1967): 34–38.

46. Ritchason, Jack, N.D. *The Little Herb Encyclopedia,* third edition. Pleasant Grove, UT: Woodland Health Books, 1995.

47. Mindell, Earl, Ph.D. *Earl Mindell's Herb Bible.* New York: Simon & Schuster, 1992, pages 104–109.

48. Lee, John, M.D. *What Your Doctor May Not Tell You about Menopause.* New York: Warner Books, 1996, page 89.

49. Wolfe, Sydney, M.D., et al. *Worst Pills, Best Pills.* New York: Pocket Books, 1999.

50. Arky, Ronald, M.D. *Physician's Desk Reference,* 1995 edition. Montvale, NJ: Medical Economics.

51. "Most asked questions about natural oral progesterone." *Women's International Pharmacy.* Your source for information by Women's Health Connection.

Lee, John, M.D. *What Your Doctor May Not Tell You about Menopause.* New York: Warner Books, 1996, page 89.

52. Regelson, William, M.D., and Carol Colman. *The Superhormone Promise.* New York: Simon & Schuster, 1996, page 178.

53. Lee, John R., M.D. "Is natural progesterone the missing link in osteoporosis prevention and treatment?" *Medical Hypotheses* 35 (1991): 316–318.

54. Lee, John, M.D. *What Your Doctor May Not Tell You about Menopause.* New York: Warner Books, 1996, page 89.

55. Prior, J. C. "Progesterone as a bone-trophic hormone." *Endocrine Reviews* 11 (1990): 386–389.

Gaby, Alan, M.D. *Preventing and Reversing Osteoporosis.* Rocklin, CA: Prima Publishing, 1994, pages 153–154.

56. Lee, John, M.D. *What Your Doctor May Not Tell You about Menopause.* New York: Warner Books, 1996.

57. *Ibid.*

58. *Ibid.*

59. Love, Susan, M.D., *Dr. Susan Love's Hormone Book,* Random House, NY, 1997, pp 120, 268.

60. Lee, John, M.D. *What Your Doctor May Not Tell You about Menopause.* New York: Warner Books, 1996.

61. Regelson, William, M.D., and Carol Colman. *The Superhormone Promise.* New York: Simon & Schuster, 1996, page 184.

Chapter 16...Osteoporosis Can be Prevented and Reversed

1. Hendler, Sheldon Saul, M.D., Ph.D. *The Doctors' Vitamin and Mineral Encyclopedia.* New York: Simon and Schuster, 1990, page 116.

2. Wade, Carlson. *Magic Minerals.* New York: Arco Publishing Company, 1967.

3. Gaby, Alan, M.D. *Preventing and Reversing Osteoporosis.* Rocklin, CA: Prima Publishing, 1994.

4. Hendler, Sheldon Saul, M.D., Ph.D. *The Doctors' Vitamin and Mineral Encyclopedia.*

New York: Simon and Schuster, 1990, page 117.
5. Bland, Jeffery, Ph.D. *Nutraerobics*. San Francisco, CA: Harper & Row, Publishers, 1983.
   Spencer, H. and D. Osis. *American Journal of Clinical Nutrition* 36 (1982): 776.
6. Wallace, W. A. "The increasing incidence of fractures of the proximal femur: An orthopaedic epidemic." *Lancet* 1 (1983): 1414.
7. *Journal of Clinical Nutrition* 117 (1987): 1929–1935.
8. *American Journal of Clinical Nutrition* 39 (June 1984): 857–859.
9. Gaby, Alan, M.D. *Preventing and Reversing Osteoporosis*. Rocklin, CA: Prima Publishing, 1994.
10. Chapuy, Marie C., Ph.D., et al. "Vitamin D3 and Calcium to Prevent Hip Fractures in Elderly Women." *New England Journal of Medicine* 327.23 (December 3, 1992): 1637–1642.
11. *Ibid.*
12. "New Reports on the Dangers of Too Little Calcium in Your Diet." *Executive Health* (November 1977).
    Lindberg, Gladys, and Judy McFarland. *Take Charge of Your Health*. San Francisco: Harper and Row, 1982, page 141.
13. Lindberg, Gladys, and Judy McFarland. *Take Charge of Your Health*. San Francisco: Harper and Row, 1982, page 141.
14. "New Reports on the Dangers of Too Little Calcium in Your Diet." *Executive Health* (November 1977).
15. *Ibid.*
16. *Ob-Gyn News* 13.16: 4.
17. *New York State Journal of Medicine* (February 1975): 335.
18. Bland, Jeffery, Ph.D. *Nutraerobics*. San Francisco, CA: Harper & Row, Publishers, 1983, page 225.
19. Lindberg, Gladys, and Judy McFarland. *Take Charge of Your Health*. San Francisco: Harper and Row, 1982, page 141.
20. *Ibid.*
21. *Ibid.*, page 225.
22. Adams, Ruth, and Frank Murray. *Minerals: Kill or Cure?* New York: Larchmont Books, 1980.
23. Adams, Ruth, and Frank Murray. *Minerals: Kill or Cure?* New York: Larchmont Books, 1980.
24. Nutrition Search, Inc. *Nutrition Almanac*. New York: McGraw-Hill, 1979.
25. Lindberg, Gladys, and Judy McFarland. *Take Charge of Your Health*. San Francisco: Harper and Row, 1982, page 225.
26. Rodale, J. I. *Complete Book of Minerals for Health*. Emmaus, PA: Rodale Press, 1977, page 105.
27. *Ibid.*, page 112.
28. "Boron Found to Have Role in Hardening Bones." *Chemical Marketing Reporter* (November 9, 1987).
    Smith, Emily T. "A New Recruit in the Battle Against Bone Loss." *Business Week* (November 23, 1987).
29. Leary, Warren E. "Role Seen for Boron in Curbing Bone Loss." *The New York Times* (1987).
30. *Chemical Marketing Reporter* (November 9, 1987, Schnell Publishing Co., Inc.).
31. *Journal of Trace Elements and Experimental Medicine* 5 (1992): 237–246.
32. Kamen, Betty, Ph.D. *Hormone Replacement Therapy: Yes or No?*, page 167.
    Journal of the American Dietetic Association 5 (May, 1991): 558–568.
33. Leary, Warren E. "Science Times." *The New York Times* (1987).
34. Melis, G. B., et al. *Journal of Endocrinological Investigation* 15 (1992): 755–761.
    Almada, Anthony L. "Ipriflavone: The New Bone Builder." *Nutrition Science News* 3.4 (April 1998).
35. Germano, Carl, R.D. *The Osteoporosis Solution*. New York: Kensington Books, 1999.
    Arjmandi, B. H., et al. *Nutrition Research* 17 (1997): 885–894.
    Chinoin Pharmaceutical and Chemical Works, Hungary, PCT patent 09703664.
36. Notoya, K., et al. *Calcified Tissue International* 53 (1993): 206–209.
    Almada, Anthony L. "Ipriflavone: The New Bone Builder." *Nutrition Science News* 3.4 (April 1998).
37. Notoya, K., et al. *Calcified Tissue International* 53 (1993): 206–209.

Benvenuti, S., et al. *Biochemical and Biophysical Research Communications* 201 (1994): 1084–1089.

Almada, Anthony L. "Ipriflavone: The New Bone Builder." *Nutrition Science News* 3.4 (April 1998).

38. Almada, Anthony L. "Ipriflavone: The New Bone Builder." *Nutrition Science News* 3.4 (April 1998).

Arjmandi, B.H., et al. *Nutrional Research* 17 (1997): 885–894.

Chinoin Pharmaceutical and Chemical Works, Hungary, PCT patent 09703664.

39. Prior, J. C. "Progesterone as a bone-trophic hormone." *Endocrine Reviews* 11 (1990): 386–389.

Gaby, Alan, M.D. *Preventing and Reversing Osteoporosis.* Rocklin, CA: Prima Publishing, 1994, pages 153–154.

40. Lee, John, M.D. *What Your Doctor May Not Tell You about Menopause.* New York: Warner Books, 1996.

41. Gaby, Alan, M.D. *Preventing and Reversing Osteoporosis.* Rocklin, CA: Prima Publishing, 1994.

42. Regelson, William, M.D. and Carol Colman. *The Superhormone Promise.* New York: Simon & Schuster, 1996.

43. "On Walking." *Executive Health* (July 1978): 1–2.

Chapter 17 . . . Let's Put It All Together

1. Harris, Seal, M.D. "Clinical Types of Hyperinsulinism." *Annals of Internal Medicine* (1934): 562–569.

Harris, Seal, M.D. "Hyperinsulinism and Dysinsulinism." *Journal of the American Medical Association* 83 (1929): 729–733.

2. Lindberg, Gladys, and Judy McFarland. *Take Charge of Your Health.* San Francisco: Harper and Row, 1982, pp 48–49.

3. Fredericks, Carlton, Ph.D., *Psycho-Nutrition*, Grosset & Dunlap, New York, NY, 1976.

4. Fredericks, Carlton, Ph.D. *Eat Well, Get Well, Stay Well.* New York: Grosset & Dunlap, 1980, pp 42–43.

5. *Ibid.*

6. Barnes, Broda O. and Charlotte W. Barnes. *Hope for Hypoglycemia.* Fort Collins, CO: Robinson Press, 1978, p 9.

7. Lindberg, Gladys, and Judy McFarland. *Take Charge of Your Health.* San Francisco: Harper and Row, 1982, p 53.

8. Balch, *Prescription for Nutritional Healing*, 2000.

9. Lindberg, Gladys, and Judy McFarland. *Take Charge of Your Health.* San Francisco: Harper and Row, 1982, p 54.

10. Morrison, Lester, M.D., "Serum Cholesterol Reduction and Lecithin." *Geriatrics* (January 1958:12–19.

11. Davis, Adelle, *Let's Get Well*, p 52.

12. Jacobs, Stanley W., M.D., *The Miracle of MSM: The Natural Solution of Pain*, 1999.

13. *American Journal of Clinical Nutrition*, 61;1058–1061, 1995.

Sports Medicine 21(2):80–97, 1996.

14. Carper, Jean, *Stop Aging Now!* New York: HarperCollins, 1996, pp 222–223.

15. *Ibid.*

16. Lindberg, Gladys, and Judy McFarland. *Take Charge of Your Health.* San Francisco: Harper and Row, 1982, p 100.

17. Murray, Michael, N.D., *Total Body Tune-Up*, p 24.

18. "Leading Sites of Cancer Incident and Deaths—1993 Estimates." *Cancer Facts and Figures.* American Cancer Society, 1993.

19. Lindberg, Gladys, and Judy McFarland. *Take Charge of Your Health.* San Francisco: Harper and Row, 1982, page 109.

20. Ritchason, Jack. *The Little Herb Encyclopedia,* 3rd ed. Pleasant Grove, UT: Woodland Health Books, 1994, pp 5–6.

21. Tenney, Louise. *Today's Herbal Health.* Provo, UT: Woodland Books, 1983, p 118.

22. Mindell, Earl, Ph.D., *Earl Mindell's Herb Bible*, Simon & Schuster, Fireside, NY, 1992.

23. "Melatonin: Its Fundamental Immunoregulatory role in Aging and Cancer." *Annals of the New York Academy of Sciences* 521 (1988): 140–148.

24. Julian Whitaker, M.D., *Reversing Diabetes*, Warner Books, New York, N.Y., 2001.

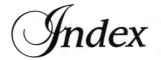

Index